Introduction to Computers for Healthcare Professionals

Fifth Edition

Irene Joos, Phd, RN

Associate Professor and Director of Online Learning
La Roche College
Pittsburgh, Pennsylvania

Ramona Nelson, PhD, RN–BC, FAAN, ANEF

Professor Emeritus, Slippery Rock University
President, Ramona Nelson Consulting
Allison Park, Pennsylvania

Marjorie J. Smith, PhD, RN, CNM

Emeritus Professor of Nursing
Winona State University
Winona and Rochester, Minnesota

JONES AND BARTLETT PUBLISHERS

Sudbury, Massachusetts

BOSTON   TORONTO   LONDON   SINGAPORE

World Headquarters
Jones and Bartlett Publishers
40 Tall Pine Drive
Sudbury, MA 01776
978-443-5000
info@jbpub.com
www.jbpub.com

Jones and Bartlett Publishers Canada
6339 Ormindale Way
Mississauga, Ontario L5V 1J2
Canada

Jones and Bartlett Publishers International
Barb House, Barb Mews
London W6 7PA
United Kingdom

Jones and Bartlett's books and products are available through most bookstores and online booksellers. To contact Jones and Bartlett Publishers directly, call 800-832-0034, fax 978-443-8000, or visit our website www.jbpub.com.

Substantial discounts on bulk quantities of Jones and Bartlett's publications are available to corporations, professional associations, and other qualified organizations. For details and specific discount information, contact the special sales department at Jones and Bartlett via the above contact information or send an email to specialsales@jbpub.com.

The authors, editor, and publisher have made every effort to provide accurate information. However, they are not responsible for errors, omissions, or for any outcomes related to the use of the contents of this book and take no responsibility for the use of the products and procedures described. Treatments and side effects described in this book may not be applicable to all people; likewise, some people may require a dose or experience a side effect that is not described herein. Drugs and medical devices are discussed that may have limited availability controlled by the Food and Drug Administration (FDA) for use only in a research study or clinical trial. Research, clinical practice, and government regulations often change the accepted standard in this field. When consideration is being given to use of any drug in the clinical setting, the health care provider or reader is responsible for determining FDA status of the drug, reading the package insert, and reviewing prescribing information for the most up-to-date recommendations on dose, precautions, and contraindications, and determining the appropriate usage for the product. This is especially important in the case of drugs that are new or seldom used.

Production Credits
Publisher: Kevin Sullivan
Aquisitions Editor: Emily Ekle
Aquisitions Editor: Amy Sibley
Associate Editor: Patricia Donnelly
Editorial Assistant: Rachel Shuster
Production Editor: Amanda Clerkin
Marketing Manager: Barb Bartoszek
V.P., Manufacturing and Inventory Control: Therese Connell
Composition: Circle Graphics, Inc.
Cover Design: Kristin E. Parker
Cover Image Credit: © Andresr/ShutterStock, Inc.
Printing and Binding: Malloy, Inc.
Cover Printing: Malloy, Inc.

ISBN-10: 0-7637-6113-3
ISBN-13: 978-0-7637-6113-4

Library of Congress Cataloging-in-Publication Data
CIP data not available at time of publication.

6048

Printed in the United States of America
13 12 11 10   10 9 8 7 6 5 4 3 2

Dedication

This book is dedicated to faculty, healthcare providers, healthcare administrators, and those corporate and government leaders who have led, and continue to lead, the effort to improve health care through the use of computers and automation.

Contents

About the Authors

Irene Joos

Irene Joos is an associate professor in the IST Department as well the Director of Online Learning at La Roche College. Prior to this position, she was the Director of Library and Instructional Technologies at La Roche College. Dr. Joos received her baccalaureate degree in nursing from Pennsylvania State University. She holds a master's degree in both medical-surgical nursing and information science as well as a doctorate in education from the University of Pittsburgh.

Dr. Joos has taught medical-surgical nursing, foundations, basic nursing concepts and theories, professional nursing role, and nursing informatics courses at diploma, baccalaureate, and 1st REVISE programs. With two FULD grants, she was instrumental in the installation of interactive video units in the skills laboratory and also managed both the microcomputer and skills laboratory at the University of Pittsburgh School of Nursing, Learning Resources Center. She teaches Office Automation, Management of Information Systems, Cyberspace, Computer Based Training, and Nursing Informatics courses to both undergraduate and graduate students in on campus and online formats. As the Director of Online Learning she was instrumental in planning and implementing the online initiative at La Roche College. She currently supports online students and faculty as well as conducts training sessions for faculty in online teaching and using Blackboard. She serves as the faculty advisor for the Web site of the student's literary journal, *Nuances*.

Dr. Joos' area of interest is the use of technology to help us do our work in an efficient and effective manner. This includes using technology in whatever arena you might find yourself—education, research, and practice. This has been the focus of her publications and presentations.

Ramona Nelson

Ramona Nelson holds a baccalaureate degree in nursing from Duquesne University and a master's degree in both nursing and information science, as well as a PhD in education from the University of Pittsburgh. In addition she completed a post-doc fellowship at the University of Utah with Dr. Judy Graves. Previous to her current position as president of her own consulting company, Ramona was a Professor of Nursing and Chair of the Department of Nursing at Slippery Rock University. As a result of her service at Slippery Rock University, Ramona was appointed professor emeritus. Her teaching at the University included courses related to healthcare informatics, community health, nursing research and school nurse courses. All of these courses were offered via Web-based distance education. Her primary area of research is nursing informatics with a focus on theoretical concepts in nursing informatics, consumer informatics, and distance education.

Her past publications include textbooks, monographs, book chapters, journal articles, WWW publications, abstracts and newsletters. Ramona has been an active member of professional organizations. She was named a fellow in the American Academy of Nursing in 2004 and was inducted into the NLN Academy of Nursing Education Fellows in 2007. Because of her pioneering work in informatics she was invited to participate as a member of the task force charged with revising the Scope and Standards of Nursing Informatics published in 2008 by the American Nurses Association (ANA). In 2008 she received the Eleventh Annual Recognition Award for Advancement of Computer Technology in Healthcare from Rutgers University College of Nursing and was elected chair-elect of the NLN Educational Technology and Information Management Advisory Council.

Marjorie J. Smith

Marjorie J. Smith, PhD, RN, CNM, is an emeritus professor of nursing at Winona State University, Winona and Rochester, MN, where she was formerly the director of the master's program in nursing. Dr. Smith received her baccalaureate degree in nursing from the University of Wisconsin, Madison. Her master's degree in childbearing family nursing and doctorate in adult education are from the University of Minnesota. She is a certified nurse–midwife and was a member of Sigma Theta Tau and the American College of Nurse–Midwives.

Dr. Smith taught medical-surgical nursing, pediatric nursing, and obstetrical nursing at the undergraduate level in diploma, associate degree, and baccalaureate programs. She has also taught advanced courses in nursing theory, research, women's health care, instruction and evaluation, nursing informatics, and healthcare technology and computers. She was chief editor of the textbook *Child and Family: Concepts of Nursing Practice*, published by McGraw-Hill in 1982 and 1987. She has also written a computer assisted learning program, *The Client Using the Birth Control Pill*, published by Medi-Sim in 1991. In 2000 she received the Outstanding Nurse Educator award from the Minnesota Association of Colleges of Nursing. In 2009 Dr. Smith was selected as one of the 100 distinguished alumni of the University of Minnesota's School of Nursing in celebration of its Centennial. Outstanding individuals were selected from some 8,500 living alumni who were deemed to have made great achievements to advance health care or were doing significant work in the nursing profession that has had a profound impact on families, communities, the school, or the nursing profession. Dr. Smith has continued her work related to CenteringPregnancy, a model of group prenatal care that is part of the Centering HealthCare Institute. She also continues her work with computers and enjoys an active travel and family life.

Preface

In order to provide safe and effective health care in today's automated health-care environment healthcare professionals must master both computer and information literacy skills. The fifth edition of *Introduction to Computers for Healthcare Professionals* provides the foundational computer and information literacy knowledge and skills needed by these professionals. In each chapter the process for using the computer is carefully explained. This information is followed by several examples and assignments where both computer and information skills are mastered. Each of these exercises and assignments are designed to be applicable in a healthcare setting. The book concludes by introducing the reader to healthcare informatics.

Each chapter has been updated and revised to emphasize foundational concepts and terms that reflect change in the computer world and provides a basis for understanding and using computers. The chapters are designed to stand alone, so that the user can order them in the sequence that meets his or her needs. Where appropriate, the user is referred to other chapters in the book that provide information related to the current chapter.

The need for computer and information literate healthcare professionals has been well documented in the professional literature of the health-care disciplines. On November 29, 1999, the Institute of Medicine (IOM) released a report called *To Err Is Human: Building a Safer Health System* (Kohn, Corrigan & Donaldson, 2000). This report estimated that medical errors kill between 45,000 and 98,000 hospitalized Americans each year. Additional fatal errors also occur in nonhospitalized patients. Automated health care information systems and electronic health records were identi-fied as a critical element in improved safety of all patients. However, the development and use of such systems requires that health professional are computer and information literate.

As a follow-up to this report, in 2002 over 150 experts attended a Health Professions Education Summit. Their goal was to assist the IOM Com-mittee on Health Profession Education Summit develop strategies to ensure that educational systems for health professionals were consistent with the principles of the 21st-century health system. Based on this summit the IOM issued a seminal report titled *Health Professions Education: A Bridge to Quality* (Greiner & Knebel, 2003).

The report stated that doctors, nurses, pharmacists and other health professionals are not adequately prepared to provide the highest quality and safest medical care possible. To meet this challenge the report called on educators as well as accreditation, licensing and certification organizations to ensure that students and working professionals develop and maintain proficiency in five core areas. These core competencies are patient-centered care, interdisciplinary teams, evidence-based practice, quality improvement, and informatics. To obtain competency in information healthcare professionals must first be computer and information literate.

The IOM publication established the need for health care professionals to be computer, information, and informatics literate and called upon the health professions to make this a reality. Several of the health professional organizations have taken up this call. The Joint Task Force of the American Health Information Management Association (AHIMA) and American Medical Informatics Association (AMIA) focused on the education of health care workforce as shown in the follow example:

> There are several important cross-cutting issues, including the wide variety of health professionals—from physicians and nurses to therapists and admissions staff—who are or will be using EHRs as part of their day-to-day activities. This, in turn, has an impact on the broad range of training needed, from basic computer literacy to more sophisticated computer applications and health. (AHIMA & AMIA, 2008, p. 5)

In nursing this call was answered by the American Nurses Association (ANA), the National League for Nursing (NLN) and the American Association of Colleges of Nursing (AACN). The American Nurses Association's *Nursing Informatics: Scope and Standards of Nursing Informatics Practice* (2008) identified informatics competencies that are required of all nurses. "These competencies are categorized in three overall areas: computer literacy, information literacy and professional development/leadership." (ANA, 2008, p. 36).

In 2008 both the NLN and the AACN documented the need for computer, information, and informatics literacy within nursing. The AACN stated in the revised *Essentials of Baccalaureate Education for Professional Nursing Practice* that "Computer and information literacy are crucial to the future of nursing" (2008, p.17). The NLN went one step further pointing out the need for nursing faculty and administration to be prepared to provide the needed education. The NLN's recommendations for faculty and administration preparation are outlined in their Position Paper, *Preparing The Next Generation Of Nurses To Practice In A Technology-Rich Environment: An Informatics Agenda.*

The fifth edition of *Introduction to Computers for Healthcare Professionals* reflects the ever-changing world of computers, their applications, and the "real" world of today. It features updated lesson material, exercises, and activities which provide more experience with the Internet, Vista and the latest version of Microsoft Office, 2007. Examples of differences in Windows XP and Vista are presented.

The first chapter incorporates information about information literacy and its importance in the work world and provides an introduction to OneNote. Chapter 2, "Computer Systems: Hardware, Software, and Connectivity," which presents basic information necessary to understand current technology, has been revised and expanded to reflect changing technology.

Chapter 3, "The Computer and Its Operating System Environment," now includes more Desktop and Windows management concepts and exercises, while still providing foundational concepts on managing files and folders. The next chapter, "Software Applications: Common Tasks," provides information and activities common to Windows software programs. These include using online help; creating, opening, saving, deleting, and copying files; and so forth.

Chapters 4–8, the software application chapters, were updated to reflect the skill set needed to use the Office 2007 suite effectively.

Chapters 9 and 10, the Internet and communications chapters were updated to reflect the evolving world of the Internet and related communication activities including the world of Web 2.0.

Chapter 11 is a new chapter focused on Distance Education Technology. This chapter was added to provide information related to successful online learning.

Chapter 12 "Information: Access, Evaluation, and Use," provides specific information literacy skills used in a health care setting. It includes concepts and exercises about search strategies and the subsequent evaluation and use of the retrieved health related information. These concepts can be used in educating patients as well as for searching the professional literature including gray literature.

Chapter 13, a redesigned privacy and security chapter replaces the legal and ethics chapter and addresses threats to and procedures for protecting privacy, confidentiality, integrity, and security of personal data including health related data.

The book concludes with a chapter called "Healthcare Informatics and Information Systems," which provides the learner with an introduction to information systems concepts and theories related to heath care informatics.

It is our sincere hope that this book will serve as a sound foundation for developing computer skills for health care professionals and in turn improve the quality of patient care delivered by these professionals.

References

AHIMA & AMIA. (2008) Joint Work Force Task Force. *Health Information Management and Informatics Core Competencies for Individuals Working With Electronic Health Records.* Retrieved December 21, 2008 from www.amia.org/files/shared/Workforce_2008.pdf.

American Association of Colleges of Nursing. (Oct. 2008) *The Essentials of Baccalaureate Education for Professional Nursing Practice.* Retrieved December 21, 2008, from http://www.aacn.nche.edu/Education/pdf/BaccEssentials08.pdf

American Nurses Association. (2008). *Scope and standards of nursing informatics practice.* Silver Spring, Maryland: NurseBooks.org.

Greiner, A., & Knebel, E. (Eds.). (2003). Institute of Medicine: Committee on the Health Professions Education Summit. *Health professions education: A bridge to quality.* Washington, DC: The National Academies Press. Available from http://www.nap.edu.

Kohn, L. T., Corrigan, J. M. Donaldson, M. S. (Eds.). (2000) *To err is human: building a safer health system.* Washington, DC: National Academy Press, Institute of Medicine.

National League for Nursing. (2008) *Position Paper: Preparing The Next Generation Of Nurses To Practice In A Technology-Rich Environment: An Informatics Agenda.* Retrieved December 21, 2008, from http://www.nln.org/aboutnln/PositionStatements/informatics_052808.pdf

Special Acknowledgment

The Publisher would like to thank Naomi R. Persinger-Baker, of Edison Community College, for her assistance in reviewing the Fourth Edition of this text in its entirety as well as creating resources for the companion Web site for this book.

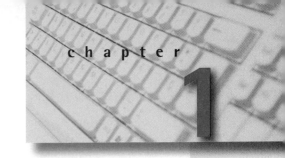
On the Way to Computer and Information Literacy

Objectives

1. Introduce the concepts of information and computer literacy.
2. Review the organization of this book.
3. Identify elements of a computer lab system.
4. Log in to a computer system.
5. Create a PDF file.
6. Compress and unzip a file.
7. Download and upload an email attachment.
8. Develop basic skill in using OneNote to explore a few computer and information literacy concepts.

Healthcare professionals increasingly rely on information systems to assist them in providing quality care. They realize that a large percentage of their practice involves the management of information. Computers are often required to perform information-related functions such as sorting and addressing patient needs and documenting care; providing remote patient care through telemedicine facilities; organizing, calculating, and managing financial data; and accessing healthcare literature. To use the tools of automation in meeting their responsibilities and take advantage of evolving computer technologies, healthcare professionals must be computer and information literate.

This book is designed to help you develop the essential computer and information literacy skills needed by all healthcare professionals. Its focus is the introduction of concepts that cross specific applications and the development of practical computer skills. In each chapter, exercises from the healthcare arena provide practice in applying the concepts and skills.

1

Literacy

Healthcare providers learn to use a stethoscope as a tool to assess patients. This practice involves understanding the function and purpose of the stethoscope as well as developing skill in using it. Just as healthcare providers learn to use the stethoscope, so they must also learn the function and purpose of computers in health care as well as develop skill in their use. In other words, healthcare providers must become "computer and information literate."

Literacy	Literacy means the ability to locate and use printed and written information to make decisions and to function in society, both personally and professionally.
Computer Literacy	Add "computer" to the term "literacy," and it refers to the ability to use the computer to do practical tasks. A variety of viewpoints exist that identify computer skills required for computer literacy, but there is general agreement that computer literacy includes the ability to use basic computer applications to complete tasks.
Information Literacy	This term describes a set of skills that enables a person to identify an information need, locate and access the required information many times by using technology, evaluate the information found, and communicate and use that information effectively. With the explosion of information, both good and bad, information literacy has taken on a major role in all educational settings. Given information literacy's growing importance, Chapter 12 provides further information on this topic.

People who are computer and information literate have the following characteristics: They

- use the computer and associated software as tools to complete their work in a more effective and efficient manner.
- recognize the need for accurate and complete information as the basis for intelligent decision making.
- find appropriate sources of information using successful search strategies.
- evaluate and manage information to facilitate their work.
- communicate information in various formats.
- integrate technology and information strategies into their daily professional lives.

Many professional organizations and accrediting agencies now include information and computer literacy requirements as part of their criteria. For example, the Association of College and Research Libraries (ACRL) produced a document defining and outlining specific criteria and standards for demonstrating information literacy (Association of College and Research Libraries, 2000). To support the development of information literacy, the ACRL has establish a Web site with links and citations to information literacy standards and curricula developed by accrediting agencies, professional associations, and institutions of higher education. Several of the healthcare professions are included in its site. The ACRL Web site can be viewed at http://www.ala.org/ala/mgrps/divs/acrl/about/sections/is/projpubs/infolitdisciplines/index.cfm.

Organization of the Book

This book consists of 14 chapters and an index that features highlighted computer terms. Most chapters are organized in the same way, beginning with a lesson that introduces the content, describes key concepts and terms, and, in application chapters, provides descriptions of common application functions and keystrokes. Each chapter also includes one or more exercises for use in the classroom or computer laboratory to practice application of lesson concepts and one or more assignments intended for you to demonstrate the knowledge and skill acquired. Additional materials for exercises and assignments can be downloaded from the book's Web site.

The first chapter provides material that is useful to understanding and using this book as well as an introduction to OneNote. Chapters 2, 3, and 4 contain content about hardware and software. Computer hardware and software terms are introduced in Chapter 2. Chapter 3 focuses on managing the computer environment. Chapter 4 covers tasks that are common to most application programs. As a consequence of this consistency, many applications in a graphic environment have common looks and functions.

The next four chapters include lessons and practice exercises for word processing, presentation graphics, spreadsheet, and database applications. Microsoft Office 2007 is used to illustrate the basic concepts of each of these chapters.

Basic Internet concepts for connecting and browsing, and related software such as Internet Explorer and Firefox, are then introduced. Tips for successful communication over the Internet and in distance education endeavors are shared in Chapters 9, 10, and 11. Means of accessing informational resources and issues of security, integrity, and ethical use of electronic data are reviewed in Chapters 12 and 13. Chapter 14 provides an introduction to the field of healthcare informatics.

Every attempt was made to select Internet sites that would exist while this book is used and that demonstrate the concepts presented. Remember, however, that Internet sites can and do change, so some of the links may not work.

Before Beginning: Some Helpful Information

Every computer system and every computer laboratory have subtle differences that can cause problems for the beginner; therefore, learning something about the computer environment used is essential. Professors or computer laboratory personnel can help to answer the following questions:

Accounts	Is an account needed to use the computer laboratory or university's resources? If so, what is the process for getting one? Some schools have at least a 24-hour wait time before the laboratories can be used. By comparison, some other schools automatically create an account when a student registers or provide facilities and directions to create an instant account. Some schools require students to own laptops, but you still need an account to sign on to the school's network. A separate account may also be needed to access course materials made available through the Internet or that reside on course management software servers.
Computer Laboratories	Where are the computer laboratories located, and who has access to them? Is an identification card needed to use the equipment and software? Are some laboratories reserved for specific student populations—for example, health professional students or engineering students—or are all laboratories general-purpose facilities that are available to all students, staff, and faculty?
Cost	Is there a user charge for accessing and using the computer equipment and software? Do the rates vary (less at night or during off-peak times)? Is a computer fee included in tuition charges? What does the fee cover?
Documentation	Does the computer laboratory have user documentation? Where is the documentation? Are handouts available in the computer laboratory, or are the documents available online to read and/or print? Which documentation is needed to begin? Most computer laboratories have user documentation that provides helpful information for starting and learning specific software programs. For example, the laboratory might have a document called "Getting Started with Outlook" or "Accessing the Network from Home."
Equipment/Storage	Which type of hardware will be used? Which types of storage devices are needed, and where can they be

purchased? How is the equipment turned on? Where can students store data files?

Laboratory Hours

What are the laboratory hours? Do they change during the term? Is the laboratory open over the weekend? Some laboratories expand their hours of operation toward the end of the term when many papers and projects are due. Does a laboratory assistant need to be present for the laboratory to be open, or is the laboratory left unattended?

Lease or Buy

Does the university have a program whereby students lease or buy a laptop computer for use at home, in the dormitory, or in the classroom? If so, how long does it take to get a computer? How does the university support this program in terms of repair, software, and other technical issues? Is a certain operating system (i.e., PC or Mac) required? Can you buy the computer at the end of the lease?

Logging In

Most resources that you will need as a student and as a professional will require you to log in to the system. Some institutions will have a universal login that provides a customized home page (referred to as a portal) with all your resources a click away; other institutions require separate accounts for each resource like the network, email, library online databases, student records, course management software, patient clinical records, drug administration systems, and so forth.

Is there a login procedure (a series of steps to access the computer software)? If so, how do you log into the system? Is there a help sheet to follow?

Mobile Devices

Are there places around campus where students with laptops can connect to the resources available on the network? Is it wireless or wired? What are the requirements for connecting your laptop to the network while on campus?

Policies

What are the policies that govern use of the computer laboratory? Policies can include anything from how often to change a password to how many pages can be printed each term to respecting the rights of other users. What are the penalties for not adhering to the policies? Penalties might range from a warning for a minor offense to dismissal or expulsion for a major offense. Most computer laboratories and organizations or businesses provide the policies to each account holder or give directions for viewing them online. If this is an employee account (rather than a student account), certain policies related to confidentiality of data and protection of a password need to be acknowledged and followed.

Printing

Which printing capabilities are available in the laboratory? Is there access to color printing? Is there a charge for printing? Some schools use a prepaid print card, keep an electronic record of printing that allows individual billing, or use a software program such as PaperCut to keep track of printing costs. When the printing credits go to zero, the student must add more print credits to continue printing. Other schools permit unlimited printing.

Rules

What are the rules that govern use of the computer laboratory? Many laboratories prohibit eating and drinking, chatting, and game playing. Laboratories can be restricted to academic use only. Some laboratories also check all removable storage devices that are brought into the laboratory for viruses.

Support/Help

What kind of support is available when help is needed? Many laboratories provide helpers to assist patrons who have questions or are experiencing problems. Others provide online help services and quick reference guides for their users. Are there orientation classes for the laboratories and/or training classes on specific software? What is the telephone number for the help desk? What is its email address?

Getting Started with Your Computer

It is wise to review the material in this section before beginning work on a computer.

Enter

Used throughout this book, Enter refers to the Enter or return key. When the word "Enter" appears in this book, do not type it. Instead, press the Enter or return key; it is usually marked with a left-pointing arrow.

Bold

Instructions in bold indicate what to click on, which keys to press, or what to type. Computers are very exacting. A misspelled word or failure to place a blank where a blank is needed may result in an error message. Make sure what is typed is exactly what is bolded.

Ctrl+*X*	When Ctrl (or Alt or Shift) appears followed by a plus sign (+) and function key number or letter, press the first key and then, while holding it down, press the correct function or letter key. Release both keys together.
Version	The specific sequence and location of commands vary with different versions of software. In this book, Microsoft Office 2007 is used for the word processing, presentation graphics, spreadsheet, and database content, and Internet Explorer (version 7) and Firefox (version 3) are used for the two browsers. If your computer is a Mac equipped with Office 2008 or Safari (browser), some of the specific commands will be different.
Windows/Mac OS	Although the exercises for Word, Excel, Access, PowerPoint, Internet Explorer, and Firefox were written using Windows Vista, Mac-based programs can just as easily be used for these exercises. Most of the keystrokes are exactly the same. A few menu items and a few keys on the keyboard are different. Although every attempt was made to replicate the windows in true form, your system may display some variations in terms of how the window "looks." Despite these minor differences, you should be able to follow along in the exercises.

Learning a Few Basic Skills

Logging In

To log in:

1. Access the system. This may mean typing an address in a browser like intranet.laroche.edu to access the main internal Web page, pressing Ctrl+Alt+Delete to access the login screen, or opening an icon on the desktop for a specific system. **Figure 1-1** provides two examples.
2. Type your UserID or user name in the appropriate textbox.
3. Type your password in the appropriate text box. NOTE: The password will not show but will have asterisks in place of the letters and numbers typed. Some system passwords are case sensitive.

> NOTE: Some systems you access may have specific settings required for them to function properly. For example, Blackboard requires JavaScript and cookies enabled while Microsoft's Web-based access to Outlook requires popups to be enabled. Your institution should provide you with how to enable these should they be required.

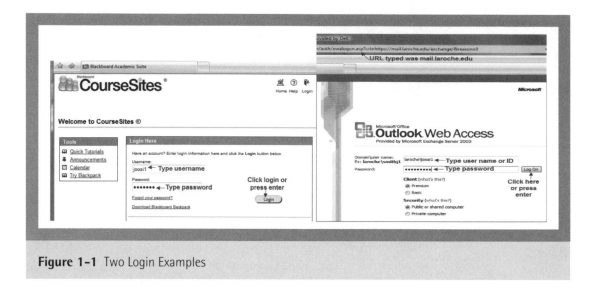

Figure 1-1 Two Login Examples

File Formats

Working in the computer environment requires some knowledge of working with files that you might need for a class or that you might need to send to your professor. Two things you might have to do are to (1) create or open a PDF (portable document format) file or (2) compress/decompress a file. PDF is a fixed-layout format often used in publishing. Two popular fixed-layout formats are Adobe PDF and Microsoft's PDF and XPS (XML Paper Specification).

To create a PDF file, you will need to install a free Office add-in utility (or plug-in) or use another program like PDFCreator that may be installed on laboratory computers.

To download the Microsoft utility:

1. Start **Internet Explorer** or another browser.
2. **Type office.microsoft.com/en-us/downloads/** in the URL or address text box and press **Enter.**
3. In the search box, type **Microsoft Office Add-in save as PDF** and **click** the **Search** button. See **Figure 1-2.**
4. **Click** the hyperlink for **Microsoft Office Add-in save as PDF.**
5. Review the System Requirements, Overview, and Instructions sections.
6. To install the download:
   a. **Click** the **Download** button **Download**. At the File Download— Security Warning dialog box, click the **Save** button **Save** and save the file to your hard disk on the desktop or download folder.
   b. At the Download Complete dialog box, **click** the **Run** button **Run**. Alternatively, you may install the utility later. To do this, **double-click** the **SaveAsPDFandXPS.exe** program file on your desktop or in your download folder to start the Setup program.

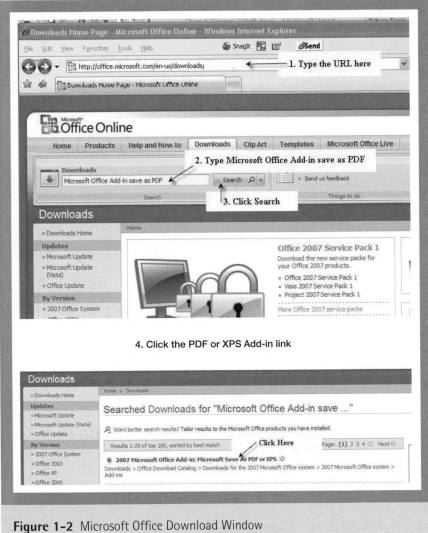

Figure 1-2 Microsoft Office Download Window

c. If selecting the Run option, follow the instructions on the screen to complete the installation. This may require accepting the software agreement and/or clicking **Continue** as those windows pop up.

NOTE: You can also click the **Office** button, **Save as**, and **PDF or XPS format** toward the bottom of the menu. Verify that you have a legal copy of Microsoft Office and follow the screen directions to download it.

To save a file in PDF format:

1. **Open** the document you want to publish.
2. **Click** the Office button and then point to **Save As**.
3. When the pop-up menu appears, click **PDF or XPS**.
4. **Type** a name and select a location for the saved file or accept the default name and location.

NOTE: The procedure for creating a PDF file may vary depending on the program you are using. Some require you to select **Publish to** or **Print, Print,** and to change the printer to Adobe PDF.

For more information, search Microsoft Office Help online for "Save a file in PDF format" or "Save a file in XPS format."

Compression Files

Both Windows Vista and Windows XP come with a compression utility that allows you to send or receive large or multiple files. Other programs that zip and unzip files include WinZip and StuffIt. Faculty may send textbook files to you as email attachments or place them on a file server. Many of these files are compressed.

To compress a file:

1. **Select** the file or folder from your storage device.
2. **Right-click** the file or folder.
3. Choose **Send To** and then **Compressed (Zipped) Folder**. (See **Figure 1-3**.) A compressed folder appears in the same place as the original folder. It may look like this if you are using WinZip.

To unzip a file:

1. **Double-click** the compressed file or folder. You may also *right-click* the compressed file or folder, choose **Open with,** and then choose **Compressed (Zipped) Folder** or **WinZip**. See **Figure 1-4**.
2. **Figure 1-5** shows the dialog window that appears with the contents of the zipped file. Note that your window might look slightly different but will function similarly.
3. **Select** the appropriate file or folder to extract and then **click** the **extract all files** text. Again, a button may be available on a toolbar that you can use to extract files, depending on the program.

Although you can view compressed files, they will *not* work properly until they are extracted.

Figure 1–3
Dialog Box for Compressing a File/Folder

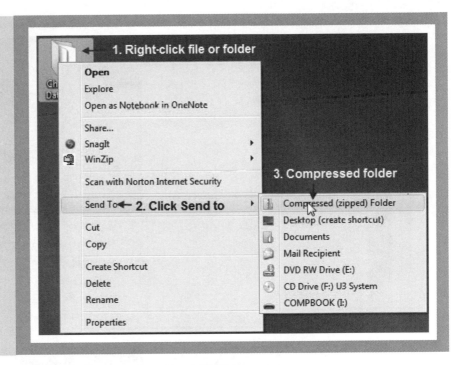

Figure 1–4
Dialog Box for Opening a Compressed File/Folder

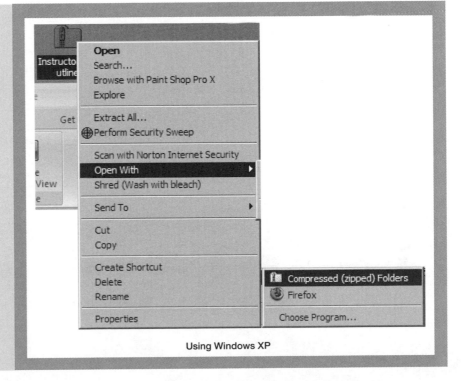

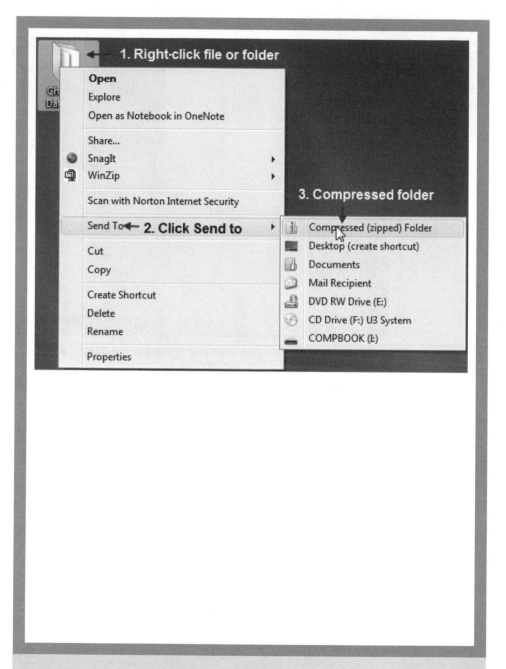

Figure 1-5 Dialog Boxes for Opening a Compressed File/Folder

Email Attachments

In addition to saving files in PDF format and extracting compressed files, you may need to download a file attached to an email message or attach one of your assignments to an email message.

To download an email attachment:

1. **Open** the email program and display the mail message.
2. Look for words or a paper clip that indicates an attachment. It should look something like this: Attachments: Flower Sales.pptx(1MB) PresentationCD.zip(12MB)
3. **Right-click** the file and **save target as** (or something similar to those words).
4. **Select** a place to download the file.

Each mail program is slightly different in terms of the location and display of the attached file. Nevertheless, all programs should give you the ability to right-click and save the file to a specific location.

To attach a file to an email:

1. Open the email program and look for words like **compose mail** Compose Mail or **new message** New . **Click** the words to start and compose a message.
2. Once the message is composed, look for a paper clip Attach a file or attachment words Attachments: . **Click** the words or paper clip.
3. Complete the window that appears asking for the location and file to attach. Make sure the attachment appears in the mail message window before you send the message.

Introduction to OneNote

Microsoft Office OneNote 2007 provides you with an electronic tool for organizing and storing information such as notes from class, reference materials, and Internet sources. Information is gathered in electronic notebooks that are equivalent to traditional three-ring binders, where each notebook has sections and pages. You can store almost any kind of electronic information in OneNote, such as photos, text, graphics, audio, Web clippings, and video clips. You can write a note with the keyboard, write a note with a "pen," or copy something from the screen and paste it into OneNote or even into another Office document. When you copy something from the Internet, the address from which you copied the information will automatically appear on the OneNote page. Many of the small figures or icons used in this book were captured using OneNote. OneNote does not use the ribbon concept of Office 2007.

OneNote Basics

Three notebooks are included when you install OneNote—OneNote 2007 Guide, Personal Notebook, and Work Notebook. When you click OneNote 2007 Guide, the first section of OneNote basic information appears. (See **Figure 1-6**.) On the right, under New Page, is a list of all pages in this section. To explore this guide, try clicking each page tab and reading its contents to get an idea of how OneNote works. Page tabs can be expanded « or collapsed » by clicking the chevrons to the right of New Page. There are also up and down chevrons on the Notebooks task pane that expands and collapses the view of each notebook. Be sure to look at **Figure 1-7**, which provides information about many of the tools available in OneNote as well as instructions about hyperlinks, audio and video recordings, tables, and use of OneNote with other applications.

Figure 1-8 shows the Personal Notebook with *Personal Information* selected. Sections in this notebook include Shopping, Books, Travel, Recipes, To Do, and Miscellaneous as noted on the tabs.

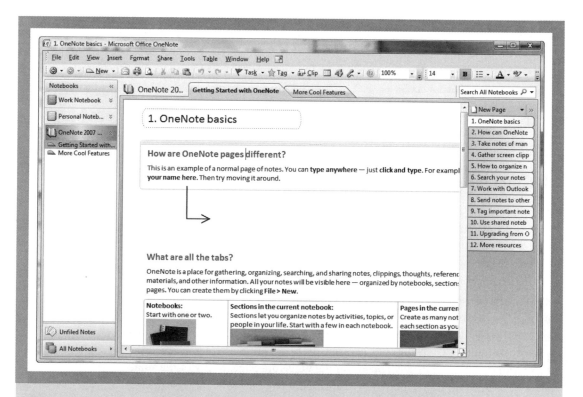

Figure 1-6 OneNote Window: OneNote 2007 Guide Selected

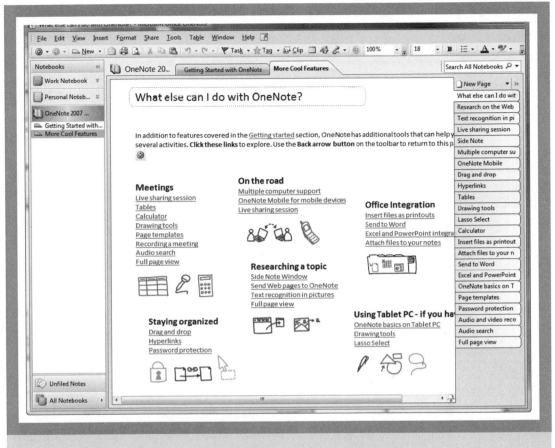

Figure 1-7 OneNote Guide: More Cool Features

The third notebook, the Work Notebook, is shown in **Figure 1-9** with the *Travel tab* selected. It includes sections for Meeting notes, Planning, Research, and Projects.

You will also find it worthwhile to review the online training available from Microsoft for OneNote. Click **Help** in the menu bar and choose **Microsoft Office Online** to discover the options available.

Using OneNote

When you open OneNote for the first time, you will see a window like that shown in **Figure 1-10**—an Unfiled note or page. You can click anywhere inside the page and write a note, draw something, or paste text or a picture. The note will appear in a "container" or text box like this: Type here. The container can be modified using traditional Microsoft protocols.

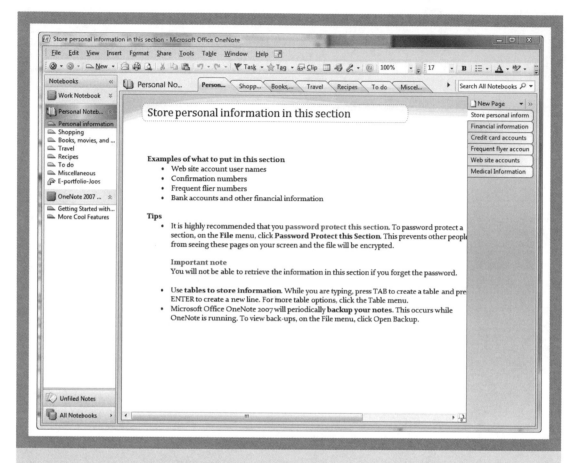

Figure 1-8 OneNote: Personal Notebook, Personal Information Selected

NOTE: If you don't see the Untitled Note Page, click the Unfiled Notes button on the bottom of the Notebooks task pane.

When you put your cursor in a container, it will change to a four-headed arrow ✛. Click the container, and you can move it anywhere on the page. If the cursor looks like a two-headed arrow ↔, you can change the width of the container.

To remove what you have typed, select the **text** and then press **Backspace**, **Delete**; alternatively, you can **right-click** and choose **Delete** from the menu that appears.

To add a new Untitled Note, click the symbol 📝 in the Navigation Pane, click the New Page command in the Page task pane, or click the New button

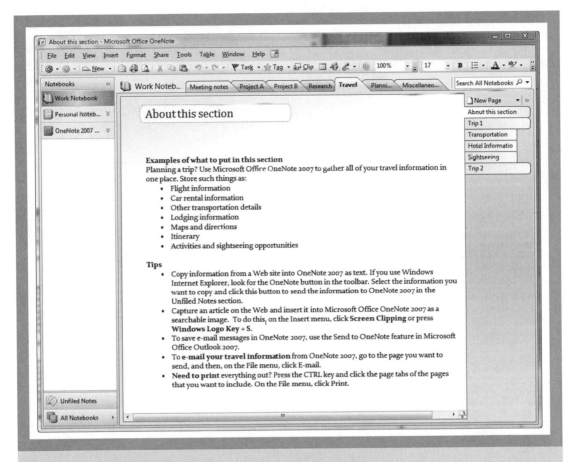

Figure 1-9 OneNote: Work Notebook, Travel Section Selected

on the toolbar. You will see more untitled note pages appearing in the Page task pane.

To see another view of the notebook sections, click the All Notebooks list in the Navigation Pane. You will then see a list similar to that shown in **Figure 1-11**.

Opening a New Notebook, Section, or Page

To open a new notebook, click **File** and place the cursor over **New**; a menu will appear, as shown in **Figure 1-12a**. If you choose **Notebook**, the *New Notebook Wizard* will appear as shown in **Figure 1-12b**. From the wizard, it is possible to select a Research Notebook, a Student Semester Notebook, or several other options. Even more templates are available online that deal with house hunting, wedding planning, school, and work, for example. Each notebook can have several sections. New

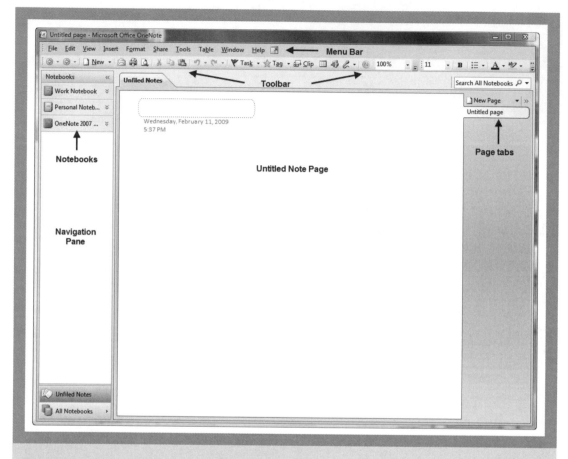

Figure 1–10 OneNote Window

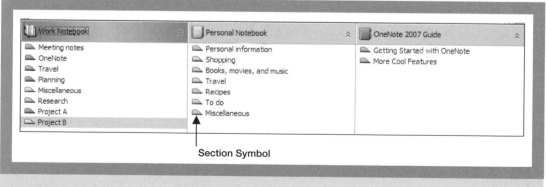

Figure 1–11 All Notebooks List

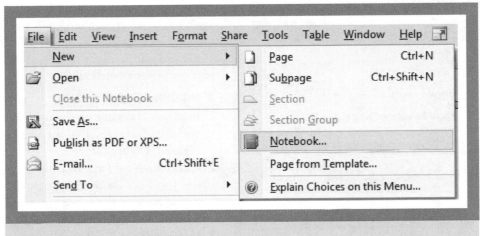

Figure 1–12a Opening a New Notebook

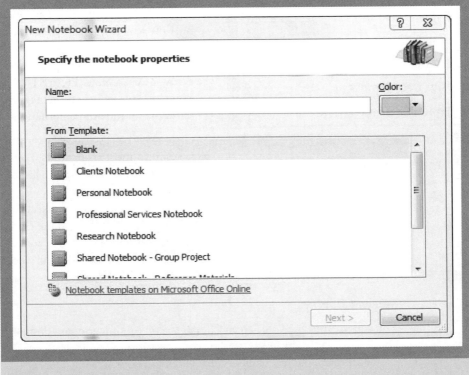

Figure 1–12b New Notebook Wizard

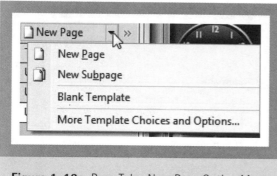

Figure 1-13a Page Tabs: New Page Option Menu

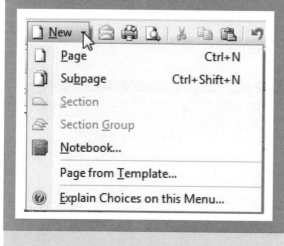

Figure 1-13b New Page Button on Toolbar: Menu Options

notebooks can be added at any time, just as new pages can be added in a section. If you opened the Notebook wizard, click the **Close** button.

Here is another way to open a notebook page, section, or notebook:

1. **Click New Page** above the page tabs task pane on the right side. Click the down arrow. The menu shown in **Figure 1-13a** appears.
2. **Click** the **New Page button** in the toolbar. Or, click the **down arrow** beside **New** on the menu bar, and a menu appears. See **Figure 1-13b**.
3. If you choose **Explain Choices on this Menu . . .** , a task pane will appear on the right side as shown in **Figure 1-14**.

Here is another way to see the task pane:

1. On the **View** menu, **click Task Pane** in the bottom row to place a check next to the command.
2. In the task pane on the **right click** the down arrow next to New. **Figure 1-15** appears. You can choose New to see Figure 1-14 or select one of the other alternatives.

Once a new page is selected, you can alter the page setup to meet your needs. For example, you can change the font, make a list, use bullets or numbers, and check spelling.

Remember that notes and sections can be added to a notebook at any time. Unfiled notes can be moved easily to sections or notebooks. However, it is wise to consider which kind of tasks you have and which kind of organizational structure will work the best for you. Remember, too, that notes and notebooks are automatically saved.

Screen Clippings

You can use the One Note Screen Clipper to copy an image of anything you see on your computer screen.

To capture a picture, icon, or *piece* of text on your screen:

1. **Press** the **Windows logo key** + **S**. The screen changes to a filmy white and the cursor changes to a plus sign.

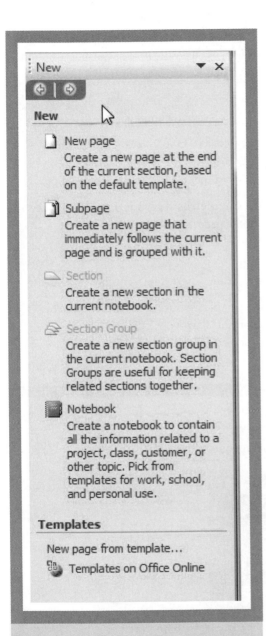

Figure 1–14 Page Explanations in Task Pane

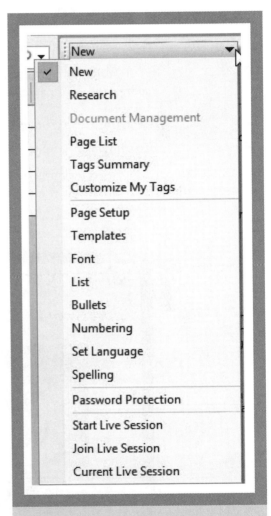

Figure 1–15 Task Pane

2. Put the **plus sign** over a corner of the object/picture you wish to copy; **click** and **drag** until you have selected the image you desire. **Release** the mouse button.

3. The image will appear on an Unfiled Notes page, along with the date and time when it was clipped.

Here is another way to prepare to take a screen clipping:

1. Click ⌧ Clip in the standard toolbar in OneNote; the screen turns white and you proceed the same way.

2. Another option is to go to the **Insert** menu and choose **Screen Clipping**.

If you captured an image off the Internet, as shown in **Figure 1-15**, the site address will appear automatically on the page as well.

Copying Text or Images

To copy an image or text from *OneNote* and insert it into another document:

1. **Select** the image or text. When you place your mouse arrow over the image/text, it turns into a four-headed arrow ⊞ ☆ Tag ⊹.

Screen clipping

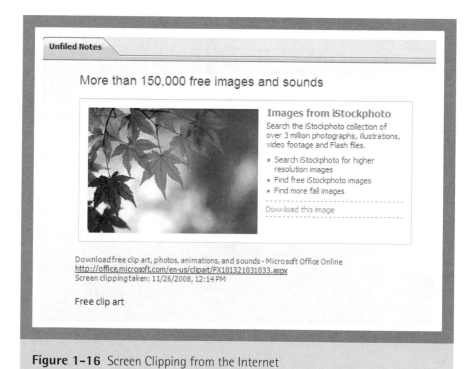

Figure 1–16 Screen Clipping from the Internet

2. **Click** the dotted-line box and it looks like this:
3. You have three ways to copy it:
   a. Under Edit on the menu bar, choose **Copy**, or
   b. **Click** the **Copy** icon in the toolbar bar, or
   c. **Press Ctrl+C.**
4. Go to the document where you want to place the image:
   a. Choose **Paste** or
   b. Press **Ctrl+V.**

Drawing in OneNote

In OneNote, it is very easy to draw images freehand or use buttons on the drawing toolbar. See **Figure 1-17.**

   If the drawing toolbar does not appear at the bottom of the OneNote window, click the **Drawing Toolbar** button . Click the **pen**, and then try to draw a figure or flower. You will find that it takes practice! If you have a tablet PC, it will be kind of fun! Practice with all the shapes and with the many pen styles. After you have drawn something, select it, and either press the backspace or delete key or click the **Delete** button. Experiment with other tools until you are familiar with what each one can do. Each image can be resized or moved around the page in the same way that other containers can.

Side Note

Side Note is a small version of OneNote. It appears in its own small window. It will stay open on your desktop when you click the **Keep Window on Top**

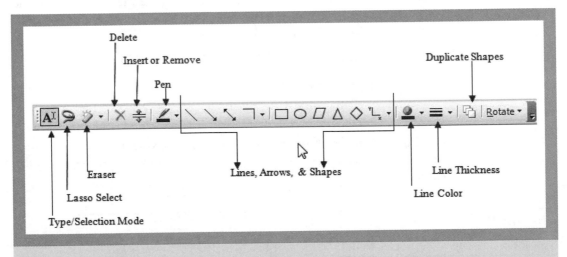

Figure 1-17 OneNote Drawing Tools

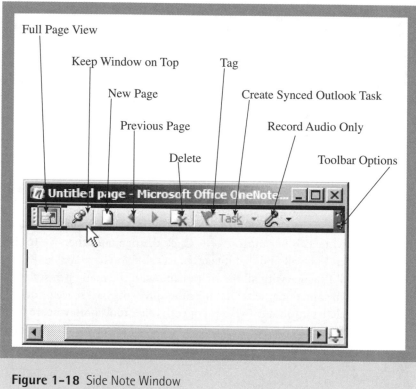

Figure 1-18 Side Note Window

button 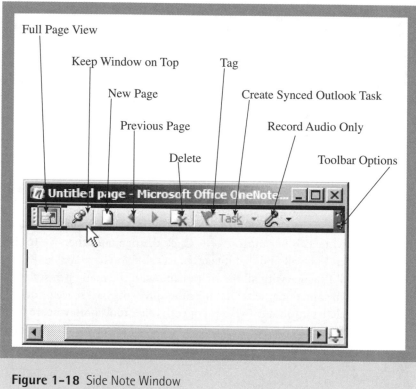 as shown in **Figure 1-18**. You can adjust the size of the window and pull up other toolbar options at any time.

To open a Side Note window:

1. Press the **Windows logo key** + **N**.

If you opened the Side Note, close it.

Moving Pages, Sections, and Notebooks

Moving large pieces of information is easy in OneNote. Following are some ways you can do this. Be aware that the target notebook must be open to move content to it.

To Move This	Do This
A page or subpage within a section	**Drag** the page tab up or down in the page task pane.
A page to another notebook	**Drag** the page tab to the desired section tab in the notebook header or in the Navigation Pane.

A section within a notebook	**Drag** the section tab left or right in the notebook header; or **Drag** the section tab to the desired location in the Navigation Pane; or **Right-click** the section tab, and then click **Move**. In the **Move Section To** dialog box, click the location where you want the section to go, and then **click Move Before** or **Move After**.
A section to another notebook	**Drag** the section tab to a new location in the Navigation Pane; or **Right-click** the section tab, and then click **Move**. In the **Move Section To** dialog box, click the notebook where you want to move the section, and then click **Move Into**.
A notebook on the Navigation Pane	**Drag** the notebook title up or down the notebook list.

Other Features

It is easy to send a piece of information, a table, or picture to another Office Program:

1. **Select** the pages or section you want to send.
2. Go to **File** and click **Send To**. You can choose one of the three options listed as shown in **Figure 1-19**.

Notes can also be tagged:

1. Pick a note to tag.
2. **Click Tag** ☆ Tag ▾ .
3. A star ☆ will appear in the note's container.

If you click the down arrow, a menu will appear as shown in **Figure 1-20**. Many more choices become available on this menu.

If you are working in Internet Explorer, you can send an image or text to OneNote.

1. **Select** an **image** or **portion of text** or even the whole page.
2. Under **Tools** ⚙ Tools ▾ , **click** the drop-down arrow.
3. Choose **Send to OneNote**.

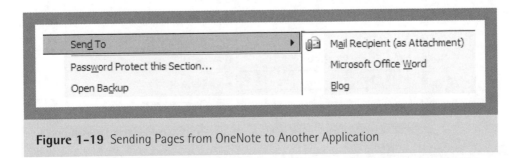

Figure 1-19 Sending Pages from OneNote to Another Application

Figure 1-20
Drop-Down
Menu for the Tag
Toolbar Button

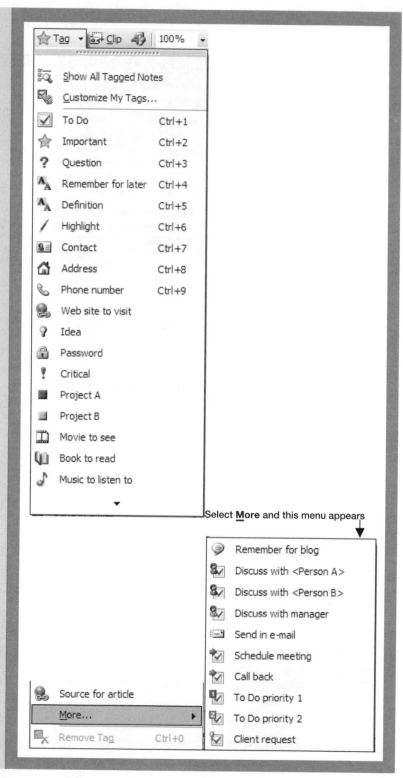

Select **More** and this menu appears

This section has highlighted just a few of the many things you can do with OneNote. If you use this program as it is meant to be used, you will end up with a large collection of information. Even if you use all the tools possible to organize your information, you may need to search for some information.

1. **Go to** the **Search** text box Search All Notebooks ; click in it.
2. **Type** the word(s) you are looking for.
3. **Click** the **magnifying glass** .
4. A list of the matches appears, highlighted in yellow. **Click View List**, and a partial description of each match appears on the right side of the window.

Additional Tips

Some additional tips described here will prove helpful as you work through this book to develop your computer and information literacy.

1. Do not try to complete all of the book exercises at once. Sometimes it is helpful to come back later, especially when the exercises are not going well or when fatigue sets in.
2. Pay attention to messages on the screen. They are the computer's way of trying to provide help.
3. Use the software sequences found at the end of each lesson on an application program to complete the exercises or assignments for that software program. It is not necessary to memorize the commands, mouse clicks, or sequences of events. Use the screen clues, prompts, and online help to guide you through the sequence.
4. Explore additional functions by referring to other reference sources such as online help, manuals, or reference books. The functions highlighted in this book were chosen to help you complete the exercises and learn some basics of how the programs work. Many more functions are available within each of the software programs presented here.
5. Always back up your files. This point is especially important for the beginner so that hours of work will not be lost. Open a document and then save it immediately; don't wait until you have finished it or finished your session on the computer.
6. Practice doing assignments from all courses using your computer. It takes practice to develop computer literacy. The more you use the computer, the easier and faster tasks will become.
7. Be patient. Learning a new vocabulary and developing new skills take time and energy.
8. Start collecting information for your e-portfolio using OneNote.

Summary

This chapter provided an orientation to computer and information literacy. It described how this book is organized and the conventions used to denote user actions. Some helpful information about getting started using the school or laboratory facilities was also presented. Instructions related to creating a PDF file and compressing files were included as well. Also described were the basics of using OneNote—getting started, opening new notebooks, adding pages or sections, using the drawing tools, and taking screen clippings. Finally, resources for learning more about OneNote were described.

References

Association of College and Research Libraries. (2000). *Information literacy competency standards for higher education.* Chicago: Author. Retrieved January 29, 2009, from http://www.ala.org/ala/mgrps/divs/acrl/standards/informationliteracycompetency.cfm

---

EXERCISE 1 Log In, Download, and Send an Email Attachment

■ **Objectives**
1. Log in to the email program.
2. Download and send an email attachment.

■ **Activity**
1. **Log in** to the mail program you will be using for this course. You will receive an email with an attachment from your professor.
2. **Open** the email and follow the instructions contained in it. It will contain a compressed file. Download the compressed file using the directions provided in this chapter. Extract the contents of the file. What was in the compressed file?
3. Send an email to your classmates and professor that contains the following information:
   a. A brief introduction of you, your interests, and so on.
   b. A picture of you attached to the email.
4. Read and respond to your classmates' emails.

EXERCISE 2 Information Literacy Competency Standards for Higher Education

---

■ **Objectives**
1. Develop a personal definition of information literacy.

■ **Activity**
1. Go to the Web site of the Association of College and Research Libraries.
   a. **Type http://www.ala.org/ala/mgrps/divs/acrl/index.cfm**
   b. **Click Standards and Guidelines** on the left side of the screen.
   c. Move down the list and **click Information Literacy Competency Standards for Higher Education (Jan. 2000).**
   d. Review the standards by selecting **Standards, Performance Indicators, and Outcomes.**

e. Review the material on information literacy and information technology at this site.

2. From this material, develop your own definition of information literacy.

3. Place this definition in OneNote for later addition to your e-portfolio. Keep a weekly journal of the skills you are developing in this course.

EXERCISE 3 Electronic Reference Formats

■ **Objectives**

1. Find sources for styling electronic references.
2. Recognize the appropriate format for electronic references used by the American Psychological Association (APA).

■ **Activity**

Use OneNote to keep a notebook of your findings regarding how to format electronic references. If necessary, review the processes described earlier in this chapter. In the Word chapter, you will learn how to use templates and the References tab to automatically format your papers and references in the correct style.

1. Go to the Dartmouth Institute for Writing and Rhetoric.
   a. **Type http://www.dartmouth.edu/~writing/.**
   b. **Click Sources & Citation at Dartmouth.**
   c. Download a copy and review it. (Note: You will need the **PDF add-in utility** on your computer. If necessary, review the process for adding the PDF utility that was described earlier in this chapter.)
2. Go to APA Style.Org.
   a. **Type http://www.apastyle.org/elecref.html.**
   b. **Click Electronic media and URLs.**
   c. Review the article.
3. Review the following sources:
   a. **Type http://www.dianahacker.com/resdoc/.**
      i. Hold the mouse pointer over **Sciences Section** and click **Nursing and health sciences.**
      ii. Review the sections on databases and indexes, Web resources, and reference books.
   b. Go to "The Owl at Purdue" and review its **APA Formatting and Style Guide.**
      i. **Type http://owl.english.purdue.edu/owl/resource/560/01/.**
      ii. Scroll down and choose **No. 10: Reference List: Electronic Sources.**
      iii. Review the materials.

EXERCISE 4   Compare Four Information Literacy Tutorials

■ **Objectives**
   1. Review three different information literacy tutorials.
   2. Compare and evaluate them.

■ **Activity**
   1. Compare the following four information literacy tutorials in terms of their ease of use, ease of navigation (i.e., ability to move around them), content, and value to you.
      a. Information Literacy Tutorial: University of Wisconsin-Parkside Library
         Type http://www.uwp.edu/
         Under **Quick Links, click Library**
         Click the **Information Literacy Tutorial** under Guides and Tutorials
         Click Start the Tutorial button
      b. Information Literacy Tutorial: Five Colleges of Ohio
         Type http://www.ohio5.org/
         Click Library Resources and Initiatives
         Click Information Literacy Projects
         Click Information Literacy Tutorial
      c. Information Literacy Tutorial: Penn State University Libraries
         Type http://www.libraries.psu.edu/psul.html
         Under **Get Help** on the right side of the screen, **click Tutorials**
         Click Information Literacy & You
         Click Searching Online Databases
         Now, **click Using Web Resources** on the left side of the screen
         Review other sections as desired.

EXERCISE 5   Explore the Uses of e-Portfolios

■ **Objectives**
   1. Describe the essentials of an e-portfolio.
   2. Describe the relationship between information literacy and e-portfolios.

■ **Activity**
   1. Go to the e-portfolio site at Penn State:
      a. Type **http://portfolio.psu.edu/**.
      b. Click the **About** link.
      c. View some of the other links such as **Collect**, **Select**, and **Reflect**.

2. What is an e-portfolio?
3. How does it relate to information literacy?
4. If you are interested in learning more about e-Portfolios, check out this site: http://www.elearnspace.org/Articles/eportfolios.htm.

ASSIGNMENT 1 Learning About Your School's Computer Policies

■ **Directions**

Use your school's intranet site to find the answers to the following questions:

1. Find your school's Web site. What is its Uniform Resource Locator (URL)?
2. Is there a technical support center? Is it known by another name?
3. What are the policies and procedures of the academic computing center?
4. Can you download these policies?
5. How does a student set up network and email accounts?
6. Which operating systems and software does the center support?
7. Is there a laptop lease/buy program at your school?
8. Does your school have an e-Portfolio system for students?
9. Is there an e-learning center? If so, which classes are available?
10. What are the hours for technical support?
11. What was the most valuable thing you learned from this assignment?

Turn in a summary of what you learned answering these questions.

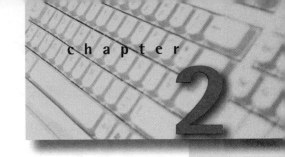
Computer Systems: Hardware, Software, and Connectivity

Objectives

1. Define inlock keysformation systems.
2. Describe the major components of computer systems and their related functions.
3. Define basic terminology related to hardware, software, and connectivity.
4. Describe the main categories of computer software.
5. Appreciate the language of information systems.

In today's "information age," people need to use information systems to manage the sometimes overwhelming wealth of information that is available. Healthcare practitioners rely on an ever-expanding body of information to provide safe, efficient client care and on technology to assist in providing that information.

A *system* is a set of interrelated parts; an *information system* is a system that produces information using an input/process/output cycle. A basic information system consists of four elements: people, policies and procedures, communication (connectivity), and data. A computer information system then adds two more elements: (hardware) and software. See **Figure 2-1.** Types of information systems include transaction systems, such as payroll and order entry systems; management information systems, which facilitate running an organization; decision support systems, which facilitate decision making; and expert systems, which provide advice or make recommendations regarding diagnosis or treatments.

The purpose of an information system is to provide information to the users so as to facilitate the work of the organization. A brief description of each of its elements follows.

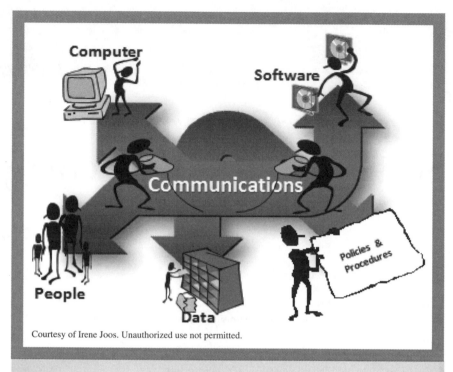

Courtesy of Irene Joos. Unauthorized use not permitted.

Figure 2-1 Components of a Computer Information System

People

People are the most important part of the system; they—and ultimately their organizations—benefit from the information provided by these systems. Three basic types of users are typically identified: end users, technical professionals, and informatics specialists. In health care, end users are the healthcare providers who use computers as tools to assist them in delivering care. Increasingly, end users also include consumers who access healthcare information on the Internet and/or store their personal health records (PHR) on Internet-accessible servers.

Technical professionals are the information technology professionals who develop, maintain, and evaluate the technical aspects of information systems. They are generally responsible for the network, databases, software and hardware updates, security, communications, and so forth. These are the people who respond to end user problems and questions.

Informatics specialists are professionals who bridge the gap between the healthcare provider as end user and the technical expert. Their education and professional experience include both health care and computer/information science. Examples of types of Information Technology personnel typically found in health care are provided in Chapter 14.

It is impossible to bridge the gap between end users and technical experts, thereby creating healthcare information systems, if healthcare providers have not achieved a basic level of computer and information literacy. Achieving the goal of computer and information literate healthcare providers is the mission of this book.

Policies and Procedures

Policies and procedures outline the guiding principles related to information and technology use and give step-by-step directions for how the system works and how things are done to accomplish the end results. Most systems have a manual or documentation—written and/or online—that includes the necessary directions and/or instructions, rules or policies, and special guidelines for using the system. Later chapters dealing with communications in healthcare systems (Chapter 10) as well as data integrity and security (Chapter 13) provide examples of specific policies and procedures for healthcare technology.

Communication/Connectivity

Communication (also known as connectivity) refers to the electronic transfer of data from one place to another. This is an area of rapid developments that change how work is done. Communication also refers to how people use the technology to enhance their communications with each other and with healthcare consumers. Chapters 9, 10, and 11 review basic concepts regarding communication, including appropriate and professional communications within the healthcare setting. This chapter deals with the hardware necessary for a computer to connect to and communicate with other computers.

Data

Data and information, along with knowledge and wisdom, are described in Chapter 14. Database concepts are presented in Chapter 8 along with an introduction to Access, a database software program, while information access is covered in Chapters 9 and 12.

Hardware, software, and connectivity are the focus of this chapter. Later chapters in this book contain more information about specific software applications and communications.

Introduction to Computer Systems: Hardware

The hardware for a computer system consists of input devices, the system unit (processing unit, memory, boards, and power supply), output devices, and secondary storage devices. The basic function of the computer is to accept data and instructions from a user, process the data to produce information, store the data for later retrieval, and display the information. More advanced functions involve the creation, communication, and storage of knowledge used in the provision of health care. Supporting the implementation of evidence-based care at the point of delivery is an example of this advanced function.

The following definitions are important to understanding the upcoming sections on hardware. Refer to these definitions as these terms appear throughout this chapter.

Common Computer Terms

A computer is a programmable machine capable of performing a series of logical and arithmetic operations. One of the most frequent uses of a computer in health care is the conversion of data into information. As an electronic device, the computer uses a series of 0s and 1s to describe data and to represent information. It does not understand the spoken word as we do, but must convert words to a sequence of 0s and 1s.

A bit is the smallest unit of data, the lowest level; the term "bit" is an abbreviation for "binary digit." A bit represents one of two states for the computer, 0 or 1; these two states are equivalent to off or on (like the two states possible for a light switch). Everything the computer understands uses combinations of 0s and 1s.

A byte is a string of bits used to represent a character, digit, or symbol. It usually contains 8 bits.

Computers come in various sizes and configurations. Over the years, the power, speed, and storage capacity of computers have increased, while their size and cost have decreased. **Figure** 2-2 illustrates several types of computers. Some common types of computers are described next.

Supercomputer	Supercomputers are the fastest, most expensive, and most powerful type of computers available. They tend to focus on running a few programs requiring a lot of computations; by comparison, other types of computers typically run many programs concurrently. Uses of supercomputers include animation graphics, weather forecasting, and research applications. Some medical-related examples include re-creating the internal architecture of bone structures to guide bone replacement in reconstructive surgery, designing new molecular compounds for drug-related therapies, and genetic mapping in understanding Parkinson's disease.
Mainframe	A mainframe is a large computer that accommodates hundreds of users simultaneously. It has a large data storage

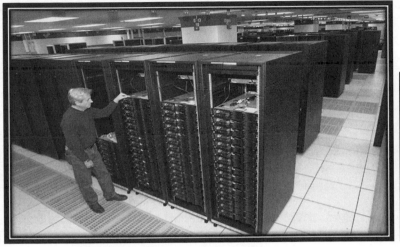

Courtesy of International Business Machines Corporation. Unauthorized use not permitted.

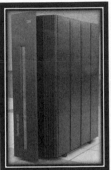

Courtesy of International
Business Machines Corporation.
Unauthorized use not permitted.

Supercomputer

Mainframe Computer

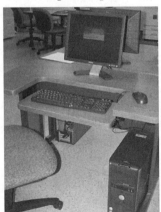

Courtesy of Irene Joos. Unauthorized use not permitted.

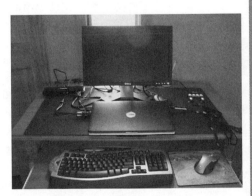

Courtesy of Irene Joos. Unauthorized use not permitted.

Desktop Computer

**Laptop with Docking Station, Monitor,
Wireless Keyboard, and Wireless Mouse**

Figure 2-2 Examples of Various Computers

capacity, a large amount of memory, multiple input/output (I/O) devices, and speedy processor(s). Many universities and hospitals run their computer systems on mainframe computers.

Midrange

The term "midrange computer" (formerly called a mini-computer) describes a medium-sized computer that is faster and stores more data than a personal computer (PC). Midrange computers are cheaper than mainframes. In terms of size, they are between mainframes and PCs. Many departments in larger companies use such computers to house specific software related to the department's function. For example, midrange computers may run pharmacy or laboratory software for that department.

Servers

A server is a computer that controls access to the software, hardware (like printers on the network), and data located on a network. Users use their personal computers to access the resources on the network and to store data on specialized servers called file servers. There is also a trend toward increased use of specialized servers, called Web servers, to host Web pages and other files accessed through the Internet.

Microcomputer

A microcomputer is a small, one-user computer system with its own central processing unit (CPU), memory, and storage devices. Also referred to as PCs and desktops, these models are growing in processing power, speed, and storage capacity.

Mobile Devices

In this class of computers are laptops, PC tablets, handheld computers (also called ultra-mobile PCs), PDAs, and smart phones like the iPhone and BlackBerry. **Figure 2-3** shows some examples of mobile devices.

Laptops, sometimes called notebooks, are generally more expensive than PCs, but have the same power and capabilities. Their small size and portability make them a good choice for use in temporary spaces such as airplanes, libraries, and homes or in small spaces such as a nurse's station. Batteries or AC outlets provide power to laptops. Laptops integrate the monitor, keyboard, and mouse into the laptop case. Users can convert laptops into a PC by using a docking station, ports, or a laptop interface that accepts a larger monitor, full-size keyboard, mouse, or printer.

Handheld computers can fit in your hand. These models have full PC functionality but include much smaller screens

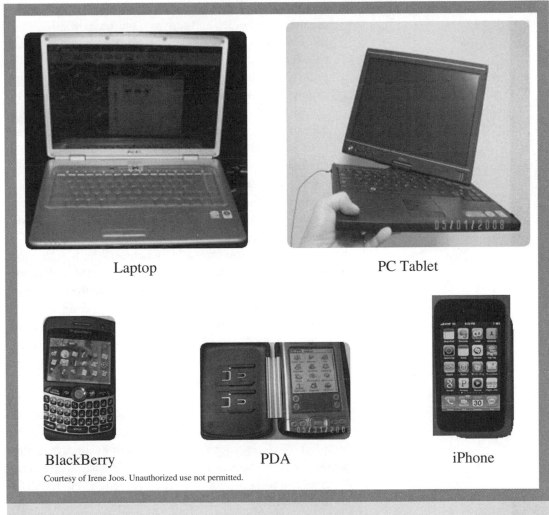

Laptop

PC Tablet

BlackBerry   PDA   iPhone

Courtesy of Irene Joos. Unauthorized use not permitted.

Figure 2–3 Mobile Devices

and keyboards (sometimes specialized keyboards). They range in size from 6 to 10 inches in width and are popular with people whose work requires them to move around.

PDAs (personal digital assistants) or palmtop computers are popular in all walks of life. They perform many of the same functions as PCs, but are meant to supplement PCs, not replace them. PDAs have a processor, an operating system (OS), memory, a power source (batteries), a display, an input device (newer ones use color touch screens), audio capability, I/O ports, and software, but no hard drive. Basic information such as a calendar, address book, contacts, and so forth is stored on a read-only memory (ROM) chip; programs added later, such as drug reference material, are stored on a random access memory (RAM) chip.

Most PDAs can access the Internet via wireless connections, and some models have Global Positioning System (GPS) capabilities. Their ability to store information such as contacts, drug references, laboratory tests, and other diagnostic reference material as well as their small size make them favorites in the healthcare field. An increasing number of nursing programs have chosen to provide their students with PDAs as quick reference sources to use in clinical rotations.

Most PDAs also have a PC synchronizing function that allows for updating a database on both the PDA and the PC. Synchronizing also prevents data loss in case the PDA is lost, stolen, or destroyed. Generally, it requires connecting the PDA to a PC with either a cable, a cradle, or a wireless connection. A sync button is then pressed on the PDA or cradle. At that point, files are compared and updated with the latest version on both the PC and the PDA.

Smart phones include devices such as the BlackBerry and the iPhone. These devices provide access to the Internet, email, phone, references, GPS, books, and games, to name a few resources. Increasing numbers of healthcare professionals are using these devices to provide quick access to references during patient care. The distinction between PDAs and smart phones is also blurring as their functions increasingly overlap.

The downside to mobile devices relates to security. Specifically, steps must be taken to secure these devices when they contain confidential information.

Before describing the four basic computer components, four more definitions are necessary.

Boot	To start the computer so that it can execute the necessary startup routines. The boot process is described in more detail in Chapter 3.
Default	The setting the computer uses unless told otherwise. This concept is important because, for example, users will have difficulty retrieving

or finding files if they do not know the default folder where the computer is storing their files. Most college laboratories require their users to store data on a removable storage device or folder on the file server and not in the Microsoft Office Documents folder (the default). Some work environments, by default, set the files to store in the user's folder on a file server so that the files will be backed up when the file server is backed up.

Toggle   To switch from one mode of operation to another. For example, pressing the Insert key toggles between insert mode and typeover mode.

Upgrade   To enhance a piece of equipment or buy the newest release of a software program. Many computers are "upgradeable," meaning that the user may add more memory, additional storage devices, and so forth.

Computer Components: Input Devices

Input devices are hardware components that convert data from an external source into electronic signals understood by the computer. The user interacts with the computer through an interface and an input device. In this interaction, the term "cursor" or "pointer" is used to describe the "visible indicator" on the screen that marks the current location and the point at which the work begins. The cursor can appear as a pointer (generally an arrow), a vertical line (), a horizontal line (), or an I-beam (). The cursor also changes to reflect processes and functions. For example, in Windows, it changes to an hourglass () when the program is processing a command. In Internet Explorer (a Web browser), it changes to a hand () when placed over linked text or objects (text or objects that can lead to more information either at this site or at another site).

The two major input devices are the keyboard and the mouse.

Keyboard

The keyboard is an input device for typing data into the computer. The most common layout includes the typical alphanumeric keys with the function keys at the top and the cursor movement keys and the numeric keypad (calculator layout) on the right. In contrast, laptop computers have a slightly different layout because of their size limitations. Mobile devices such as smart phones and PDAs have fewer keys, with each key representing multiple characters that the user cycles through. For example, the number 2 also represents the letters A, B, and C. Newer keyboards may also include additional keys for Internet access and media controls. Mac keyboards have many of the same keys, but they may be called by another name. Some have fingerprint and card readers. **Figure 2-4** shows a wireless, ergonomic keyboard, a wired keyboard, and a laptop keyboard.

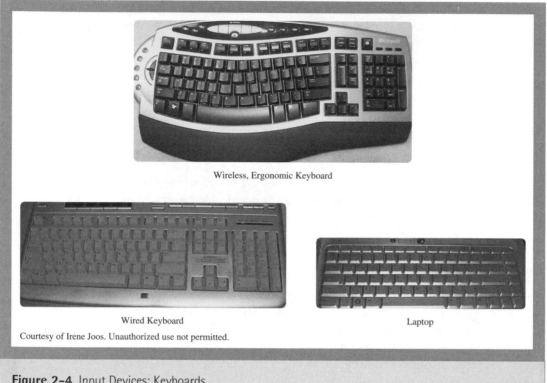

Wireless, Ergonomic Keyboard

Wired Keyboard

Laptop

Courtesy of Irene Joos. Unauthorized use not permitted.

Figure 2–4 Input Devices: Keyboards

Most keyboards connect to the system unit through the keyboard port, although some use the serial port or the USB port. Cordless keyboards use radio waves or infrared light waves to communicate to the system unit via an IrDA or Bluetooth port in the system unit. Laptop keyboards are integral to the top of the system unit. The design of some newer keyboards is intended to reduce the chance of wrist and hand injuries; they are referred to as "ergonomic" keyboards.

Some of the keys used on keyboards are described next.

Main Keyboard Keys

Letters, numbers, and **punctuation** keys enter the corresponding symbol into the software program that is currently in use. Some of the keys have dual functions when they are pressed in conjunction with the Shift, Ctrl, or Alt key. For example, letters become capital letters when pressed along with the Shift or Caps Lock key; numbers become symbols such as $, %, and * when pressed along with the Shift key.

Use the **Caps Lock** key to switch or toggle between all uppercase and lowercase letters. This key is helpful when large amounts of text need to be in all caps.

Use the Backspace key to delete characters to the left of the cursor.

Use the **Delete** key to delete text to the right of the cursor. Sometimes labeled "Del," this key is located above the arrow keys on most full-sized keyboards.

The **Insert** key is found above the arrow keys on many full-sized keyboards and above the Backspace key on a laptop. The default is to insert characters at the location of the cursor, moving all other characters to the right. In many programs, the Insert key serves as a toggle switch to move between typeover and insert modes. When typing replaces characters, press the Insert key to toggle back to insert mode. Some of the newer keyboards have eliminated this key.

The **Tab** key moves the cursor along the screen at defined intervals or to the next field in a dialog box. For example, pressing the Tab key moves the cursor five spaces at a time in many application programs.

Alt, Ctrl, F4, and **Shift** are special keys that modify normal operations. These keys, in combination with other keys, initiate commands or complete tasks. They also provide keyboard shortcuts to some commands. For example, Ctrl+S is equivalent to the Save command in many applications; the F4 key closes a program or active window in Microsoft Windows. By themselves, the Alt, Ctrl, F4, and Shift keys usually have no function.

Pressing the **space bar** enters a space between words, while pressing the **Enter** key sends the text to the next line. The space bar may also have other functions when used in combination with a control key. For example, it may close a window. Use the Enter key to end paragraphs and to accept the highlighted or outlined button in a Windows dialog box (a special window that expects the user to make some selections before the command is implemented). Some texts use symbols (such as <CR>) to represent the enter key. This book uses Enter to mean "press the Enter key."

Cursor Keys

Cursor movement keys, also known as arrow keys, generally take the form of a cluster of four keys that have directional arrows on them. On most full-sized keyboards, they are located on the lower-right side. Press an arrow key to move the cursor on the screen in the direction of that key's arrow.

Use the **Page Up/Down, Home,** and **End** keys to move quickly from one place in the document or on the screen to other locations. These keys are found above the arrow keys on most full-sized keyboards.

Additional Keys

The **Esc** key generally backs out of a program or menu one screen or one menu at a time.

The name of the **Fn** key is an abbreviation for "function." Use this key in conjunction with other keys to produce special actions that vary with applications. The Fn is commonly found on laptops that lack full-sized keyboards.

The Function keys are special keys that application programs use to complete tasks. They are most frequently found at the top of the keyboard, and their specific functions vary for each software program. These keys typically carry labels such as F1, F2, and so on, usually up to F12. With the advent of windows-based environments, the use of these keys has diminished in favor of mouse clicks and shortcut keystrokes such as Ctrl+P for "print" and Ctrl+O for "open." Some newer keyboards list the command above the function key number.

The Print Screen key, when used either in combination with the Alt key or alone, places an image of the screen or active window onto the clipboard. Once on the clipboard, the user can paste the image into an application program.

Lock keys lock part of a keyboard. Their location varies with the different keyboards. Use the Num Lock key to toggle the numeric keypad on and off.

The power management key provides the ability to place the computer in sleep mode and to power up the computer when it is currently in sleep mode.

Numeric Keypad

The numeric keys function like a numeric keypad to enter numbers. Some keyboards require the Num Lock indicator light to be on when using the numeric keypad numbers because the numbers function as cursor movement keys when the Num Lock light is off. On PCs the numeric keypad and the number keys across the top of the keyboard can operate differently to produce American Standard Code for Information Interchange (ASCII) characters when in combination with the Alt key and numbers. For example, pressing the Alt+0176 on the numeric keypad produces the degree symbol when working in an application; doing the same thing with the numbers across the top of the keyboard results in a window opening.

Special Windows Keys

The Application key 📋 displays the shortcut menu for the selected item. For example, it will display the shortcut menu for this text if pressed while the cursor is in this paragraph. This key was introduced on extended keyboards.

The Windows logo key 🪟 displays or hides the Start menu. It is also used in combination with other keys to execute commands. For example, pressing the Windows logo key + F opens the "Search for a file or folder" dialog window. Windows 95 and extended keyboards introduced this key, which is located on the bottom-left side of the keyboard between the Ctrl and Alt keys and also on the bottom-right side between the Alt and application key of some keyboards. This location may vary on some keyboards.

Special Application and Media Controls

Internet/application buttons, generally found on the left side of enhanced keyboards, control selected application functions such as email, documents, photos, gadgets, and Web access.

Media control buttons make it easier to control the media player, access the DVD drive, and control the speakers. See **Figure 2-5**.

Mouse

Currently, most computers come with another input device in addition to the keyboard—namely, a mouse. See **Figure 2-6**. The traditional mechanical mouse has a ball on the underside of the unit. To use such a device, the user slides it over a mouse pad or desktop. Most of today's mice are "optical" models that do not have a ball on the underside but rather sense changes in light reflection to detect mouse movement. An optical mouse has no moving mechanical parts. It can be used on almost all surfaces, thereby decreasing the need for a mouse pad. The optical mouse also requires no cleaning and is more precise than a traditional mechanical mouse.

Some laptops have a trackball, pointing stick, or touch pad that serves as the mouse or pointing device. A trackball is a stationary mouse with the ball on the top part of it; the user moves the ball instead of the mouse. A pointing stick looks like a pencil eraser and uses pressure to detect mouse movement. A touch pad is another stationary pointing device for which the user moves a finger around on the pad to move the cursor. These devices were designed for mobile computers, in recognition of the fact that there may not be desktop space to move the mouse along.

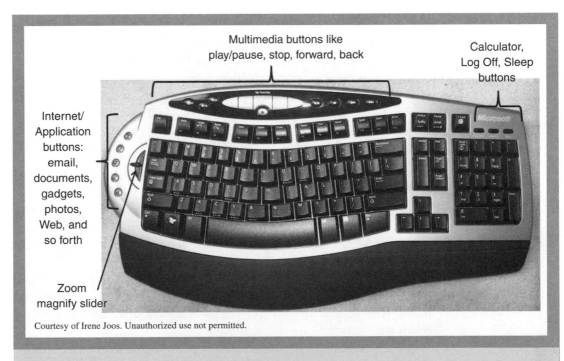

Courtesy of Irene Joos. Unauthorized use not permitted.

Figure 2-5 Special Buttons Found on Some Keyboards

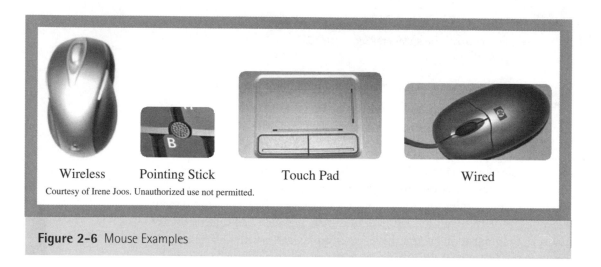

Wireless   Pointing Stick   Touch Pad   Wired

Courtesy of Irene Joos. Unauthorized use not permitted.

Figure 2-6 Mouse Examples

The mouse connects to the computer via a cord plugged into the mouse port. Alternatively, radio waves and infrared light waves may be used as a mode of communication between the system unit and a wireless mouse.

The mouse is used to access menus or functions, open application programs, and create graphic elements without using the function or cursor keys. A button is a place on the mouse that the user presses to invoke a command or activity; it clicks when pressed. A mouse generally has two buttons, denoted as left and right. Some models also have programmable thumb or side buttons that enable the user to perform additional functions. For example, on the Microsoft wireless mouse, the left thumb button activates the magnifier. In addition, a mouse may have a scroll wheel in the center for scrolling in windows or on Web sites.

Common mouse operations are described next:

Point means to move the mouse so that the cursor is on or over a particular command or icon on the screen.

Click (press) means to press and hold the mouse button down, as on a menu item to see the commands, or to scroll through a window until the desired command is selected. Often, this term is inappropriately used to mean single-click. Click requires the user to hold down the mouse button.

Single-click means to press and release the left mouse button once to activate a command or to select an icon or menu option. Use a single click to insert the I-beam (cursor in the shape of a capital I) at the point in the document where typing is to occur.

Double-click means, with the cursor on an icon or option, to press and release the left mouse button twice in quick succession. Use a double-click to start an application program, to open a file or folder, or to select a word for editing.

Right-click means to press and release the right mouse button once. This operation is used to activate the shortcut menu. Make sure to right-click the appropriate place, because different shortcut menus appear depending on the object and place clicked. Use this operation when instructed to "right-click"; otherwise, use the left mouse button.

Triple-click means to press and release the left mouse button three times. In word processing programs, this operation selects an entire paragraph.

Drag means to left-click an icon, menu option, or window border; then, without lifting the finger off the mouse, roll the mouse to move the object to another place on the screen. This operation can change a window's size, copy a file or document, select text, or take something to the trash.

Right-drag means to hold down the right mouse button, move the mouse to a different location, and then release the mouse button. This operation generally results in the appearance of a shortcut menu from which to select a command. The commands vary depending on the object that is right-clicked by the user.

Rotate wheel means to move the wheel forward and backward. Use this action to scroll up and down in a document or at a Web site.

Press wheel button means to click the wheel once and move the mouse on the desktop. This action causes the mouse pointer to scroll along the document automatically until the user presses the wheel button again.

Other Input Devices

A variety of other devices is used to input data to the system. See **Figure 2-7** for some examples of these input devices.

Gaming input devices such as light guns, joysticks, dance pads, and motion sensing controllers are not covered here. Nevertheless, a number of these devices have become increasingly important tools in the rehabilitation and maintenance of patients with limitations or disabilities. For example, gaming systems such as the Nintendo Wii, with its bowling and tennis games, are a big hit in nursing homes as a means of having fun while participating in some exercise.

Cradles or docking stations are input devices primarily used with PDAs, laptops, iPods, and cameras to input data from the mobile device to the desktop computer, and vice versa. Connecting them to the computer facilitates the movement of data from one device to the other. To use this input strategy, the user places the mobile device in the cradle or on the docking station. Some cradles require the user to press a button to perform the data transfer between the mobile device and the desktop computer.

A **digital camera** is used to take photographs and then upload them to the computer or to a special picture printer. Digital cameras eliminate the need for both film and film development. Some of these cameras are stand-alone units that look much like traditional film-based cameras; others are built into smart

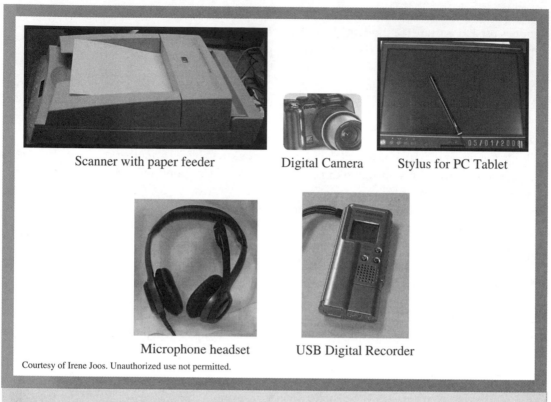

Scanner with paper feeder   Digital Camera   Stylus for PC Tablet

Microphone headset   USB Digital Recorder

Courtesy of Irene Joos. Unauthorized use not permitted.

Figure 2-7 Examples of Other Input Devices

phones or other mobile devices. Increasingly, digital and video cameras are being used to monitor people from remote places.

A light pen is a light-sensitive, pen-like device often used in hospital clinical information systems. Some models require a special monitor to enter data. Light pens and electronic pens are not the same thing, however; electronic pens permit the construction of electronic signatures and require the user to hold the pen and write on a special pad. In contrast, light pens enable the user to enter data only with special screens.

A microphone (voice input device) permits the user to speak into the computer so as to enter data or give instructions. A quadriplegic might use this device to give commands to computer-controlled robots that help the person complete activities of daily living or do work. Healthcare providers use these applications in settings such as the operating room where they are using their hands to provide patient care.

A PC video camera is an input device that the operator uses to capture video. It may be used to send video images as email attachments, to make video telephone calls (video conferencing), and to post live, real-time images to a Web server. A PC video camera that captures and displays images on a Web server is called a Web cam.

RFID (radio frequency identification) uses radio signals to communicate information found on a tag attached to an object or person first to an RFID reader and then to the computer. In health care, RFID technology may be used to track confused patients, control inventory, and monitor staff movements. New passports are equipped with this technology to aid in going through customs.

A scanner is an input device that converts character or graphic patterns into digital data (discrete coded units of data). Such a device can scan a picture and then display the image on the computer screen. Software programs can then import this converted data. Two main types of scanners are used: image readers (for text and graphics) and bar code readers (for database work). Growing in popularity are data collection devices that collect data at remote places and then upload these data to the main computer. In high-security areas, some scanners now collect biometric (body-specific) data such as a fingerprint, voiceprint, or retinal scan to verify the user. Many hospitals use bar code scanners to input data related to supplies or medications used by patients.

A stylus or digital pen is used with a tablet to create an image on the tablet surface. The tablet then converts the marks or images to digital data that the computer can use. A special stylus, used to select options from a screen, is the main input device for many PDAs, for example.

A touch screen allows commands or actions to be entered by pressing specific places on a special screen with a finger. Many PDAs, smart phones, and inter-active video programs use touch screens as the main input device. Some computer manufacturers are now offering this option on their home PCs.

Computer Components: System Unit

The system unit is contained in a case, which varies in size and shape. It may be a separate unit, found inside the display screen, or tucked into a mobile device. In any event, the system unit contains the control center or "brains" of the computer; it is not visible to the eye on most computers unless someone removes the cover of the computer. For most computers, the input and output devices reside outside the system unit; for most mobile devices, the input and output devices and the system unit are contained within one unit.

Motherboard	The motherboard (also referred to as the system board) is the main circuit board of the system unit. It contains slots for the processor chip, memory slots, and slots for adapter cards for video, sound, and connection to peripheral devices.
Processor	The processor is the central unit in a computer that contains the circuitry for performing the instructions that computer

programs provide. An older term for the processor is "central processing unit" (CPU); both the older and current terms are sometimes used interchangeably. A **microprocessor** is a processor that fits on one integrated circuit chip.

The processor has two parts: the control unit and the arithmetic/logic unit. The control unit coordinates the computer's activities. It receives, interprets, and implements instructions. The arithmetic unit performs math functions such as addition, subtraction, multiplication, and division. The logic unit compares two values of data to determine whether they are equal or whether one is greater than or less than the other. The arithmetic/logic unit temporarily uses registers and memory locations to hold data being processed.

Microprocessors have specific names and are produced by manufacturers such as Intel, AMD (Advanced Micro Devices), IBM, and Motorola. Most processors today use multi-core chips—hence the names Core 2 Extreme and Core 2 Duo. A dual-core processor contains two independent cores (usually two processors) placed within a single package. The idea underlying this combination is to streamline processing by making it more efficient.

Laptop processors, which have names like Centrino Pro and Centrino Duo, generally use a lower voltage and clock speed to reduce heat output and conserve power when running on a battery. This balancing act entails a trade-off between performance and conservation of power.

Specially designed processors are also available for smaller mobile devices such as portable media players that use the system on a chip (SoC) processor. These processors integrate the functions of a processor, memory, and video into a single, small unit.

The important point to remember here is that processor names, speed, and size inevitably change over time, but the basic functions of processors remain the same.

Chip A chip is a tiny piece of semiconducting material (usually silicon) that packs many millions of electronic elements onto an area the size of a fingernail. The circuit boards found in computers consist of many chips. The specialized chip called a processor or CPU contains an entire processing unit; in contrast, memory chips hold only programs and data.

Memory Memory is a form of semiconductor storage that resides inside the computer, generally on a motherboard, and that takes the form of one or more chips. It stores operating system commands, programs, and data. Primary memory storage is fast but has low density (amount of data stored per square inch) and costs more per unit of storage than does secondary storage (discussed later). Other terms used to describe memory include main storage, internal storage, main memory, and primary storage.

Read-only memory (ROM) is memory that has been burned on the chip at the factory; the computer can read instructions from it but cannot alter them. This memory is permanent. Computer startup instructions reside in ROM; these instructions tell the computer what to do when it is turned on (see Chapter 3 for more on the startup process). Other types of ROM include programmable read-only memory (PROM), which permits instructions to be programmed on the chip only once, and erasable programmable read-only memory (EPROM), which permits a user to program the instructions many times.

Random access memory (RAM) stores data that the computer needs to use temporarily. This type of memory is volatile—the data disappear from RAM when the power is off. The most common unit of measurement for RAM is the byte, which is the amount of storage space it takes to hold a character. The more RAM a computer has, the greater its computing capabilities. When a software program starts, the computer loads the necessary program and user data files into RAM. As additional functions are requested, the computer loads the required software files. If the memory is not large enough to hold all of these files simultaneously, software files are swapped in and out of the system as needed, slowing down the work.

Just as with ROM, several variations of RAM are available. For example, dynamic RAM (DRAM) must be reenergized constantly or else will lose its contents. By contrast, static RAM (SRAM) does not need to be reenergized, so it is much faster— and more expensive—than DRAM. Double data rate synchronous dynamic random access memory (DDR2 SDRAM) is a type of RAM in common use in personal computers today. It is normally packaged in dual inline memory modules (DIMM) that are mounted in memory slots in the computer. Generally, the size requirements for RAM increase with each new version of software released.

Flash memory is a type of nonvolatile memory that the user can erase and rewrite, making it easier to update the memory contents. Some computers hold their startup instructions in this type of memory so that the user can upgrade the instructions. This type of memory is used with mobile devices, digital cameras, and digital voice recorders.

Cache memory stores frequently used instructions and data. The computer accesses cache memory before RAM memory, thereby speeding up processing.

Ports

Ports are the highways that lead into, out of, and around the computer. They take the form of plugs, sockets, or hot spots that are found on the back, front, and sides of most system units. Ports allow the computer to communicate with peripheral devices, carrying information to and from these devices. For example, many computers have built-in game, mouse, keyboard, card reader, and monitor ports that allow the computer to "talk" with these devices. The ports described here are also considered external data buses, where a bus comprises a series of connections or pathways over which data travels. Computers today generally come with multiple USB (universal serial bus) ports. Some computers can be configured with FireWire, IrDA, and/or Bluetooth ports that connect to peripheral technologies such as digital cameras, PDAs, and MP3 players. **Figure 2-8** shows some examples of ports. Many manufacturers configure computers with multiple ports on the front of the computer to facilitate access to them.

The term "jack" is often used to refer to connections for audio and video ports. On some multimedia computers, audio and video ports are color coded to match the cable tip so that there is no confusion about which device plugs into which port.

Serial ports, also known as "com" ports, arrange data in serial form, sending it to the destination one bit at a time. This strategy allows data to move from the internal, parallel form in the computer to external devices. Because serial ports allow two-way communication, the reverse data flow also occurs, from the external devices back to the computer. Most keyboards, mice, and modems connect to serial ports.

Parallel ports are unidirectional ports that send data in parallel—that is, as groups of eight bits (one byte) of information in a row much like a parade. Parallel ports commonly connect the computer to a printer (one-way communication).

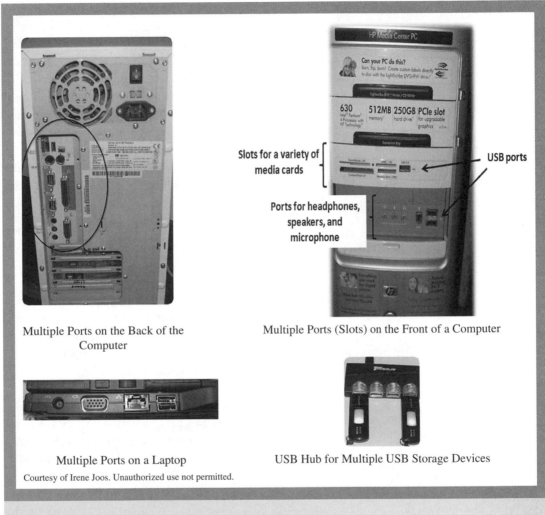

Slots for a variety of media cards

USB ports

Ports for headphones, speakers, and microphone

Multiple Ports on the Back of the Computer

Multiple Ports (Slots) on the Front of a Computer

Multiple Ports on a Laptop

USB Hub for Multiple USB Storage Devices

Courtesy of Irene Joos. Unauthorized use not permitted.

Figure 2-8 Ports/Slots

Another version of this port is the enhanced parallel port (EPP), which permits bidirectional communication. Parallel ports are largely being replaced by USB ports.

USB (universal serial bus) is a port standard that supports fast data transfer rates (12 million bits per second). It can support as many as 127 peripheral devices simultaneously as well as plug-and-play technologies. Devices that can connect to a USB port include the mouse, printers, cameras, microphones, PDAs, USB removable storage devices, and game consoles. In recent years, the USB port has virtually replaced audio, mouse, keyboard, serial, and parallel ports.

FireWire is a special-purpose port that is similar to a USB port in that the user can attach multiple devices to it. A variety of devices that require faster data transmission than is possible with normal ports, such as cameras and camcorders, connect to FireWire ports. A FireWire port can support a maximum of 63 devices simultaneously. In recent years, this type of port has largely replaced audio, parallel, and SCSI ports.

The following list describes special-purpose ports that the computer does not generally include unless the user specifically orders or installs them.

SCSI: A Small Computer System Interface (pronounced "scuzzy") is a parallel port that supports faster data transfers than are possible with traditional parallel ports. SCSI ports permit attachment of as many as seven peripheral devices in a linked chain fashion. This kind of interface also contains a set of command protocols or instructions for data transfer. Many varieties of SCSI ports exist, ranging from SCSI-3 to SAS (Serial Attached SCSI); they vary in terms of their pin connectors and data transfer rates.

IrDA: An infrared light beam port connects wireless devices to the computer using light waves. For this scheme to work, the wireless device must line up with the port on the computer, just like a remote control must line up with a television. Wireless keyboards, a mouse, and PDAs may use IrDA technology.

Bluetooth: Bluetooth ports compete with IrDA ports, although Bluetooth uses radio waves to communicate between the devices instead of infrared light waves. The advantage over the IrDA port is that it eliminates the line-of-sight requirement. Many electronic devices today, such as PDAs, cell phones, baby monitors, and garage doors, are Bluetooth enabled.

MIDI: A MIDI port permits the connection of musical instruments to the computer.

Expansion Slots

Expansion slots are places on the system board where one can add cards, adapters, or other computer boards. They enable the computer to accommodate additional devices such as scanners, sound cards (containing synthesizers for playing sound files), network cards, and hard drives (secondary storage devices).

Power Supply   A power supply box converts the power available at the wall socket (120-volt, 60-MHz, AC current) to the power necessary to run the computer (+5 and +12 volt, DC current). The power supply must ensure a high-quality, steady supply of both 5- and 12-volt DC power for the computer to operate effectively. It includes a built-in fan that cools the system (computer processing generates lots of heat). Laptops and many external peripherals, such as wireless routers and modems, have their own AC adapters. Many laptop power adapters can use both 110 and 220 volts, which is most advantageous in other countries such as Europe when 220 volt power is common.

In addition to the processor found in the computer, other factors in the system unit affect how fast the computer works. They include the computer's registers, the RAM, the clock speed, the internal data bus, and the cache. Registers are temporary, high-speed storage spaces that the processor uses when it processes data. They are part of the processing unit, not the memory. The size of the registers affects processing speed: Put simply, the larger the register, the faster the processing. For example, a 64-bit register is faster than a 32-bit register.

The amount of RAM available (discussed earlier) also has implications for the speed of processing. A program runs faster when more of it fits into RAM simultaneously.

Cache memory (described earlier) also affects how fast the computer works. It is time-consuming to move data back and forth between the processor registers and the memory. Data stored in a cache can be accessed much more quickly than other data, so more cache memory means faster processing.

The clock speed is a function of the quartz crystal circuit that controls the timing of computer work. The faster the internal clock (which is used to time processing operations) runs, the faster the computer works. The unit of measurement for the clock speed is gigahertz (GHz; 1 GHz = 1 billion cycles per second). Theoretically, the higher the clock speed, the faster the computer works.

Data buses, which comprise a collection of wires, move data around in the computer. As mentioned earlier, a data bus is the path that connects internal computer parts such as the processor, memory, and other devices. The wider the bus (determined by the number of wires or pins), the faster it can move data. All buses consist of two parts: an address bus (where the data is going) and a data bus (the actual data). The most important factors for the bus are its width (either 16, 32, or 64 bits) and its speed. The width determines how much data the bus can move at a time, and the speed determines how fast it moves the data.

Expansion buses permit users to insert various types of expansion cards onto the motherboard. They also affect the speed at which data transfer occurs from one device to another. Several types of expansion buses are discussed here.

PCI/PCI-E: The Peripheral Component Interconnect (PCI) bus and the PCI-Express (PCI-E) bus are relatively new standards for connecting higher-speed devices such as the local hard drive, network cards, sound cards, and video cards. PCI-E is intended to replace the PCI and AGP buses.

AGP: The accelerated graphics port (AGP) bus is the default internal bus between the graphics controller and the main memory. It is dedicated to, and designed specifically for, video systems.

USB and FireWire: The USB and FireWire buses eliminate the need to install a card on the motherboard. Instead, they provide a hub for connecting multiple devices with only one cable going into the computer's USB port.

PC Card: The PC card bus is used to move data from a digital camera through a PC card slot into the computer. Figure 2-8 shows an example of this type of expansion bus in the top right computer, media cards.

Computer Components: Output Devices

Output devices take the processed data, which is called *information,* and present it to the user in display (text or graphics), print, or sound form. **Figure 2-9** shows some of the most popular output devices.

Monitor

Monitors display graphic images from the video output of a computer. Other terms used for this device include display screen and flat panel. In recent years, flat panel LCD (liquid crystal display) monitors have begun replacing cathode ray tube (CRT) monitors. Flat panels have a smaller footprint, smaller power

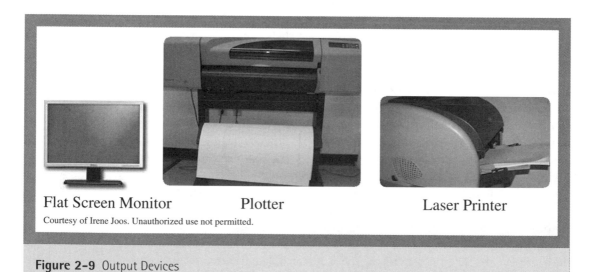

Flat Screen Monitor   Plotter   Laser Printer

Courtesy of Irene Joos. Unauthorized use not permitted.

Figure 2-9 Output Devices

requirement, and no-flicker effect. As a consequence, most computers now use LCD technology for the display device. Computers in many industries, including health care, are rapidly moving to adopt touch screen technologies. Large businesses or industrial process entities sometimes use gas plasma monitors that display images and run simulations on a larger screen display like those seen in convention centers.

Monitors vary in terms of their size, footprint, color, resolution, response time, dot pitch, brightness, and contrast ratio. The ability of a monitor to project an image that can be used for diagnostic purposes is of key importance in health care. The following factors determine the quality of the monitor.

Size refers to the diagonal measurement from corner to corner of the display unit. The active viewing area refers to the actual measurement from left to right and top to bottom of the screen. The appropriate monitor size depends on the proposed usage and application. Commonly encountered computer display sizes are 15, 17, and 19 inches; larger sizes are appropriate for desktop and Internet publishing as well as for diagnostic imaging in healthcare facilities. Mobile devices typically have smaller viewing areas, ranging from a few inches for PDAs and smart phones up to 17 and 20 inches for larger laptops.

Footprint refers to how much space the monitor takes up on the desktop. Flat screen monitors require far less space than older traditional monitors and have all but replaced them in recent years.

Color refers to whether the monitor is monochrome (one color, usually green or amber, on a black background) or colored. The number of displayed colors ranges from 256 to much higher numbers. Most monitors today are colored monitors.

Resolution describes the number of horizontal and vertical pixels (dots) found on the screen. Monitors display images by projecting tiny dots of light on the screen, and they vary widely in terms of the number of pixels per screen (resolution). The more pixels on the screen, the sharper the image. A common resolution today is 1440×900 pixels, but many monitors are capable of a much higher resolution.

Response time refers to the time (in milliseconds) it takes to turn a dot on or off. Response times vary with monitors and can range from 3 to 16 milliseconds.

Dot pitch is a measure (in millimeters) of the distance between the red, green, and blue phosphors that make up the colors of the monitor. The closer together they are, the sharper and denser the screen colors are. The smaller the dot pitch number, the better the colors.

Brightness refers to the visible light intensity of the screen and is measured in nits. The more nits, the brighter the picture.

Contrast ratio is the ratio of the brightest color (white) to the darkest color (black) on the screen. Today's monitors produce contrast ratios of 20,000:1. Higher ratios provide better representation of colors.

A last key point to consider with monitors relates to their conformance to two standards. First, a monitor should be energy efficient and should conform to the Energy Star guidelines established by the U.S. Environmental Protection Agency. To do so, the monitor must meet certain energy standards when it is on, in standby mode, in suspended mode, and off. In July 2007, new energy-efficiency standards were adopted.

Second, the amount of electromagnetic emissions produced by the monitor must be considered. Specifically, the monitor should comply with the Swedish MPR-II or TCO emissions standard.

Printers

Printers produce either black-and-white or color output. Use black-and-white printers for papers, correspondence, handouts, and reports. Use color printers for overheads, poster presentations, and documents in which color enhances the message. Printers connect to the computer via cables or radio signals through wireless technologies.

With **nonimpact** printers, the printing mechanism does not touch the surface of the paper. Examples include laser, thermal, and ink jet printers. Laser printers are the most expensive of these types of printers. They produce high-quality print, are fast, and generate little noise. Thermal printers press heated pins against special paper to produce the printed image; the quality of this output is low, so such printers are generally used in sites such as retail sales and gas pumps. Ink jet printers are usually reasonably priced and less expensive to purchase than laser printers. They produce a better-quality output than do dot matrix printers and serve as an excellent middle ground between laser and dot matrix printers. However, depending on the printing requirements, laser printers can be cheaper than ink jet printers. Growing in popularity are photo printers, which use ink jet technology to produce color pictures in varying sizes. Some **plotters** also use ink jet technology to produce large banners and architectural drawings.

With **impact** printers, the printing mechanism touches the surface of the paper; that is, a mechanism strikes against a ribbon. Common examples include dot matrix and line printers or plotters. Dot matrix printers are the least expensive of these models, but are noisy and produce low-quality documents. Use dot matrix printers when printing on carbon forms such as invoices and statements.

Some cameras come with docking stations that serve as printers. Other compact mobile printers attach to PDAs or laptops and may, for example, be used by nurses in patients' homes.

Other Output Devices

As end users have become more adept at using technology, the demand for other output devices has increased.

Speakers and **headsets** (headphones) come with most computers today and usually reproduce high-quality sound. Speakers can be integral to the monitor, be mounted on the monitor, or stand separately on the desktop. Some high-level multimedia computers also come with a subwoofer to handle bass sounds. Most computer laboratories now require users to wear headphones so that computer-generated sounds do not disturb other users; if no headphones are used in the labs, users may need to turn off the sound capability.

Data projectors display graphic presentations to an audience. Such a device takes the image on the computer screen and projects it onto a larger screen. Data projectors may be either portable or ceiling mounted. As with all electronic devices, the price and quality of these output devices vary dramatically, ranging from low-end to high-end models.

Multifunction devices are all-in-one I/O devices. They typically incorporate a printer, scanner, copier, and fax machine into a single unit. Usually they are cheaper than purchasing each device separately and take up less space. However, if the device breaks down, all functions are gone. In addition, stand-alone devices may offer more advanced features.

Interactive whiteboards are display devices that connect to a computer and permit the user to interact with the computer through the whiteboard. This interaction can take place through remote controls, special pens, a writing tablet, or a finger.

Computer Components: Secondary Storage

Storage comprises a place or space for holding data and application programs. The computer has both primary (memory storage—covered earlier in this chapter) and secondary (e.g., hard drives, optical drives, USB storage devices) storage spaces.

Secondary storage media hold application programs and user data when these are not in use. It takes longer to access data held in secondary storage. Secondary storage has a higher density (amount of data per square inch) and is less expensive than primary storage. Data storage uses the same units to measure size as memory does—for example, bytes, kilobytes, megabytes, gigabytes, and terabytes. A byte is equal to one character. One kilobyte is 1024 bytes; one megabyte (MB) is 1 million+ bytes; one gigabyte (GB) is 1 billion+ bytes; and one terabyte is 1 trillion+ bytes.

A notable trend for data storage is the use of smaller physical sizes to hold larger amounts of data. **Figure 2-10** shows examples of storage devices.

Storage Devices

Hard disks (also known as **hard drives**) are fixed data storage devices in sealed cases that read stored data on platters in the drive. These magnetic storage devices store data in sizes ranging from gigabytes to terabytes. Hard drives are generally slower than primary memory (RAM). They are either external to the system unit (portable) or internal to the system unit (fixed). Hard cards are hard disks that are

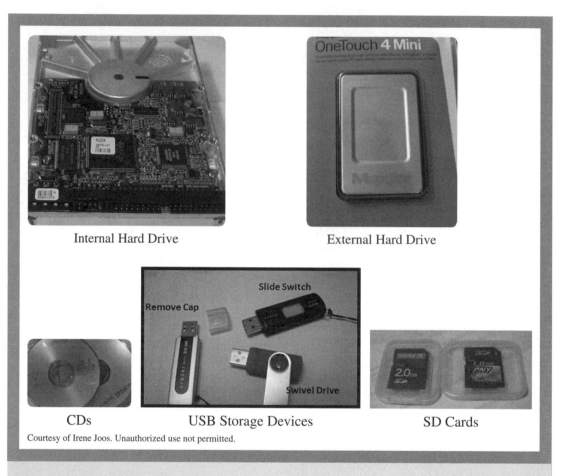

Internal Hard Drive   External Hard Drive

CDs   USB Storage Devices   SD Cards

Courtesy of Irene Joos. Unauthorized use not permitted.

Figure 2-10 Storage Devices

inserted in an expansion slot; portable drives are inserted in a bay or connect to a USB or FireWire port. Both PCs and laptops generally come with one hard disk drive. Most hard drives last at least three to five years or more. Proper maintenance of the hard disk drive requires periodic defragmentation and periodic disk scans.

Tape drives are secondary storage devices that allow the backup or duplication of stored data on a hard disk. They store data sequentially (one bit right after the other) in magnetic form, much like an audiotape. The popularity of tape drives is generally declining, except in larger computer systems and for use in lieu of optical backup devices.

Optical drives are an alternative to magnetic storage. They hold large amounts of data, which are usually written (pressed) once and accessed many times. Almost all computers come with at least one optical drive. The most common example is the CD-ROM (compact disc read-only memory). This storage device typically holds 650 MB of data, although the capacity of some models goes as high as 1 GB. Other variations of optical drives include CD-R (compact disc–recordable) drives, which permit users to write data only once (but not erase data), and CD-RW (compact disc–rewritable) drives, which permit users to write and erase data many times. Optical drives can store digital audio, full-motion video, graphics, and animation in addition to text data.

The latest addition to the CD-ROM storage line is DVD technology. The design of earlier DVDs accommodated video—hence the name "digital video discs." As use of these discs increased as data storage media, DVD has come to mean "digital versatile disc." These discs can hold more data, such as a full-length movie, than can CDs. Variations of DVDs include DVD-ROM; BD-ROM (Blu-Ray disc), with a storage capacity of 100 GB; and HD DVD-ROM (high definition), with a storage capacity of 60 GB. RW DVDs are rewritable. Multimedia-ready computers generally come with at least one DVD drive that determines which type of DVD the drive will accept. DVDs can last anywhere from 5 to 100 years with proper care. Proper care includes storing the disc in a case and holding the disc only by its edges. Discs should not be stacked but rather should be stored on their edge; it is best not to touch the underside, expose the disc to excess temperatures, or eat or smoke around a DVD.

Solid-state media such as **flash memory cards** and **USB storage devices** consist of electronic components and have no moving parts. The life expectancy of solid-state media is in the range of 10–100 years, depending on the manufacturer. Currently, the maximum storage capacity of these devices is 16 GB, but like any storage device the capacity is moving toward 32 and 64 GB. Flash memory cards are commonly found in digital cameras, smart phones, and PDAs; they are more expensive than other storage media. USB storage devices are popular for portable storage because of their capacity and size. **Figure 2-11** gives the appropriate care instructions for a USB storage device.

Smart cards store data on a credit card–sized card that contains a microprocessor, input and output functions, and storage. Increasingly, various industries are using smart cards to store personal information such as a person's medical record and credit card information. Smart cards are already in extensive use in Europe for storing healthcare information.

Labeling Disk Drives

Operating systems assign letters to storage drives. The use of drive letters and drive icons with letters allows users to access stored information on a specific drive. The letters "C" and "D" usually refer to hard disk(s); the default hard drive is C. Other drives and devices use the letters "D," "E," "F," or "G." The computer reserves the letters "A" and/or "B" for floppy drives, if they are present. In the Windows

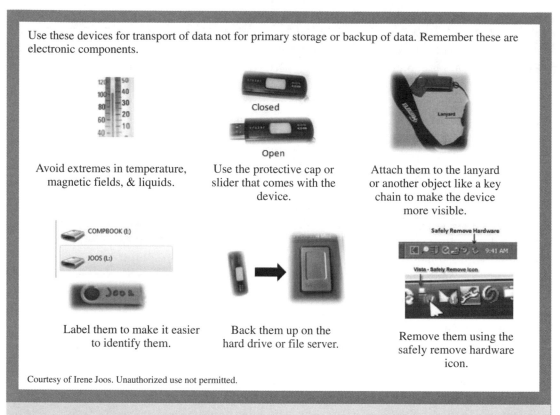

Use these devices for transport of data not for primary storage or backup of data. Remember these are electronic components.

Avoid extremes in temperature, magnetic fields, & liquids.

Closed

Open

Use the protective cap or slider that comes with the device.

Lanyard

Attach them to the lanyard or another object like a key chain to make the device more visible.

COMPBOOK (I:)

JOOS (L:)

Label them to make it easier to identify them.

Back them up on the hard drive or file server.

Safely Remove Hardware

9:41 AM

Vista - Safely Remove Icon

Remove them using the safely remove hardware icon.

Courtesy of Irene Joos. Unauthorized use not permitted.

Figure 2–11 Care of USB Storage Devices

environment, words appear next to the letters describing the nature of that storage device as well as the assigned letter. As an example, **Figure 2-12** shows disk drive labeling on a network using Windows XP versus disk drive labeling on a stand-alone computer using Windows Vista. Because many variations for drive labeling exist, consult the laboratory assistant or instructor for the applications of conventions in your laboratory.

Other Peripherals

Two other peripheral devices to consider when looking at hardware are the surge protector and the uninterruptible power supply.

A **surge protector** is a device that sits between the electrical outlet and the computer supply source. It protects the computer from low-voltage surges in electrical power by directing the extra power to the outlet's grounding wire. Although it offers protection from normal surges in voltage, it cannot protect the computer

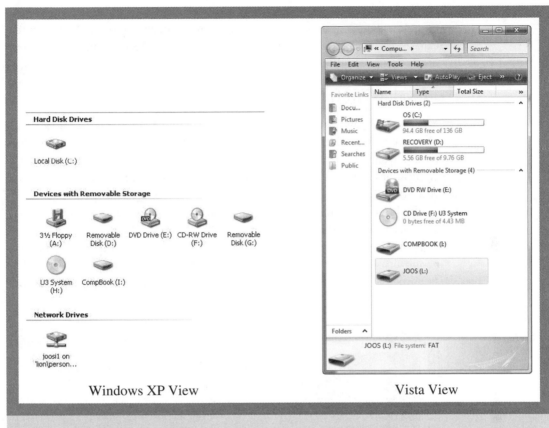

Windows XP View   Vista View

Figure 2-12 Labeling Storage Devices

from lightning strikes. Surge protectors are also referred to as power strips and surge suppressors, but be careful when making assumptions about their capabilities: Not all power strips include the surge protection feature.

An **uninterruptible power supply (UPS)** device provides electrical power generated by a battery in the event of a power outage. The battery keeps the computer going for several minutes after the outage occurs. During this time, the user can save data and properly shut down the computer. Two types of UPS systems are available: standby and online. Standby devices monitor the power line and switch to battery power when they detect a problem. Online devices constantly provide power even when the power line is functioning properly, thereby avoiding the momentary lack of power that may occur when the UPS switches from power to battery. Online devices are the more expensive units. Think of UPS devices as standby generators, much like hospitals use in case of a power outage, albeit on a much smaller scale.

Generally one should plug printers, speakers, and scanners into surge protectors, and plug computers, monitors, and storage devices into the UPS. Printers can cause a large drain on the battery of a UPS. Many UPS units also bundle surge protection in one device. See **Figure 2-13.**

Introduction to Computer Systems: Connectivity

Most people now assume that a computer has the ability to communicate with other computers. **Communication** refers to the process of moving data and information from one computer device to another. Today's users expect to be able to communicate from a PC to a laptop to a handheld device to a Web server with very little effort on their part.

The basic communication process includes a sender and receiver, a channel, and a communication device. Chapter 9, Using the World Wide Web, and Chapter 10, Computer-Assisted Communication, discuss some of the services people use when communicating using the Internet. Relevant terms for understanding basic computer communications or connectivity are discussed in this section.

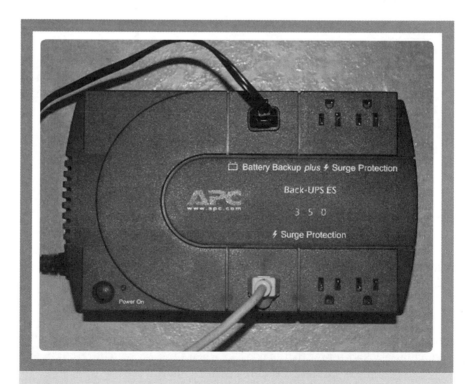

Figure 2-13 UPS and Surge Protector

Networks

A network is a collection of computers and other hardware devices such as a printer, scanner, and file server that are connected together using communication devices and transmission media.

A local area network (LAN) is a type of network with distance limitations. A building or small campus environment might use a LAN. Some departments within healthcare institutions use LANs to connect various types of equipment for the purpose of communicating and sharing information. LANs typically use a communications standard called **Ethernet**.

A wireless local area network (WLAN) does not use wires for communication between the server and the client computer or mobile device. Most WLANs physically connect to a LAN for the purpose of accessing resources on the LAN. Many campuses now have a WLAN for use with mobile devices such as laptops and PDAs. Access points are scattered around the building or facility that provides the local computer with access to the LAN. Communication standards or protocols in the wireless world include Wi-Fi (wireless fidelity), Bluetooth, IrDA, and RFID. Wi-Fi permits two Wi-Fi devices to communicate with each other or with a Wi-Fi–enabled network. Bluetooth enables communication with laptops, PDAs, microphones, and similar devices. IrDA provides line-of-sight communications between two devices. RFID (radio frequency identification) allows the reading of tags on objects as varied as supplies and passports. One of the key problems with wireless connections in hospitals are dead spaces caused by interference to the signal by such things as lead-lined rooms or doors.

The metropolitan area network (MAN) and wide area network (WAN) are high-speed networks that cover larger geographic distances. MANs may include a city or Internet service provider (ISP) that provides the connection for city agencies or individual users with access to the Internet. The best example of a WAN is the Internet, which uses the Transmission Control Protocol/Internet Protocol (TCP/IP) communications standard. These networks may also use Worldwide Interoperability for Microwave Access (WiMAX) when the network includes use of wireless towers. Wireless Application Protocol (WAP) is a standard used by mobile devices such as smart phones and BlackBerries when they are communicating with Internet services.

Wireless home networks are growing in both popularity and simplicity, and are now part of the broadband services that many telecommunications companies offer. With this type of network, each computer or device that connects to the wireless network must have a wireless network card or built-in wireless networking capabilities (found on many laptops). The network also must have a wireless access point or a combination router/wireless device that connects to one of the desktop computers in the home. **Figure 2-14** shows an example of a wireless router for a home network connected to a FiOS connection and wireless access points in a library.

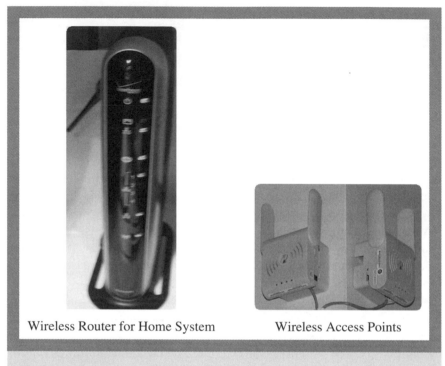

Wireless Router for Home System   Wireless Access Points

Figure 2-14 Wireless Router and Access Points

Communication Devices

A communication device is any type of hardware capable of transmitting data and information from one computer to another. This section discusses some types of modems and cards commonly used to communicate with a network. Computers and mobile devices must have a communication device to communicate with a network.

A cable modem is a device that connects to the network using television cable services. The cable company that provides the connection service supplies the cable modem.

A dial-up modem is a device that prepares data for transmission over a telephone line. It converts digital data into its analog (wave) form and then reverses the process at the other end of the connection. Although dial-up modems are quickly disappearing, some people continue to use this means of connecting to the Internet when other choices are either not available where they live or are too expensive.

A DSL modem is a device that connects to the network over a DSL connection. The telecommunications company that provides the connection service generally provides or sells this modem.

An **Ethernet card** fits into a computer slot and provides connectivity to an internal network. Schools, offices, and businesses often use Ethernet cards to connect computers and peripheral devices to their network.

A **wireless card** fits into a computer slot and permits the computer to access a wireless network via radio-based connection. The computer must be in range of the wireless access point to access the network. See Figure 2-14 for an example of an access point.

A **wireless modem** is a device with an external or built-in antenna for use with mobile devices such as laptops and cell phones. Some mobile phones, smart phones, and PDAs can function as data modems. These modems use the cell phone network to connect to the Internet. The wireless modem device is generally available as a PC card, flash card, or ExpressCard. It either fits into a PC slot or uses the USB port.

Communications Channels

A **communications channel** is the transmission pathway that data take to arrive at the other end of a connection.

Bandwidth describes the amount of data that can travel over a communications channel at one time. The larger the number, the more data the channel transmits at one time. Remember that music, video, and graphic files take up more bandwidth than plain text. Healthcare systems typically need a larger bandwidth because they often transmit data-intensive images such as CAT scans and MRIs along with text.

Broadband refers to the ability to transmit multiple signals at the same time. DSL, cable, and satellite are examples of broadband connections.

Dial-up service is also referred to as plain old telephone service (POTS). It uses telephone wires to access the network. This type of access is much slower than use of other media, with the top speed for dial-up data transmission being 56 Kbps. When a computer is connected to a network via dial-up service, the phone line is tied up with the connection and cannot receive telephone calls at the same time.

Transmission media refers to the materials or substances capable of transmitting a signal. They are of two types: physical media and wireless media. Physical media include twisted-pair cable, which is widely used but slow; coaxial cables, which are common in cable TV connections and offer faster data transmission than twisted-pair; and fiber-optic cables, which connect large networks as well as private homes through some telecommunication company media. Fiber-optic cable is the fastest of these media. Wireless transmission media include infrared, broadcast radio, cellular radio, microwaves, and satellites. Wireless media is more convenient in that the user does not have to install cables to make a connection and it provides more flexibility in moving equipment.

Connection Options

Dial-up connections use traditional telephone lines to access the Internet and other networks. They are very slow and will probably soon disappear as an option for connecting to the Internet. For some people, however, dial-up service is a low-cost option for accessing the Internet and email.

A DSL connection makes a faster connection than dial-up service, usually through the phone system. DSL connections have severe distance limitations. The user must be within 18,000 feet of a phone switching station; as computers move farther away from the switching station, the data transmission rate declines. Data transmission rates via DSL range from 128 Kbps to 9 Mbps. These connections provide both voice and data signals simultaneously.

The **cable** lines coming into most homes provide another option for a communications channel. This type of communications channel is faster than either dial-up or DSL, but degrades in speed as more people access the cable lines at the same time.

Fiber-optic cables, such as those used in Verizon's FiOS service, are a broadband option for connecting to a network using the fiber-optic cable run to the home and businesses by some phone companies.

T1 and T3 are communication connections used by large businesses. A telecommunications company generally provides these services. Larger healthcare facilities and some colleges and universities may connect using this connection service.

Wireless connection employs a microwave dish generally located outside the house. This data transmission option is subject to noise interference during rain and snow storms, but may be the only option for people who are located in rural areas.

The important point to remember here is that for a computer to communicate with other computers, it needs a communication device, a communications channel, and media and network service. Most ISPs provide these tools and services to enable their customers to connect to the Internet. Most larger organizations provide these tools and services through their Information Technology (IT) department. The IT department typically provides the hardware specifications for connecting individual laptops to the organization's network (either wired or wireless).

Introduction to Computer Systems: Software

Computers are multipurpose machines. They are, however, unable to complete any task without directions from software programs. Software programs consist of step-by-step instructions that direct the computer hardware to perform specific tasks such as multiplying, dividing, fetching, or delivering data. All computers require software to function. When the computer is using a specific program, users say they are *running* or *executing* the program.

The three major categories of software are operating systems (OSs), languages, and applications.

Operating Systems

The operating system (OS) is the most important program that runs on a computer: It tells the computer how to use its own components or hardware. No general-purpose computer can work without an OS.

Operating systems perform some functions necessary to all users of the computer system. These basic functions include keeping track of files and folders, communicating to peripheral devices such as printers, receiving and interpreting input from the mouse or keyboard, displaying output on a screen, and managing how data move around inside the computer. In other words, operating systems coordinate the computer hardware components and supervise all basic operations.

The most common operating system for PCs is the Windows family (Windows Vista, XP, and Windows 7). Apple computers use the Macintosh operating system (OS 10). Some computers also use variations of UNIX called Linux and Xenix. Portable computers may use Windows CE. Larger computer systems or networks and workstations may use Windows Server 2008 and UNIX or a UNIX variation such as Solaris. Mobile devices use such variations as Windows Embedded CE, Windows Mobile, Palm OS, BlackBerry, and Symbian OS, which is an open-source OS.

The important point to remember here is that all computers need an operating system to work and that operating systems inevitably change over time to reflect changes in technology and user needs. Chapters 3 and 4 provide more detail about working in the Windows environment.

Languages

Language software presents a simplified means to execute a series of instructions, called a **language**. Specifically, a language consists of a vocabulary and an accompanying set of rules that tell the computer how to work. Languages permit the user to develop programs to perform specific tasks. Popular languages include C, C++, C#, COBOL (Common Business Oriented Language), Java, and Visual Basic. Users do not need to be programmers to use the computer; however, understanding programming concepts and developing programming skills are helpful when trying to do more advanced work on the computer.

Several types of programming languages exist. Machine-level languages are the lowest level and consist of numbers only; this type of language is the only one that the computer recognizes directly. Assembly languages are the next generation of languages, and they give the programmer the ability to use names instead of numbers when telling the computer what to do. Procedural or 3GL (third-generation level) languages are what users normally think of when they say "programming language." They include the previously mentioned languages such as Visual Basic and C. Object-oriented programming languages include the ever-popular Java, C++, and Visual Basic. The 4GL (fourth-generation level) languages include SQL (Structured Query Language), which is used when working with large relational databases.

Although many people include HTML (Hypertext Markup Language), SGML (Standard Generalized Markup Language), and scripts such as PERL (Practical Extraction and Report Language) and PHP as programming languages, in reality they are not. These standard protocols are considered organizing and tagging languages that are designed to manage the layout and formatting of documents between different computer systems or scripting languages.

Applications

Application programs meet specific task needs of the user; running these programs to complete your work in an efficient and effective manner is the primary use of any computer system. Programmers use language software to write application programs. Major types of applications or programs include the following:

- General-purpose software such as word processors, spreadsheets, database managers, presentation graphics, communications programs, and Web page authoring programs
- Educational programs such as simulations or computer-assisted learning
- Utility programs such as virus scanners, personal firewalls, screen savers, spyware and adware removers, hard disk managers, media players, and Internet filters such as antispam programs, pop-up blockers, and phishing filters
- Personal programs such as calculators, calendars, and money managers
- Entertainment programs such as games and simulations

This book covers the more commonly used general-purpose application software.

General-Purpose Software

Electronic mail (email) software permits the sending and receiving of messages from one person to one or many other people. The computers send and receive these messages by using standard communication protocols (rules and procedures that govern the communication between the computers).

Database software helps organize, store, retrieve, and manipulate data for the purpose of later retrieval and report generation.

Desktop publishing software permits the user to create high-quality specialty publications such as newspapers, bulletins, and brochures. It handles page layouts better than word processors and can import a variety of text and graphic files from other application programs.

Graphics software facilitates the creation of a variety of graphics. Three types of graphics programs exist. **Presentation** graphics permit the user to create or alter symbols, display a variety of chart styles, make transparencies and slides, and produce slide shows. **Paint** programs permit users to create symbols or images from scratch. **Computer-aided drafting** programs meet the drawing needs of architects and engineers.

Integrated software includes in one program multiple capabilities, such as word processing, database, spreadsheet, graphics, and communication programs.

Spreadsheet software permits the manipulation of numbers in a format of rows and columns. Spreadsheet programs contain special functions for adding and computing statistical and financial formulas. Use them for financial functions and number crunching.

Statistics software permits statistical analysis of numeric data.

Suites are value packages that include a word processor, a spreadsheet, a database, a presentation graphics program, and sometimes a personal information manager. The main advantage of these suites is their cost (lower than buying each program individually) and the ability to share data easily between each program.

Word processing software permits the creating, editing, formatting, storing, and printing of text. Most have spelling and grammar checkers.

Education

Computer-assisted instruction software comprises a set of programs that help users learn concepts or specific content related to their discipline or area of study. In some circles, developers refer to this type of program as training software. The Internet is a natural means for delivering computer-assisted instruction.

CD-ROMs and DVDs hold educational programs that provide integrated sound and motion to provide a lesson.

Utilities

Utilities are a group of software programs that help with the management or maintenance of the computer and protection of the computer from unwanted intrusion. Examples include hard disk managers, virus detectors, compression/decompression programs, spyware removers, firewalls, spam blockers, and viewers.

Personal

Personal software programs help people manage their personal lives. Examples include appointment calendars, checkbook balancing applications, money management applications, and calculators.

Entertainment

The class of software programs that the industry has designed for fun is called entertainment software. Many games exist to provide diversion, including golf and football. Others challenge the user's problem-solving abilities. Some programs are more like arcade-type games. Still others are strategy-based programs in which players takes turns and the game unfolds in real time.

When discussing software developments, the trend is toward easier-to-use, graphic interactive programs with certain built-in intelligence that anticipate the preferences of the end user.

Summary

This chapter presented the terminology and concepts necessary to become an intelligent computer user. To that end, the tenets underlying an information system were described. The major components of computers and connectivity were presented, as networking is clearly a key trend with all computer systems. Software basics were presented by describing the three major classes: operating systems, languages, and applications. Although some of the specifics of computer systems will undoubtedly change as technology evolves, the basic concepts will remain the same. Users will always need to follow the input–process–output cycle and use some form of software.

References

AMSA. Overview of handheld devices. Retrieved December 14, 2008, from http://www
.amsa.org/resource/pda.cfm.

How computers work: The CPU and memory. Retrieved July 22, 2008, from http://
homepage.cs.uri.edu/faculty/wolfe/book/Readings/Reading04.htm.

Minasi, M., Wempen, F., & Quentin, D. (2005). *Complete PC upgrade and maintenance
guide* (16th ed.). Alameda, CA: Sybex.

White, R., & Downs, T. (2008). *How computers work* (9th ed.). Indianapolis, IN: Que.

Online Resources

How Stuff Works (http://www.howstuffworks.com) is an excellent site for learning about
computer hardware and connectivity.

Online Computer Directory for Computer and Internet Terms and Definitions (http://
pcwebopedia.com/) is a great site for finding definitions and understanding basic concepts. It has a wonderful interface and is simple and easy to use. Another site of this
type is Tech Target (http://whatis.techtarget.com/).

PC Magazine (http://www.pcmag.com) is an excellent site for reviews and the latest hap-
penings regarding hardware and connectivity.

PC Tech Guide (http://www.pctechguide.com) covers a lot more detail and technical
issues regarding technology.

EXERCISE 1 Identify Computer Components[1]

■ **Objectives**

1. Identify the specific computer hardware being used.
2. Use the proper terminology to describe the computer and related components.

■ **Activity**

Use the computer in front of you to answer the following questions.

1. Computer.
   a. Which type of computer is being used?
      Make: Model:
      (*Make* refers to the company that manufactures the computer. Some
      examples are Dell, Hewlett-Packard [HP], and Apple. *Model* refers to
      the specific computer manufactured by the company.)
   b. Why is this important to know?
   c. How does one turn the computer on?
2. Monitor.
   a. Is the monitor part of the system unit or separate from the system unit?
   b. What size is it?

---

[1]This exercise is also available as a Word document downloadable from the book's Web site.

      c. Does it need to be turned on separately from the system unit? If so, how is it turned on?

3. Storage.
   a. Which storage devices are available on this computer? (Describe them here.)
   b. Is there access to a network file server?
   c. Where are users permitted to store data?
   d. Which type of removable storage devices can be used?
   e. Why is this information important to know?
   f. Which letter is used to describe the DVD/CD drive? Which letter(s) is (are) used to describe the USB ports? Which words are used to describe the file server?

4. I/O devices.
   a. Which types of input devices are available with this computer?
   b. Which types of output devices are available with this computer?
   c. Does the computer share a printer?

5. Connectivity.
   a. Are there places to plug in a mouse, modem, printer, or other peripheral devices?
   b. Is the computer connected to another computer that serves as a file server? (A file server is a computer that contains software and data shared by those using the system.) Is the computer networked?
   c. Turn on the equipment. Are a user identification (name) and password needed to access the system? If so, do you know your user identification and password? If not, where would you obtain that information?

6. Software. List the software available for use on this computer.

EXERCISE 2   Using Your USB Storage Device[2]

■ **Objectives**
   1. Identify the rationale for each safety tip in caring for a USB storage device.
   2. Insert a USB storage device into the computer properly.
   3. Save a file to the USB device.
   4. View the contents of the USB device.
   5. Remove the USB device safely.

■ **Activity**
   1. Match the safety tip in column A with that explanation from column B.

---

[2]This exercise is also available as a Word document downloadable from the book's Web site.

A. Safety Tip	B. Rationale
___ Avoid extremes in temperatures.	A. Files might become corrupt if the "safely remove" feature is not used.
___ Use the cap or slider when finished with the device.	B. This makes it easier to see and not leave the device in the computer unintentionally.
___ Attach the lanyard (strap) or key chain to the device.	C. This protects the metal part of the device that is inserted into the USB port.
___ Label the device.	D. Electronic devices can be damaged when exposed to extremes.
___ Back up the device	E. USB devices are storage devices for transport; they cannot be reliable permanent copies. They can become corrupt during transport or exposure to the elements.
___ Safely remove the device.	F. This makes it easier to identify if lost or left in the computer.

2. Insert a USB storage device into the computer.
   a. Locate the USB port on the computer. It has the USB symbol above or below it.
   b. Depending on the USB device, **remove** the cap, **push** the slider button, or **swivel** the device to expose the metal tip.
   c. **Line up** the metal tip with the USB port and **push it** gently into the port. The ends should match, as shown in **Figure 2-15**. The USB ports can be found on the front of many computers, on the left and/or right side of laptops, on the left side of some monitors (see **Figure 2-16**), and in the back of other computers.

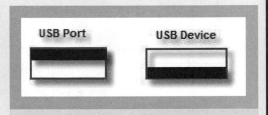

Figure 2-15 End of the USB Device to Match the USB Port

NOTE: Some devices may require the installation of a device driver, as indicated by a message that appears at the lower-right side of the screen. The message will go away once the device driver is installed.

   d. Once the USB storage device is engaged, the AutoPlay dialog box appears. See **Figure 2-17**.

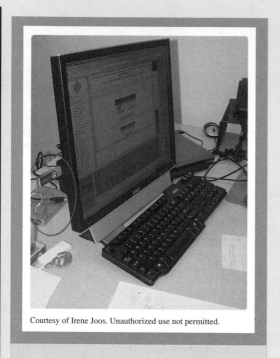

Courtesy of Irene Joos. Unauthorized use not permitted.

Figure 2-16 USB on Side of Monitor

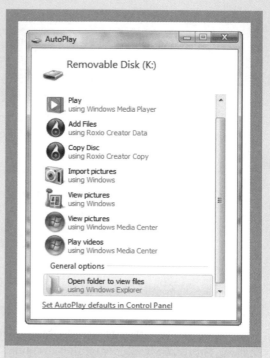

Figure 2-17 AutoPlay Dialog Box

NOTE: Depending on the computer, the user may see a message such as "This device can perform faster . . ."; click **X** to close the message balloon on the lower-right side of the screen. The user may also see another balloon on the upper-right side of the screen. If it is present, click **Cancel.**

    e. **Click Open Folder to view files** and **click OK.** You will now see a list of files or folders, if there are any, and the device letter in the computer window. The device is now ready to be used.

    f. If a folder or file is present, **double-click the file or folder** to open it. The folder or file opens.

    g. If the screen in **Figure 2-18** appears, it means the device was *not* removed FIG 18 properly the last time it was used. Choose **Scan and Fix (recommended)** and **click Close.** You are now ready to work with the USB storage device.

3. Save a file to the USB device.

    a. Open Word (**Start, All Programs, Microsoft Office, Microsoft Office Word 2007**). There are other ways to open the program, which you will learn later.

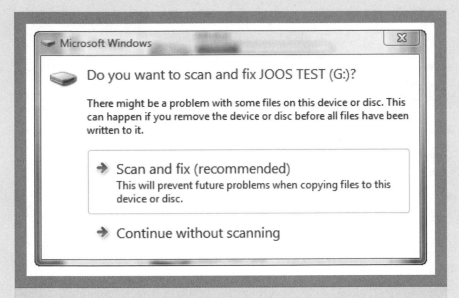

Figure 2-18 Improper Removal of a USB Device

  b. Type **This is a test document for learning how to save a document to the removable USB storage device.**

  c. **Click** the **Office** button and then the **Save** option. The screen shown in **Figure 2-19** appears.

  d. **Click** the **Computer** option on the left.

  e. **Click** the correct **USB storage device.**

  f. Type **Test document** for the file name.

  g. **Click** the **Save** button. The file is now saved to the USB device. You can repeat the process to see that it was saved. Chapter 3 describes the process of saving files in more detail.

 4. View the contents of the USB device.

  a. **Click** the **Start** button on the taskbar.

  b. **Click Computer** in the gray area on the right under the user identification.

  c. **Double-click** the **USB storage device.** The file should now appear in the window.

  d. **Click** the **Close** button on the USB storage device window. The window closes.

 5. Remove the USB device safely.

  a. When finished using the USB device but *before removing* the USB device, **click** the **icon** in the lower-right taskbar known as "Safely Remove

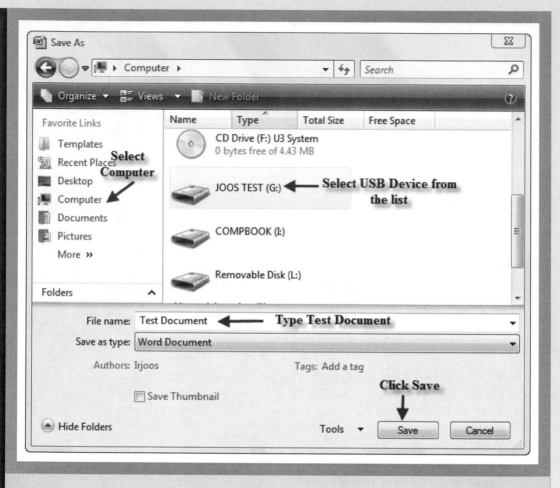

Figure 2-19 Save As Dialog Box

Hardware": 🔲 for Vista or 🔲 for Windows XP. The Safely Remove balloon appears as shown in **Figure 2-20**.

b. **Click** the **USB device**. A message appears stating that it is safe to remove the USB storage device.

c. **Click OK** and **remove** the device. **Replace** the cap, **retract** the metal tip on the slider, or **swivel** the metal tip closed.

> NOTE: If you double-click the Safely Remove Hardware icon, the Safely Remove dialog box appears as shown in the Figure 2-20. Select the device and click **Stop.** The "Stop a Hardware Device" dialog box appears. Click the correct USB storage device and then click **OK.**

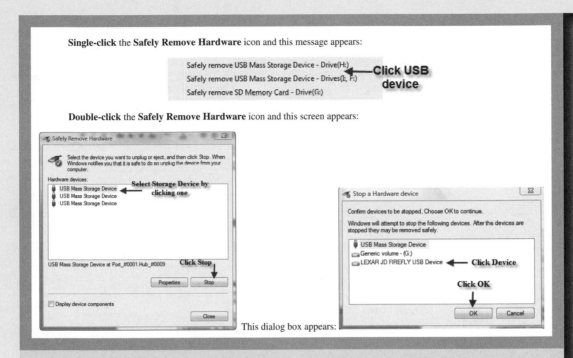

Figure 2–20 Safely Remove USB Device

EXERCISE 3 Computer Configuration

■ Objectives
1. Identify questions to ask and information needed when buying a computer.
2. Relate information from a newspaper computer advertisement to the material presented about hardware.

■ Activity
1. Using the following advertisement information, fill in the blanks below:

Dell Inspiron Laptop with Intel Pentium Dual-Core Processor T2390 with 1 MB L2 cache and 1.86 GHz processor speed; 2 GB DDR2 memory expandable to 4 GB, 1 MB cache memory, multiformat DVD-RW/CD-RW; 15.4″, glossy XGA HD widescreen (1280 × 800), 160 GB ARA serial hard drive, digital media card reader, Intel graphics media accelerator ×3100, built-in 10/100 Ethernet card, built-in Dell 1395 wireless mini-card, 4 USB 2.0 ports, 1 FireWire port, audio and S-video output, built-in speakers, weight 5.5 lb, lithium ion battery, touch pad with vertical/horizontal scroll pad, Windows Vista Home Premium, Microsoft Works 9 and Roxio Creator Basic.

Microprocessor:	Memory:
Computer Speed:	Memory Expandable:
Storage Devices:	
Monitor Type and Size:	Keyboard:
Mouse:	Ports:
Connectivity:	
Sound System:	Operating System:
Weight:	Battery:

2. Additional Information
    a. Which type of removable storage devices can be used?
    b. Can the memory be expanded?
    c. Which software is provided?
    d. Does a Web cam come with the laptop?
    e. Does a carrying case come with the laptop?
    f. Will Vista be an effective OS on this machine?
    g. List additional questions that a user should ask before buying this laptop.

EXERCISE 4 Computer Specifications

■ **Objectives**

1. Specify minimum hardware requirements for different scenarios.
2. Identify software needs.
3. Justify the recommendations for the requirements for both hardware and software.

■ **Activity A**

You are the nurse practitioner charged with opening a First Care center in the local pharmacy. You have been asked to identify the computer equipment needed to run the First Care center, which will have one full-time nurse practitioner, several part-time nurse practitioners, one full-time and several part-time nurse technicians, and an intake receptionist covering the hours of operation (Monday through Friday, 8 A.M.–11 p.m., and Saturday and Sunday, 9 A.M.–6 p.m.). You need to identify which equipment (stationary or mobile), which functionality, and which software this center will need. The system(s) will be used to help with the center's management duties, patient records, and reference resources. Itemize and justify your request. Who would you consult and what software would you recommend? Explain your thinking.

■ Activity B

You are the systems analyst in the center for research in your institution. The director decides to purchase computers for the center. You must now specify the hardware and software required to meet the computing needs for the center. The center staff consists of a director (PhD), two associate directors (PhDs), three research associates (master's degree prepared), one statistician, and three members of the clerical staff.

■ Activity C

You want your parents to purchase a laptop, a printer, docking station, wide-screen monitor, wireless keyboard, and mouse with related software as a present for you. They need some help from you to determine which type of laptop system and software you need and whether the cost is reasonable. Itemize what you want and justify it to your parents. Use hardware and software advertisements from newspapers, computer magazines, computer retailers, and the Internet to obtain hardware and software specifics as well as prices.

EXERCISE 5 Accessing Application Software

■ Objectives
1. Start application programs using a variety of techniques.
2. Identify the software programs available on the computer.
3. Identify the operating system.
4. Shut down the computer.

■ Activity
1. Start an application using the double-click method.
   a. **Turn** the computer system on if necessary. (Some computer labs leave the systems on all the time.) Text appears on the screen as the computer goes through startup routines.

      If necessary, **press Ctrl+Alt+Del** to obtain the login screen. (In other words, hold down the Ctrl key, hold down the Alt key, and then press Del.) Release all three keys.

If necessary, **type your login** (**user ID**) and **password** and press **Enter**. Use the **Tab key** to move between the user ID text field and the password text field.

b. **Double-click** the **Internet Explorer** icon on the desktop. The browser program opens. Alternatively, you can press the **Start** button and select **Internet Explorer** from the menu. UNFIG 15 TO 23

c. **Click** the **Close button** on the browser window to close the application.

2. Start an application using the Start button on the taskbar.

a. **Click** the **Start button** on the taskbar. A menu appears.

b. **Select All Programs**, **Accessories**, and **WordPad**. WordPad, a word processing program that comes with Windows, now starts.

c. **Click** the **Close button** on the WordPad window to close the application.

3. Start an application using Computer.

a. **Double-click** the **Computer** icon . Alternatively, you can click the **Start** button and then the **Computer** option. The Computer window opens.

b. **Double-click** the **local (OS) drive** icon (usually **C:**), the **Windows** folder, and then the **System32** folder. You will need to scroll through the window to find the calculator icon, as shown in **Figure 2-21**. FIG 21

c. **Double-click** the **Calc** icon . The calculator program opens.

d. **Click** the **Close** button on the calculator window to close the application.

4. Identify application programs on the system.

a. **Click** the **Start** button on the taskbar.

b. **Select All Programs**.

c. List the application programs that are accessible on this computer.

5. Identify the operating system.

a. **Click** the **Start button** , and **select Control Panel**. The Control Panel window opens.

b. **Click Getting Started with Windows** under the **System and Maintenance** option. The System and Maintenance window opens. If you are using a different version of Windows, look around the Control Panel for system information.

Which version of Windows are you using? _____

What is the processor for this computer? _____

What are the speed and RAM for this computer? _____

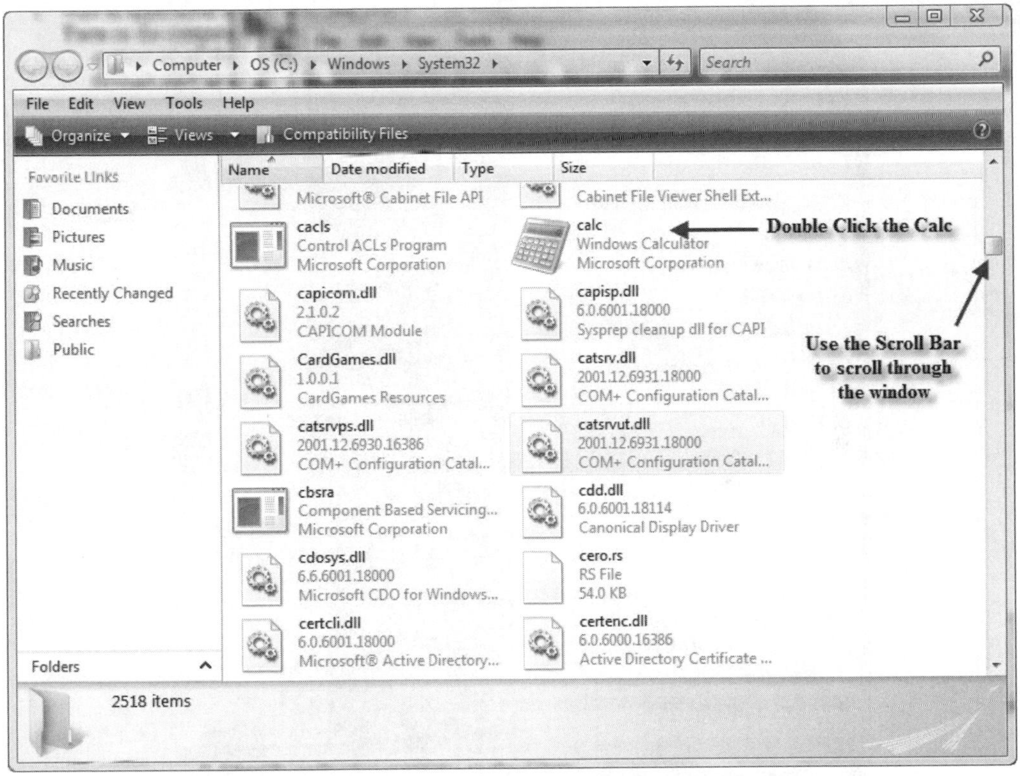

Figure 2-21 Using Computer to Start an Application

---

   c. **Click** the **Close** button on the upper-right side of the System Properties window.

   d. **Close** all remaining **open windows**.

6. Shut down the computer.

   a. **Click** the **Start** button.

   b. **Click** the **Save Session and Turn Off the Computer** button [image] or **click** the **Log Off menu** button [image] and **select** an **option**. **Figure 2-22** shows your options.

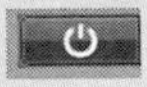

      At work and in some laboratories, users do *not* turn off the computer. In that case, select the option for logging off. At home, you might want to choose the option to save the session and turn off the computer. When you return, Windows will restore your session. Some computers automatically turn themselves off when shutting down; others require the user to turn them off physically. The same applies to the monitor.

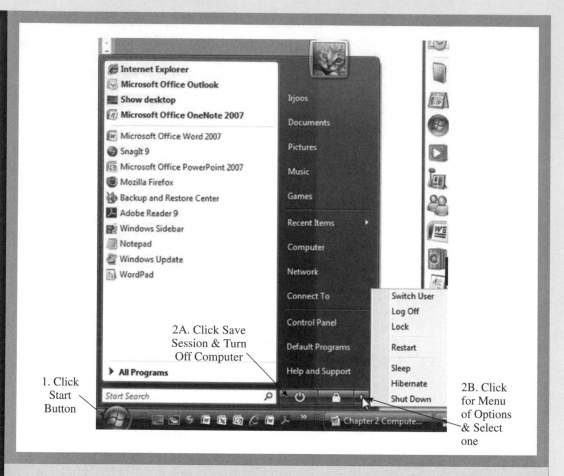

Figure 2-22 Logging Off

ASSIGNMENT 1 Compare Two Computers, Surge Protectors, and UPS Devices[3]

■ **Objectives**

1. Obtain two advertisements for a microcomputer from the newspaper, from computer magazines, or from a store that sells computers.

2. Compare the two computers by filling in the form provided in this assignment.

3. Make a recommendation for one of the computers.

---

[3]Note: This form is available online in Word 2007 format.

4. Turn in both the form and the computer advertisements.
5. Recommend a surge protector and UPS.

■ **Directions**
1. Find two advertisements for a microcomputer. These ads can be from a retail store such as Best Buy, a newspaper, or an online Web site such as the Dell or HP site.
2. Complete the following form, making a recommendation and explaining why your selection will be best.
3. Look for some information on surge protectors and UPS devices. Complete the remaining part of the form.
4. Submit the assignment to your professor in either print or electronic form.

Name: _____

Features/Specifications	Computer 1	Computer 2
System Unit		
Make/model		
Microprocessor type		
Speed	GHz	GHz
RAM	GB	GB
RAM expandable	Yes or No	Yes or No
Number of expansion slots		
Number and type of ports		
Sound and video enabled?		
Secondary Storage		
Hard drive	GB	GB
DVD-RW/CD-RW		
USB devices		
I/O Devices		
Keyboard included	Yes or No	Yes or No
If yes, type		
Mouse included	Yes or No	Yes or No
If yes, type		

Monitor included	Yes or No	Yes or No
If yes, type and size		
Printer included	Yes or No	Yes or No
If yes, make and type		
Connectivity		
Ethernet card	Yes or No	Yes or No
Wireless enabled	Yes or No	Yes or No
Additional Information		
Operating system included	Yes or No	Yes or No
If yes, which one		
Additional software	Yes or No	Yes or no
If yes, list it		
Cost	$	$

Recommendation:

Rationale/Comments:

■ **Surge Protector and UPS**

Because computers and their peripherals are an investment, users need to protect them. Evaluate two surge protectors and two UPS devices. You may include an all-in-one model that handles both power surges and power outages. Recommend which one you would purchase and why.

Surge Protectors

Criteria for selecting:

- Response time (less than 10 nanoseconds)
- Joules (How much electricity can be absorbed—at least 600)
- Indicator light (unit is working)

- Reputation of manufacturer
- Cost

Compare two models using the preceding criteria.

UPS

Calculate which size of device is needed (add the amps used by the monitor, CPU, and storage devices and anything else intended to be plugged into the UPS. Multiply that total by 110 volts).

Find a site that evaluated the UPS devices and support your decision with a review for the unit recommended.

ASSIGNMENT 2 PDA or Smart Phone

■ **Objectives**

1. Compare two PDA or smart phone products based on specific criteria.
2. Identify how you might use the product to support your healthcare education.
3. Identify two software programs that would be needed to assist you in your clinical experiences.

■ **Directions**

PDAs have been used in health care to aid in diagnosis and drug selection, provide instant access to references, record patient information, and support clinical research. Some services that might be helpful are provided by AvantGo, WardWatch, and Pendragon. Newer developments may lead to monitoring users, as sensor technologies for mobile devices develop. The trend seems to be the merging of PDAs and smart phones. For this assignment, you need to complete the following activities.

1. Compare the functionality of a PDA to that of a smart phone. What can you do with each? What are their similarities? What are their differences? Provide one reference source citation for each type of device.
2. Interview a faculty member or staff member who uses either of these devices. How is this person supporting his or her practice with it? What is this person doing with the device? Also determine how your school incorporates this type of technology in your education. List some ways that you might use either a PDA or a smart phone in your education.
3. List the most important criteria you will use in making a decision about which device is best for you. For example, consider functionality, software available for tasks intended to be used with the device, cost, compatibility with school or clinical equipment, and so forth. Next, compare one specific PDA and one specific smart phone using those criteria.

4. Select two software programs that you might use with the device you selected. To help identify some sources for such software, try these links:

AvantGo (http://my.avantgo.com/home/; type **health** in the search box)
Epocrates (http://www.epocrates.com/)
Medical PDA Software (http://www.medspda.com/)
pdaMD (http://www.pdamd.com/home)
Pendragon (http://www.pendragon-software.com/)
PEPID (http://www.pepid.com/)

List your two software programs and their cost here:

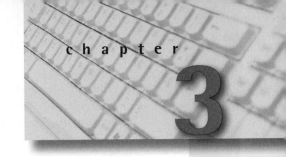
The Computer and Its Operating System Environment

Objectives

1. Describe the Windows operating system environment.
2. Perform the boot process.
3. Explain a graphical user interface.
4. Describe operating system trends in end-user design and functions.
5. Start Windows and log off from Windows.
6. Manipulate windows and manage the desktop.
7. Identify the basic concepts underlying file and disk management, including file naming conventions.

Every computer relies on an operating system to function. Computers without a functioning operating system (OS) are just pieces of hardware (with the exception of simple, single-purpose computers like those that control microwave ovens). Although many operating systems are available for different types of computers, such as Mac OS for Apple computers and UNIX/Linux for workstations and larger computers, this chapter describes the operating system environment that is used by the majority of personal computers (PCs and laptops): Microsoft's Windows. Many Mobile devices have an abbreviated Windows-type operating system.

Every three to four years, Microsoft issues a new operating system, making modifications to that OS based on users' needs, changes in technologies, and changes in the computer world. All operating systems give users the ability to manage the operating system environment and the user's own files and folders. With each version of the operating system, more functionality is added, but learning the basic concepts will help in adjusting to the new looks and functionality of each new version.

The next Microsoft operating system after Vista is Windows 7. This new version includes a redesigned taskbar that closely resembles Apple's Dock, a new version of Internet Explorer, a new Windows Media Center and Windows Media Player, revised interfaces in Paint and WordPad, improved wireless support, pervasive touch screen support, and the removal of the side bar.

Windows is designed to provide a friendly interface between the user and the hardware. This graphical user interface (GUI) is intended to take advantage of the computer's graphic and mouse capabilities and make it easier to use the commands and applications. The user employs the mouse in a point-and-click approach to issue commands and manage the interface.

Critical to working in any operating system environment is the ability to manage files and folders. Files contain data and information, whereas folders are storage places for files. This chapter includes information on managing files and folders using the Computer feature (formerly called My Computer in earlier versions of Windows). Windows Explorer, an alternative option for managing files, is now subsumed in Computer under the Folders feature.

The Operating System Environment

Operating systems are responsible for many of the computer's "housekeeping" tasks. The operating system "wakes" the computer through a set of commands and routines that make the computer recognize the central processing unit, memory, keyboard, disk drives, and printers. The purposes of the operating system are to supervise the operation of the computer's hardware components and to coordinate the flow and control of data. Without the operating system, the user cannot run language or application software.

Today, most operating systems (platforms) come preinstalled on the hard drive of the computer. Several versions of the Windows operating system are in use: 2000, NT, XP, Vista, and Windows 7. There are also versions of operating systems designed for mobile devices such as PDAs, where the operating system resides on a ROM chip. General trends noted with these versions include the integration of Internet capabilities, the ability to perform multiple tasks at the same time, the ability to work in network environments, and increased inclusion of security and multimedia capabilities.

To become proficient in using the computer, a basic understanding of how the system works and how the desktop environment can be managed is needed. This means learning how to customize the desktop, manipulate the windows, switch between applications, and manage files and folders.

Starting the Computer: The Boot Process

The boot process refers to turning on the computer or using the restart button if the computer has one and initiating a series of actions. A cold boot means starting the computer when it has been powered off. A warm boot is the process of restarting a computer that is already on in one of two ways: (1) by pressing the **Ctrl+Alt+Del** keys together and then selecting the **Shut down options button** down arrow on the lower-right side of the screen or (2) by selecting the **Start** button, selecting the **Menu option** button, and clicking the **Restart** option on the menu. See **Figure 3-1** for these two examples. Some computers may have other options for a warm boot depending on the edition and settings of that OS. Use a warm boot when you are installing new software or when the computer stops responding.

POST

When the computer is turned on, the power supply sends an electrical signal to the processor, causing it to reset itself and find the basic input and output system (BIOS) instructions on the ROM chip. The BIOS performs a power-on self-test (POST), which analyzes the buses, clock, memory, drives, and ports to make sure that all of the hardware is working properly. The results of this test are compared with data stored in the complementary metal-oxide semiconductor (CMOS) chip.

System Files and Kernel

Once the POST test is completed, the software loaded in ROM activates the computer's disk drives and looks for a bootable sector of a disk—the part of the disk containing a program that loads the system files into memory. Generally, this activity involves checking the hard drive. Once found, the system files are loaded into memory. This central module of the operating system is referred to as the kernel; it is the part of the operating system that loads first and remains in memory as long as the computer is turned on. The operating system in memory is now in control of monitoring system resources.

This startup procedure runs very quickly on new computers. If problems are found, the computer makes beeping sounds and then stops running. If all goes well, the user will be asked to log in or, on PCs, to select his or her account. The desktop will then appear.

This information is not critical to using a computer. It does, however, make problem solving easier when something goes wrong during the boot process. If the On button is pressed and nothing happens, the computer may have been unplugged. It cannot initiate the startup process because it needs electricity to trigger the boot process Thus, it does nothing.

Graphical User Interface

Both Windows and Macintosh OS use GUIs as the means for the user to interact with the operating system. **Figure 3-2** shows a typical Windows desktop with its graphical interface. Your desktop may have all or few of the items shown in Figure 3-2, as individuals and companies often customize the GUI.

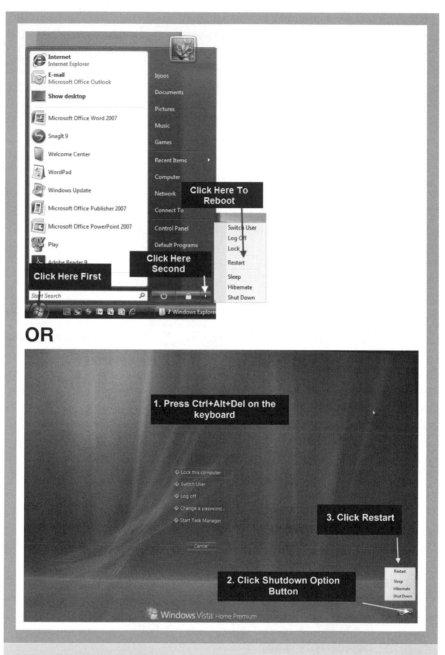

Figure 3–1 Warm Reboot

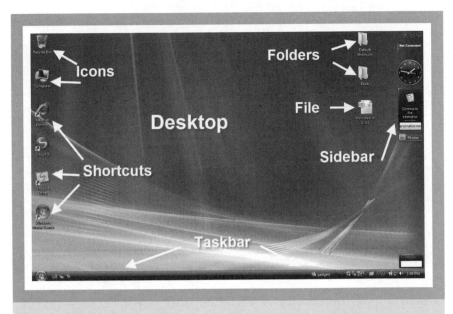

Figure 3-2 Vista Desktop

Although the focus of this chapter is the Windows operating system, some features common to both the Windows and Mac operating systems are listed here.

Desktop	The desktop is the area on the screen that displays the icons, sidebar, and taskbar. In the Windows environment, it is the primary workspace that fills the screen. The monitor displays the desktop when the computer is turned on or, if necessary, when the user logs in. The desktop may be customized to suit the user—that is, the colors and the location of objects can be changed, images can be added to the background of the desktop, and screen savers can be installed. The default look of the desktop changed with Windows Vista to include the sidebar and a different default background.
Dialog Box	The dialog box is a special window that requires the user to make selections from options to implement the commands. Making a selection may require typing information into a text box (such as a file name), selecting from a list box (such as selecting fonts and sizes in the Print dialog box), clicking a square or circle to make a selection (such as to print all pages, current pages, or just certain pages in the Print dialog box), or clicking a button. See **Figure 3-3** for an example.

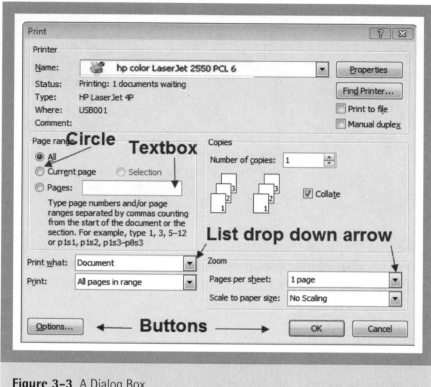

Figure 3–3 A Dialog Box

Menus	Menus are lists of commands or tasks that become available when the user selects a command category from the menu bar. See **Figure 3-4** for an example of a menu and its drop-down menu.
Mouse	One device used to select objects and issue commands is the mouse. The idea behind the use of a mouse is to make issuing commands faster, especially for the nontypist. GUIs depend on the mouse or another pointing device to select objects or commands from menus, ribbon, and toolbars. Most of the commands accessed with the mouse can also be issued by using the equivalent keyboard strokes. Refer to Chapter 2 for a description of mouse actions.
Objects	Small pictures or graphic representations of icons, files, folders, and shortcuts located on the desktop are referred to as objects. Placing the pointer on an object and clicking selects it. Double-clicking the object opens it. Right-clicking an object opens a shortcut menu, sometimes called a context-sensitive menu. See Figure 3-2 for examples of objects found on the desktop.

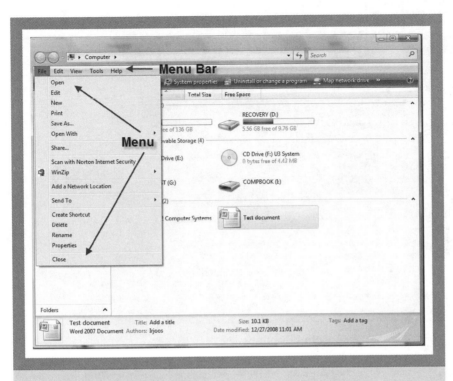

Figure 3-4 Menu Bar and a Drop-Down Menu in a Typical Window

Pointer	A pointer is the symbol used to represent the mouse location on the screen. Many application programs change the look of the pointer to reflect the process the system is expecting. For example, the pointer changes to a double-headed arrow (↖ ⟷) when it is hovered over a window border, indicating readiness for resizing the window. Use the pointer to select commands from menus and toolbars. Different pointer shapes will be presented in this book as they occur in discussions about application programs.
Sidebar	The long vertical bar on the right side of the window is the sidebar. It contains small programs called gadgets, which permit easy access to frequently used tools such as slideshows of pictures, newsfeeds, or the weather. Figure 3-2 shows an example of a sidebar, while **Figure 3-5** shows the gallery of options that comes with the operating system. The bottom of Figure 3-5 shows the gallery of options that are available when using the Google sidebar. More gadgets are available on Microsoft's Web site.
Taskbar	The taskbar is generally the long horizontal bar at the bottom of the desktop. It is used to access applications and files. All open windows become items on the taskbar. The default look of the taskbar changed in Windows Vista; it is no longer blue with a green Start button, but rather gray with a multicolor Start button.

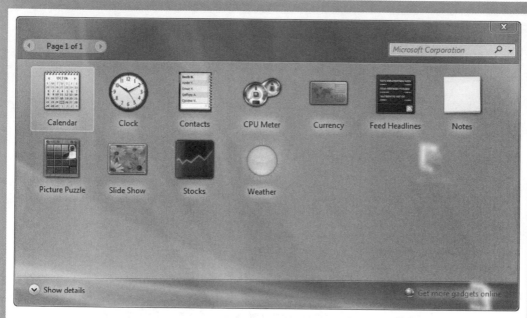

Default options

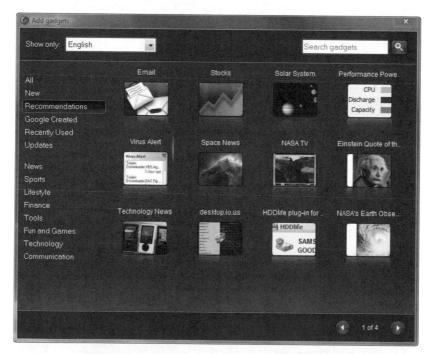

Enhanced options using the Google sidebar

Figure 3-5 Add Gadgets Gallery Screen

Window A window is a place on the desktop where the contents of application programs, files, or folders are displayed. Each program or file has its own window. Each window may contain a title bar, menu bar, one or more toolbars, an address bar, and a status bar. If the window is too small to display all of the contents, the window will also contain scroll bars. Additional window controls include those to close, maximize, minimize, and restore windows. **Figure 3-6** shows the windows component parts.

With Vista, most windows also include an address bar, a search box, and a ribbon.

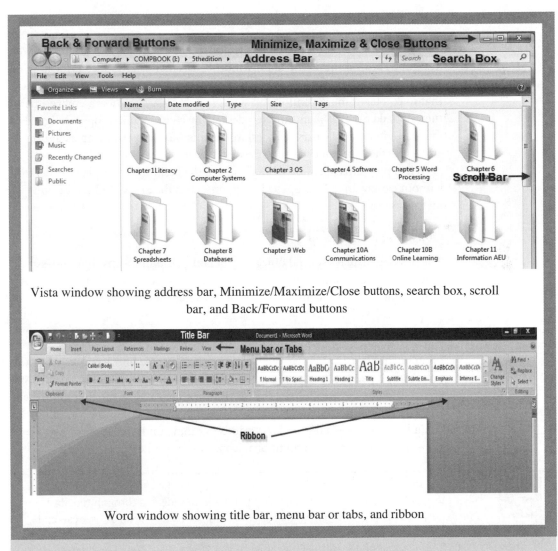

Vista window showing address bar, Minimize/Maximize/Close buttons, search box, scroll bar, and Back/Forward buttons

Word window showing title bar, menu bar or tabs, and ribbon

Figure 3-6 Components of a Window

The GUI provides the user with a consistent look and easy-to-use commands. The common features and looks enable the user to adjust quickly to other applications and to move between applications easily.

Managing the Desktop

> NOTE: In the clinical environment and school labs, you may not have permissions to alter the desktop, taskbar, or sidebar.

This section discusses the layout of the desktop and explains how to manage the desktop. The desktop is the main window or screen that is seen after logging on to the computer. Most workers enjoy arranging their desks in a specific way that makes them more comfortable and productive in their work environment; they also add personal items to their desks. The computer desktop is designed to mimic an individual's personal desktop in this way, by permitting each user to customize the computer screen as desired.

When programs open, they run on top of the desktop. To display the desktop without closing any of the opened programs, click the Show Desktop button ▦ on the taskbar.

Objects on the Desktop

The desktop displays several objects by default. *Default* means that, unless told otherwise, the computer uses a certain setting or configuration. Figure 3-2 shows some of these objects: icons, folders, shortcuts, files, and the taskbar.

Icons

Icons represent applications, such as Internet Explorer and MSN, and special programs, such as the Recycle Bin. In Windows Vista, the only icon placed on the desktop by default is the Recycle Bin. All other programs are located through the Start button or the Quick Launch area of the taskbar unless the user adds them to the desktop when a new program is installed on the computer or unless the default settings are changed. Every computer may not have all of the following icons; also, some may have additional icons not shown here.

In earlier versions of Windows, My Computer appeared on the desktop. In Windows Vista, My Computer is now called Computer and it is located through the Start button. Click the Start button and select Computer on the menu. A user can add the Computer icon to the desktop by right-clicking the entry on the Start menu and selecting **Show on desktop.** Use this icon for viewing and accessing all storage drives and devices connected to the computer.

The Recycle Bin temporarily stores deleted files until it is emptied. Files deleted from external storage devices (such as USB storage devices) are not temporarily stored here; instead, they are deleted immediately. This icon is placed on the Windows Vista desktop by default. The top view is a nearly empty Recycle Bin and the bottom view is one with files in it. The user should empty the Recycle Bin periodically.

Documents

The Documents folder stores Microsoft Office documents by default. In Windows Vista, it is located through the Start button under the user name on the right side of the menu. You may place it on the desktop for easy retrieval of your work. The picture to the left shows the folder on the desktop, which contains the Documents, Pictures, Music, and Games subfolders.

To add the user folder to the desktop, right-click the user name (that is your account user name) on the Start menu and select **Show on desktop.**

This icon starts Internet Explorer. Use it to access the World Wide Web (WWW or Web). In earlier versions of Windows, this icon may be found on the desktop; in Windows XP, it appears on the Quick Launch area of the taskbar; in Windows Vista, it is pinned to the Start menu.

If the computer is connected to a network, the user has access to the Network icon. It may or may not be placed on the desktop. Use it for viewing and accessing network resources.

Other icons may be added to the desktop or Quick Launch area of the taskbar.

Folders

Folders are holding places for files and may also be located on the desktop or other places on the hard drive or removable storage devices. Pictures of yellow file folders represent them. Folders provide a way to organize work—for example, by storing similar programs and files in them. Folders may be embedded within other folders (subfolders) to create a hierarchical structure to the system. The process of creating folders is discussed later in this chapter.

Files

Files contain data and are created in applications such as Word, Excel, and PowerPoint. They hold or store the work we do. Icons representing each file type assume the look associated with the application that created them. For example, a Word file looks like a piece of paper with a W symbol on the icon representing the file. Files are created when work is saved in an application or when the Create, New File command is selected from the shortcut menu.

Shortcuts 	Shortcuts are pointers to an actual application, folder, or file. They contain the path to the executable file for the application, to the folder, or to the file, respectively. Deleting one simply deletes the shortcut, not the application, folder, or file. Shortcuts have a right curved arrow on the bottom left of the icon. Use shortcuts to provide quick access to commonly used applications, folders, or files. A later section in this chapter describes the process of creating them. The shortcut shown to the left accesses Adobe Reader.
Taskbar	The taskbar, by default, is located at the bottom of the screen and may be moved to any screen edge. It is actually four separate components, although it looks like one object. **Figure 3-7** shows the four parts of the taskbar. Use the Start button to open the Start menu and to access programs, documents, settings (Control Panel), help, and shutdown features. The Find feature is not part of the taskbar in Vista; instead, Vista includes a built-in search field in almost all menus, including the Start menu, as shown in Figure 3-6.

The Start menu now contains the user name at the top with an icon next to it that can be changed or customized. On the left side are the most recently accessed programs and a list of favorite programs. See **Figure 3-8**. This setup represents Microsoft's attempt to unclutter the desktop. A practice exercise at the end of this chapter demonstrates how to customize the Start menu.

To the right of the Start button is the *Quick Launch* area. Frequently used applications are placed on the Quick Launch area to provide quick access to them and to keep the desktop uncluttered. In Figure 3-7, the toolbar has a Show Desktop icon, a Switch between Windows icon, a SnagIt9 icon (a screen capture program used to capture many of the screens in this chapter), and a chevron for a menu to start Office applications.

To the far right of the Start button is the *notification area.* It contains the clock and (sometimes) icons for programs that usually run in the background and need only occasional user input. Examples of these types of programs are antivirus programs, the battery charge indicator, the Safely Remove Hardware utility, and the volume control. If the mouse-controlled pointer pauses over one of these icons, the function or name of that icon appears. Periodically a small pop-up window will notify you of something (e.g., "Your virus protection software needs to be updated.").

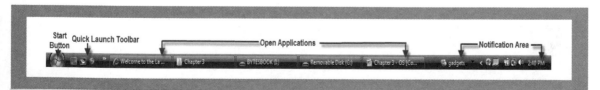

Figure 3-7 Taskbar Parts

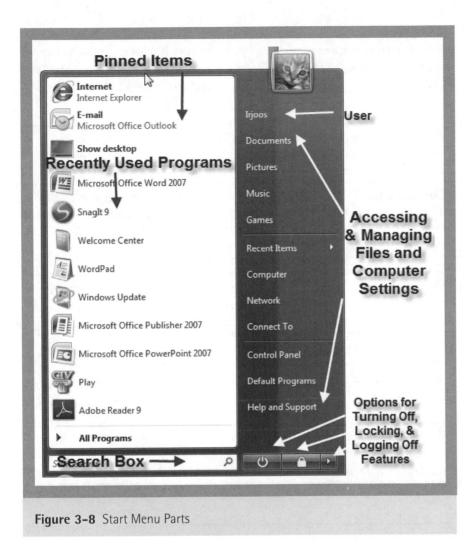

Figure 3-8 Start Menu Parts

The *Open Applications* area is in the middle and takes up the largest space on the taskbar. Most programs place a button on the taskbar when they open. Similar applications are located nearby one another. Clicking one of these buttons allows the user to bring that application's window to the foreground and make it the active window. The taskbar helps the user to switch from one application to another. In Figure 3-7, you will see Internet Explorer, a folder, two drive icons, and a Word document opened.

Sidebar	New to Vista is the sidebar. You can use the Gadget gallery to add items such as a calendar, weather, stocks, and headlines to the sidebar. This provides quick access to information based on the tasks that are important to the user. In Windows 7, the sidebar is removed, but the gadgets remain.

Pointer Shapes

As mentioned earlier, pointer or cursor shapes may change while the user is working in the Windows environment. When the pointer changes shape, the computer expects to complete certain operations and responds accordingly.

	The ready arrow means that the computer is waiting for commands. Use it to select objects, double-click objects, right-click objects, drag objects, or choose menu or icon commands.
	Use the I-beam to insert text. It appears when the user pauses over a text field, along with the insertion point (blinking vertical bar). Any text entered will be inserted at the location of the vertical bar or insertion point, not the I-beam location (which could be over any text field).
	Window-sizing pointers appear when the cursor is over a window border. There are four versions: left–right, up–down, left slanted, and right slanted. Left–right arrows widen the window. Up–down arrows lengthen the window. Slanted arrows can widen and lengthen the window simultaneously.
	The hourglass indicates that the computer is processing and cannot execute any further commands until it finishes processing. Wait. Do not type or click the mouse button until the hourglass disappears. If the user clicks anything before the ready arrow appears, the computer may freeze, stop working, or crash.
	The hand means that the mouse pointer is over a linked object or linked text. Clicking the text or object will bring more information from this site or another site. Use the hand pointer to obtain additional information.
	When the mouse pointer looks like this, the action attempted is not available.

Additional pointer shapes are discussed as they appear in specific applications.

Changing the Appearance of the Desktop

By default, computers running Vista will have the Windows Vista theme installed. Each person with an account on the computer can set up the computer to display his or her own theme. In addition, users may customize or personalize the background (also called wallpaper) or color scheme. Some users never change the theme, color, or background; others like change and stimulation in the workday world, so they change it regularly. Windows provides for both types of users by letting the user choose the theme, desktop background, and color. If the user changes the default settings, the new settings will be used until the user changes them again. A variety of digital pictures designed to be used as desktop backgrounds, as well as in complete theme packs, can be found on the Internet. Personal digital pictures can also be used as background wallpaper.

> HINT: To see additional themes, you must first install them from Microsoft's Web site or from the Internet.

To change the default theme:

1. Right-click a **blank area** of the desktop. A shortcut menu appears.
2. From the shortcut menu, select **Personalize**. The screen shown in **Figure 3-9** appears.
3. Click **Themes** and select one of the themes from the drop-down menu.
4. Click **Apply** and then **OK**. The new theme appears.

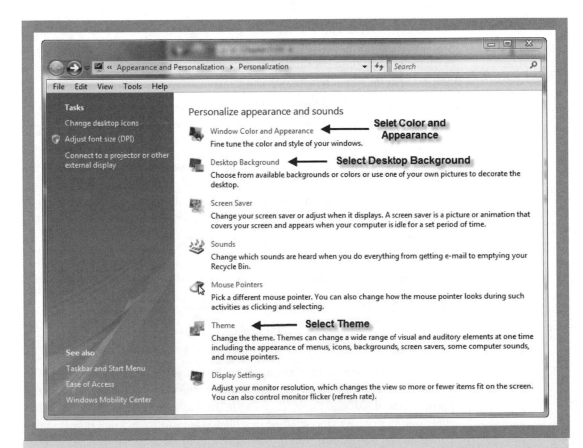

Figure 3-9 Changing the Window Color and Appearance, Desktop Background, and Theme

To change the desktop background or color scheme:

1. Right-click a **blank area** of the desktop. A shortcut menu appears.
2. From the shortcut menu, **select Personalize**. The screen shown in Figure 3-9 appears.
3. **Click** the **Desktop Background** or **Window Color and Appearance.**
4. **Select** a **background or window color and appearance** from the options presented.
5. When satisfied with your choice, **click OK.**

A user can also change the desktop from the Control Panel. To access the Control Panel, select the Start button on the taskbar, the Control Panel option, the Appearance and Personalization option, and Personalization. Again, Figure 3-9 shows the available choices. Note also that this is the same place to alter the appearance of the mouse pointer, to add sounds, and to add screen savers.

Moving Objects on the Desktop

Windows provides an option to change the location of any object on the desktop. The taskbar can be located on any of the four edges of the screen. The default is to place the taskbar on the bottom of the screen.

To change the location of the taskbar:

1. **Place** the mouse pointer on **a blank area** of the taskbar.
2. **Drag** the **taskbar** to the left, right, bottom, or top of the screen.
3. **Release** the **mouse button.**

When you drag the taskbar, it initially appears not to move. Keep dragging the mouse toward the edge of the screen, and eventually the taskbar will move unless it is locked into place. To unlock it, right-click a blank area of the taskbar and select Lock the taskbar to remove the check mark next to it.

To change the location of an icon, folder, shortcut, or file:

1. **Select** the **object.**
2. **Drag** it to the **new location.**

To arrange by name, size, type, and date modified:

1. **Right-click** a **blank area** of the desktop.
2. From the shortcut menu, **select Sort By** and **select one** of the options.

There are four choices in the "Arrange Icons By" menu: name, size, type, and date modified. Depending on which option is chosen, the icons will be arranged on the left side of the desktop in the order selected. The disadvantage of using this method of organizing icons is that every time new objects are added, they will appear in different spots on the desktop. Most people like their objects to be found in a consistent place on the desktop so that they do not need to spend time looking for them.

To align icons in a grid so they are evenly spaced:

1. **Right-click** a **blank area** of the desktop.
2. From the shortcut menu, select **View, Align to Grid option** (**Figure 3-10**).

The objects (icons) will now be in the general area where they were moved, but will appear in a straight column or row. The screen is actually organized as an invisible checkerboard. When the command "Align to Grid" is issued, the icons are snapped into the closest square to produce straight rows and columns. If the objects (icons) snap back into place when they should be moveable, right-click a blank area of the desktop, select Arrange Icons By and Auto Arrange to remove the check mark for that selection. See Figure 3-10. The check mark causes the icons to snap back into place.

Choosing a Screen Saver

Screen savers are moving or static pictures displayed on the desktop when no activity takes place for a specified period of time. They were initially designed to protect the monitor from having images burned into it. Today, they are primarily used for decoration. Many screen savers come with the operating system, and others may be obtained free from the Internet or purchased at computer software stores. Make sure you pay attention to security issues when downloading anything from or over the Internet.

To set up a screen saver:

1. **Right-click** a **blank area** of the desktop.
2. **Choose Personalize** from the shortcut menu.

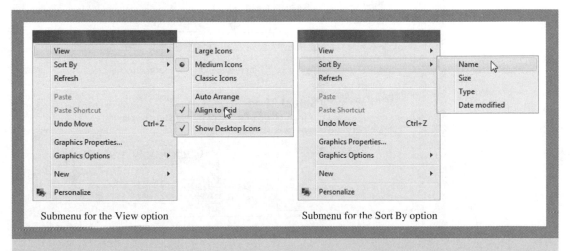

Figure 3-10 Arrangement of Icon Options

3. **Click** the **Screen Saver** option.
4. **Click** the **Screen Saver down arrow,** and select a **screen saver image**.
5. Set the **amount of time** to wait before activating the screen saver.
6. **Click Apply** and **OK.** See **Figure 3-11** for the Screen Saver Settings dialog box.

Working with the Sidebar and Gadgets

To Close the Sidebar: **Right-click** the sidebar and select **Close**

To Open the Sidebar: **Click** the **Windows sidebar button** in the notification area of the taskbar.

To Use a Gadget on the Sidebar: **Place** the mouse over the **gadget** and click.

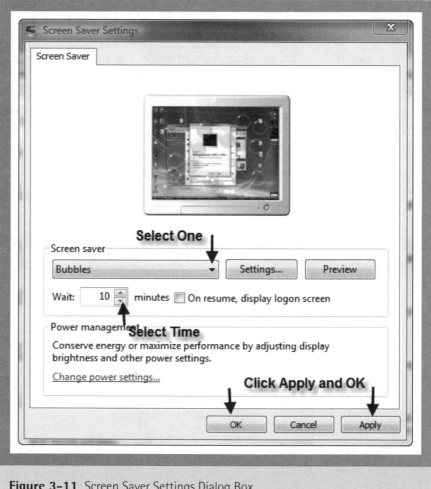

Figure 3-11 Screen Saver Settings Dialog Box

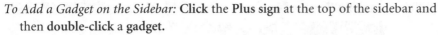

To Add a Gadget on the Sidebar: **Click** the **Plus sign** at the top of the sidebar and then **double-click** a **gadget.**

To Close a Gadget on the Sidebar: **Click** the **Close** button on the top right of the gadget.

Shutting Down the System

When you finish working with the computer, it is important to shut down the system before turning off the computer. Shutting down the computer saves the current settings and prevents the corruption of files (see **Figure 3-12**).

To shut down the system and save your session:

1. Click the **Start** button on the taskbar.
2. Click the **Save your session and turn off the Computer** button .

> HINT: If you turn on the computer after using this option, it will restore your Windows session. It isn't a good choice for shared computers, and some labs may not permit this option.

To shut down the computer without saving the session:

1. Click the **Start** button on the taskbar.
2. **Select** the **Menu Options** button ▸ and **click Shut Down** from the menu options.

To log off and prepare the computer for another user:

1. **Click** the **Start** button on the taskbar.
2. **Select** the **Menu Options** button ▸ and **click Log Off** from the menu options.

Most of the time, the appropriate option will be either Log Off or Shut Down. In most computer laboratories, the user logs off and does not turn off the computer. The computer saves all of the current user settings, closes all programs, and then prepares to receive another user. The computer remains turned on, and a login window appears with instructions (press Ctrl+Alt+Del) for how to log in. When the next user presses Ctrl+Alt+Del, the login screen appears for the user to type a user ID and password.

On a nonnetworked computer, a message appears on the screen asking the user to click the user name. The Switch User option lets another user log on while keeping the previous user's programs and files open. This is a helpful feature when two people share a computer.

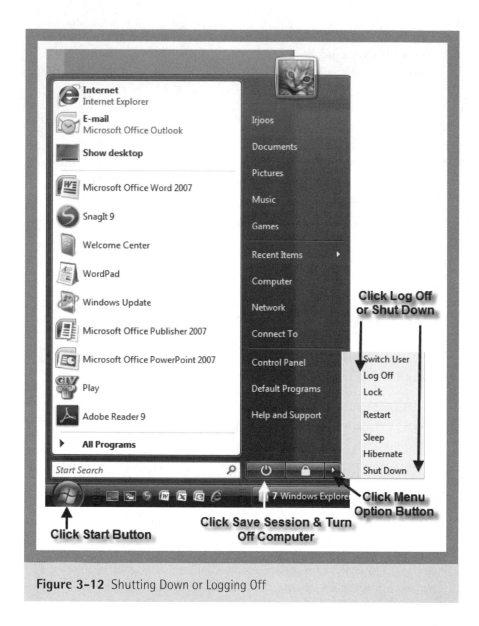

Figure 3–12 Shutting Down or Logging Off

At the end of the workday, or as appropriate at home, the best choice is to select Shut Down. The computer then proceeds to shut down. Most computers today will turn off their system units automatically, but the monitor may need to be turned off separately.

The Stand By option puts the computer into a low-power state, but will let the user quickly resume working. With this option, the computer looks like it is turned off, but the power lights remain on. To restart the computer, press the power button quickly on the computer or, in some laboratories, press the spacebar key. For some laptops, pressing the power button will wake up the computer if it is hibernating or in sleep mode.

Use the Restart option when you are updating or installing new programs. The computer will turn off and then restart itself.

Managing Windows

This section describes the layout of most application windows and the process of controlling the windows and changing the windows display options. All applications, files, and folders are displayed in a window, and each window shares similar attributes. To be able to work in the Windows world efficiently, users need to be able to manage the windows.

Common Windows Layout

Title Bar	This horizontal bar appears at the top of the window in most windows. The title bar displays a graphic button that can be used to access a menu and the name of the window or open file; on the far right are the window control buttons that minimize, maximize, and close the window. Use the title bar to move (drag) the window to another location on the desktop.
Tabs	In some newer versions of software such as browsers and Microsoft Office 2007, tabs are used instead of menu bars. They are part of the ribbon in Office 2007. Tabs function just like menu bars, in that they give the user access to commands. Tabs for specific applications are described more fully in later chapters of this book.
Menu Bar	If the window has a menu bar, it contains the names of available commands. Use the menu or horizontal bar with words on it to obtain additional drop-down options. For example, clicking File brings up such choices as New, Open, Create Shortcut, Delete, Rename, Properties, and Close, depending on the open program. Any command not available at this time appears dimmed.
	Vista hides the menu bar by default; in other words, the menu bar is available but hidden. To display the menu bar, press the **Alt** key; the menu bar then appears on the screen. Pressing the Alt key again makes the menu bar disappear.
	To make the menu bar appear in the window by default:
	1. **Open Computer** or a **Folder**; **select Organize**, **Layout**; and then **select Menu bar** from the menu.
	2. Alternatively, display the menu using the **Alt** key plus letter, **select Tools**, **Folder options**, **General** tab; **click Use Windows classic folders; click Apply** and then **OK**. See **Figure 3-13**.

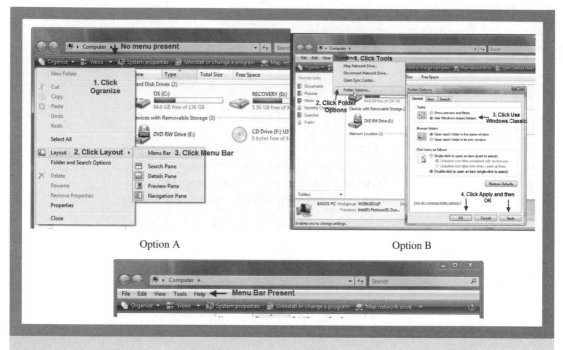

Figure 3-13 Permanently Display the Menu Bar in Vista

If three periods (an ellipsis) appear after the option, a dialog box will appear when that option is selected. A dialog box is a window that requests additional information from the user before the command can be implemented. For example, in **Figure 3-14**, selecting the Choose Details and Customize This Folder commands open a dialog box. Complete the information as appropriate in the dialog box or accept the defaults. Click OK to execute the command.

If an option has a right arrow, another menu will appear when that option is selected. In Figure 3-14, the commands Toolbars, Explorer bar, Sort by, and so forth all open another menu. This additional menu is sometimes called a nested menu or a submenu.

Ribbons	In Office 2007, the ribbon is the control center for the application. It consists of tabs, groups, and commands.
Toolbars	Some windows display one or more toolbars. The standard toolbar provides access to commonly used commands such as Create a new file, Open a file, Save a file, Print a file, and Cut/Copy/Paste data or images. See **Figure 3-15**. Chapter 4 describes these commands in more detail. Additional or different commands may appear in some applications because of the nature of particular programs. For example, Web browsers (discussed in Chapter 9) require a different set of commands. The standard toolbar in this type of application contains access to commands such as Back, Forward, Stop, Refresh or Reload, Home, and Search.

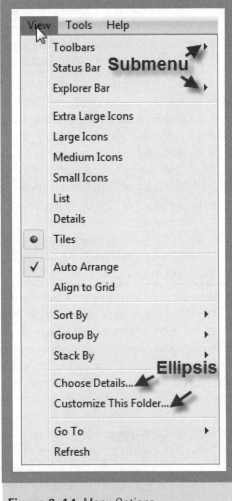

Figure 3-14 Menu Options

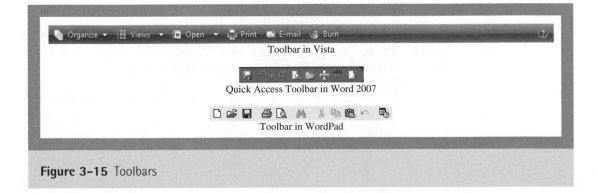

Figure 3-15 Toolbars

If there is a second toolbar, it generally relates to specialty functions such as formatting, using the ruler, and drawing. The second toolbar provides quick access to commands associated with that task. Windows also gives the user the ability to display additional toolbars as needed.

Status Bar

Some applications use a horizontal bar at the bottom of the window to display information such as the number of objects in the window, a description of menu commands, the number of pages in a document, the location of the cursor, and special toggle switches such as Overwrite, Num Lock, and Caps Lock. The contents of the status bar depend on what is important in the application. For example, in Excel, the status bar displays the Cell Mode indicator, the View shortcut, the Zoom, and the Zoom Slider; in Word, it indicates the current page number, the total number of pages, and the word count as well as the View shortcut, the Zoom, and the Zoom slider. When the user right-clicks the status bar, the Customize the status bar menu appears. The check marks on this menu show the current features that are turned on and provide an opportunity to turn on other features of the status bar.

Scroll Bars

Located along the right and bottom of the window are the vertical and horizontal scroll bars; they appear when there is more data than can be displayed in the window. Figure 3-6 shows a vertical scroll bar. Use scroll bars to move through a document or to view data when the entire document is not visible at once. Arrows appear at the top and bottom of the vertical scroll bar on the right and at the left and right sides of the horizontal scroll bar on the bottom, with a box somewhere between the arrows. Clicking the arrow buttons moves the user slowly through the window. The box or elevator in the scroll shaft indicates the current location relative to the total document. Dragging the elevator in the scroll bar gives the user more control over the process of viewing the contents of the window. The elevator shaft may also be clicked to go to an approximate location in the document.

At the bottom of the vertical scroll bar are up and down chevrons and a select object button (round circle). By default, the down chevron moves through the document one page at a time and the up chevron displays the previous page. The default can be changed by selecting the round circle and choosing an option.

Opening a Window

A window or program can be opened in several different ways:

- **Double-click** the icon representing the window to open it.
- **Right-click** the icon representing the window to be opened, and select **Open** from the menu.
- Click the **Start** button from the taskbar, and then select the window to be opened. For example, to open a recently used file, click **Start**, **Recent Items**, and the **name of the file**. To open the Control Panel folder, click **Start** and **Control Panel**.

Once the window is open, the user can perform the appropriate tasks. Because more than one window may be opened at a time, the user will need to control the window display.

Controlling the Window

Several controls are available for working with windows. Use these controls to move a window to another location on the desktop, change the size of a window, or close a window. The resize features permit the user to control the actual size of the window (see Figure 3-6). The Maximize and Minimize buttons use default standards to control the size of the window. Clicking the Maximize button expands the window to fill the screen. Clicking the Minimize button places a button for the application on the taskbar and removes the window from the desktop; with this option, the program remains open, but runs in the background. Clicking the Restore button returns the window to the size it was before it was maximized.

These buttons are helpful for controlling windows when the user is running multiple programs, opening multiple windows, or opening several files. They permit the user to view or work in each window while placing the others in the background.

In addition, the user may arrange windows on the desktop in cascade, stacked, or side-by-side style. When many windows are open, the cascade option works well if it is necessary to see all the open windows. With this option, all open windows will be cascaded from the top of the screen down, with the title bar of each open window visible to the user. Use the stacked and side-by-side arrangements to partition the screen into quadrants depending on the number of open windows. These options are useful when the user wants to drag and drop data from one window to another.

Function	Directions
Move a window	Click a **blank area** in the title bar of the window to be moved.
	Hold down the mouse button while dragging the window to a new location, and then release the mouse button.
Resize a window	Select the window to resize by clicking the **title bar**.
	Point to a window **border** or **corner**.
	When the cursor becomes a double-headed arrow (↔ or ↕), drag the **corner** or **border** until it is the desired size.
	Release the mouse button.
Enlarge a window	Select the window to enlarge by clicking its **title bar**.
	Click the **Maximize** button ▫ in the upper-right corner of the title bar. This button is a toggle switch and shares space with the Restore button.
Reduce a window	Select the window to reduce by clicking its **title bar**.
	Click the **Minimize** button ▬ in the upper-right corner of the title bar.
Restore a window	Select the window to restore by clicking its **title bar**.
	Click the **Restore** button ▣ in the upper-right corner of the title bar. This button is a toggle switch and shares space with the Maximize button.
Close a window	Select the window to close by clicking its **title bar**.
	Click the **Close** button ✕ in the upper-right corner of the title bar.
Arrange a window	Right-click a blank area of the **taskbar**.
	Select the arrange option: **Cascade**, **Stacked**, or **Side-by-Side**.

Managing Files and Folders

This section deals with the management of files and folders. The file system is a key element for working efficiently and effectively with a computer. As a consequence, knowing how to find, access, and manage files is important to managing the computer system as a whole. Use **Computer** (in Windows XP it is called My Computer) to access files and folder options and to see all the folders and sub-folders (which indicate the structure of the storage devices). **Figure 3-16** shows the Computer window without the folder option expanded on the left, and with the folder option expanded on the right.

This section first introduces some basic file and folder management concepts. The specifics of creating, renaming, moving, copying, and deleting files and folders then follow.

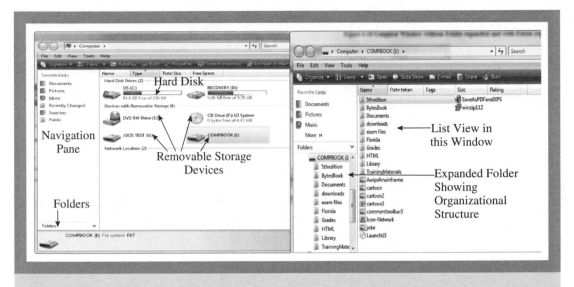

Figure 3-16 Computer Window without Folder Expanded and with Folder Expanded

Designating Default Disk Drives

The default drive is the drive that the program uses to find and save files unless told otherwise. Recall from Chapter 2 that the drive letter designation for the hard drive is generally C, and sometimes D; for a USB device and DVD or CD-ROMs, the default letters are D, E, F, G, and so forth. Most programs use a default folder on the C drive to store newly created files. For example, Microsoft Office stores all Microsoft Office files in the Documents folder on the C drive under the user's account.

All programs provide the ability to change the default storage drive and folder. To do so, find the preferences or options command. This command is accessed from the Office button ⊕ and Application Options button ⊞ Word Options in Microsoft Office 2007; in other programs, it is located in the Tools menu or the Edit menu.

If you are not permitted to alter these settings (e.g., if you are working in a computer laboratory or restrictive work environment), use the File or Office button followed by the Save As command to change the location of files each time you access the program. In Office 2007, in the Save As dialog box, click the down arrow on the Save button and select the correct storage device or computer in the Navigation Pane.

Creating Folders

Users can organize and manage their files by creating folders and then saving their work in those folders. A folder is a storage place for files and other folders. How folders are best organized depends on what you want to do. For example, one folder might contain all files related to a specific course, another folder might contain personal items, and yet another folder might contain articles or publications. Storing files in the appropriate folders allows for easy retrieval and backup of data. Associating files with projects or tasks allows for easier cleanup upon completion of projects or tasks. By comparison, saving all files in Documents or My Files folders makes retrieving and deleting more difficult and time-consuming. An icon █ represents each folder.

To create the folder:

1. **Point to** a **blank area** of the desktop or the open storage device window.
2. **Click** the **right mouse button**. A shortcut menu appears.
3. **Click** the menu item **New**. Another shortcut menu appears.
4. **Click** the menu item **Folder**. A new folder appears on the desktop or in the storage device window. The folder name is highlighted.
5. **Type** a **name** for the folder and **press Enter**. The folder now has the new name.

> NOTE: When a storage device is displayed in the Computer or Documents window, you can create a new folder by clicking the **Organize** button on the toolbar, selecting **New Folder**, and typing the name of the folder. When the menu option is present, select **File**, **New**, **Folder** from the menu. In addition, some applications include the New Folder button ▩ New Folder on a toolbar in the Save As dialog box. Use this same process to place folders within folders (subfolders) to further organize your work.

Naming Files and Folders

All files and folders have names. There are three parts to the file nomenclature: the file name, a delimiter, and a file extension. For example, in "My Smiley Face .bmp," the file name is "My Smiley Face", the delimiter is a dot (period), and the file extension is "bmp". Folders have a name, but no delimiter or extension.

File Name	In the preceding example, the portion to the left of the period ("My Smiley Face") is the file name. File names may include letters, numbers, or certain special characters, up to a maximum of 255 characters. Legal characters are letters of the alphabet (A–Z), digits (0–9), and all of the special characters except these: *, ?, <, >, \, /, ", :, and |. Although Windows permits the use of blank spaces between the characters of the file name to make the file name more readable and understandable, use blanks with caution: Some programs cannot handle file names with spaces or names longer than eight characters. File names are not case sensitive. They may be typed in all lowercase, a combination of uppercase and lowercase, or all uppercase. Use a unique file name for each file; there can be no duplicate file names in the same folder.

Delimiter	The delimiter is the period that separates the file name from the extension. Its inclusion is optional; users do not need to use the delimiter unless they are typing an extension to the file name.
Extension	The portion of the file identifier found to the right of the delimiter is the extension. Extensions indicate the nature of the file. For example, "docx" is the extension attached to files created with Word 2007. In most cases, the default option in the Windows environment is to hide the extensions. As a consequence, the user does not need to type either the extension or the delimiter; instead, the application used to create the file assigns the extension by default. In this environment, Windows uses the extension to identify which application created the file. When the file name is double-clicked, the file opens inside the appropriate application. The extension can also be used by users to determine what application was used to create a specific file.

Before working with files, think about which standards should be applied when naming files for personal work, for a clinical area, or for a department. File names can be structured in many ways, depending on the nature of the work, who does it, what users are sharing, how they are sharing it (on a network or hard drives), how they access it, and who retrieves it. The important point here is to use an understandable convention that will enable users to readily recognize what information the file holds over time— say, after 6 to 12 months has passed.

To name files, follow the directions given here. Folders are given names when they are created as noted in the previous section.

Function	Directions
Name file (application)	Start an application such as Word or Excel. **Create** the file. **Click** the **Office** button, or **File** command from a menu bar, **Save** or click the **Diskette** icon on the Quick Access toolbar. **Select** a **location** from the Navigation Pane on the left or from the **Save in** text box. **Type** the **file name** in the File name text box. **Click Save**, **OK** or **press Enter** on the keyboard. You can also use the Save as command to give a file another name. For example, Ethics in Nursing–draft, Ethics in Nursing–draft2.
Name file (on desktop)	**Right-click** a **blank area** of the desktop or in a window. **Select New**. **Select** the **Type of file** (e.g., Word, Excel). **Type** the **file name**. **Press Enter**.

Viewing Files and Folders

Once the user creates and names the files and folders, those items will need to be accessed. In Vista, users view files and folders through the Computer window.

Computer Icon without Folder View	Double-clicking the Computer icon opens a window that displays the storage devices and folders stored on this computer (Figure 3-16). If the icon does not appear on the desktop, **click** the **Start** button, **Computer** option. The screen then divides into several areas and lists the appropriate content for each area. Double-clicking a storage device or folder results in the current folder being replaced with the new folder. Repeat the double-clicking action to display the correct file or folder.
With Folder View	Clicking the **Folder** button ⌐Folders ^⌐ at the bottom of the Navigation Pane displays the organizational structure on the lower-left side and the contents of the active folder on the right side. 　　An arrow next to a folder means that there are more objects below it that are not displayed. When the arrow turns dark and rotates, all of the subfolders are displayed. This look can be changed by clicking each level of the structure to either expand or collapse it.

The display of the icons in the window depends on the view selected. See **Figure 3-17**. There are seven options for displaying icons in a window: extra large, large, medium, small, tiles, list, and details. The view used is a matter of personal preference. Use the list and small icons options to see more of the information on the storage device; use the details view to see information about the size and type of file; and use the large, medium, and extra large icons to see a thumbnail of the document.

To use Computer with or without the folder option, follow these directions:

Function	Directions
Without Folder option	**Double-click** the **Computer** icon on the desktop or click **Start, Computer.** **Double-click** the **storage device** where the file is located. **Double-click** the desired file or double-click the folders until the correct file appears. **Double-click** the file.
With Folder option	**Open** the **Computer** window. **Click** the **Folder** option. **Click** the **storage device.** **Click Folders** until the file is found. **Double-click** the file.

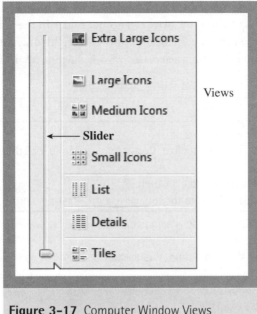

Figure 3-17 Computer Window Views

To change how files and folders look in the window, follow these directions:

Function	Directions
Change the view	Select the **View down arrow** from the toolbar bar. Click the desired view.

The slider on the left side of the menu may also be used to change views. Clicking the View button will rotate the display through the view options. Which view you choose is a personal preference, although some views are better for specific tasks. For example, the detail view is better when you are looking for details about files or folders, such as data modified and size. The list view is best for seeing a lot of files at one time without having to scroll through them.

Copying Files and Folders

The Copy command copies one, several, or all of the files from one place to another. That means there will be two copies of each file. There are several ways to copy files and folders: use menu systems, use drag and drop, or use the shortcut menu. The process for copying files and folders is the same. When using drag and drop from the F drive to another drive such as C, the default is to copy. When using drag and drop from the F drive to another folder in the F drive, the default is to move. You can override the default option by right-dragging the file. When dropping it in its new location, select Copy from the pop-up menu.

Function	Directions
Copy one file: toolbar or menu bar	**Click** the **file** to be copied. **Select Organize** from the toolbar, **Copy** from the menu, or **Edit, Copy** from the menu bar. Go to the **new location** and click there. **Select Organize, Paste** from the toolbar or **Edit, Paste** from the menu bar.
Copy one file: drag and drop	This works only when the file is being copied from one storage device to a different one: Both the file and the destination must be visible. **Select** the **file**. **Drag** it to its new location. **Release** the mouse button. When copying a file from one folder on a particular drive to another folder on the same drive, follow these directions: **Right-drag** the file to its additional location. **Release** the mouse button. **Select Copy here** from the shortcut menu.
Copy one file: shortcut menu	**Select** the **file**. **Right-click** the file. **Select Copy**. Go to the new location. **Right-click** in the new location. **Select Paste**.
Copy adjacent files	List view works best for implementing this technique: **Click** the **first file** in the group. **Hold down** the **Shift** key. **Click** the last file in the group. **Release** the **Shift** key. Follow any of the first three sets of directions when all files to be copied have been selected.
Copy nonadjacent files	**Hold down** the **Ctrl** key. **Click** each file to be copied. **Release** the **Ctrl** key. Follow any of the first three sets of directions when all files to be copied have been selected.

An alternative method for selecting multiple files is to draw a box around the files needed. To do so, go to the upper-left corner of the group of files. Hold down the left mouse button. Drag the mouse to the opposite corner, and release the mouse button. Once the files are highlighted, follow any of the first three sets of directions to copy them.

Moving Files and Folders

Moving files and folders is similar to copying files and folders. The Move command takes a file or folder from one place and puts it in another; it does not duplicate the file in the process. There are several ways to move files and folders: use menu systems, use drag and drop, or use the shortcut menu. When moving a file from one storage device to another storage device, use the right-drag option and select Move from the pop-up menu. Remember that the default for dragging and dropping a file between different storage devices is to copy the file. When moving a file from one place on the same storage drive to another place on the same storage drive, the default is to move the file.

Function	Directions
Move one file: toolbar or menu bar	**Select Organize** from the toolbar, **Cut** from the menu that appears, or **Edit**, **Cut** from the menu bar. Go to the **new location** and click there. **Select Organize** from toolbar, **Paste** from the menu, or **Edit**, **Paste** from the menu bar.
Move one file: drag and drop	This method works only when the file is going from one folder on a storage device to a different one on the same storage device: Both the file and the destination must be visible. **Select** the **file**. **Drag** the file to its new location. **Release** the mouse button. If the file is to be moved from one storage device to another storage device, follow these directions: **Right-drag** the file to its new location. **Release** the mouse button. **Select Move here** from the shortcut menu.
Move one file: shortcut menu	**Select** the **file**. **Right-click** the file. **Select Cut**. Go to the new location. **Right-click** in the new location. **Click Paste**.

Function	Directions
Move adjacent files	**Click** the **first file** in the group. **Hold down** the **Shift** key. **Click** the **last file** in the group. **Release** the **Shift** key. Follow any of the first three sets of directions after all files to be moved have been selected.
Move nonadjacent files	**Hold down** the **Ctrl** key. **Click** each **file** to be moved. **Release** the **Ctrl** key. Follow any of the first three sets of directions after all files to be moved have been selected.

Deleting Files and Folders

The Delete command removes files from the storage device. Use this command to clean storage devices and discard unneeded files. Several versions of this command are available, as noted in this section.

When you delete files from a removable storage device such as a USB storage device, the files are not moved temporarily to the Recycle Bin but instead are deleted immediately. Only files from the hard drive are moved temporarily to the Recycle Bin when deleted. Thus, if a user accidentally deletes files from the hard drive, those files may be recovered if the Recycle Bin has not been emptied. Deleted folders appear as empty folders in the Recycle Bin but actually still contain the old files. Thus, when a user restores a folder in the Recycle Bin, all of the original files are restored as well.

Function	Directions
Delete: toolbar or menu bar	**Select** the file. **Select Organize** from the toolbar, **Delete** from the menu, or **File**, **Delete** from the menu. **Click Yes** in response to the message "Are you sure you want to permanently delete this file?" *or* click **Yes** in response to the message "Are you sure you want to move this file to Recycle Bin?"
Delete: drag and drop	Make both the file or folder and the Recycle Bin visible. **Drag** the file or folder on top of the Recycle Bin icon. When the icon turns greenish-blue, release the left mouse button. If deleting the file or folder from a removable storage device, **click Yes** to confirm the deletion.

Function	Directions
Delete: Delete key	**Click** the **file or folder** to highlight it. **Press** the **Delete** key. **Click Yes** to confirm its deletion or its move to the Recycle Bin.
Delete: shortcut menu	**Right-click** the file or folder to be deleted. **Select Delete** from the shortcut menu. **Click Yes** to confirm the file or folder's deletion or move to the Recycle Bin.

Multiple files and folders may be selected, as noted in the earlier discussion of the copy and move operations. Use this same technique to delete multiple files or folders at once.

After files have been sent to the Recycle Bin, you will periodically need to empty the Recycle Bin. How often it should be emptied depends on how often files and folders are deleted and how many files and folders are deleted.

To empty the Recycle Bin:

1. **Double-click** the **Recycle Bin** icon.
2. **Select Empty Recycle Bin** from the toolbar.
3. **Click Yes** to confirm the emptying of the Recycle Bin.

To restore a deleted file or folder:

1. **Double-click** the **Recycle Bin** icon.
2. **Select** the **files or folders** to restore (if you want to restore only selected items).
3. **Select Restore all items** from the toolbar.

Renaming Files and Folders

The Rename command gives a file or folder a new name. Use this command to reorganize and change the names of files to be consistent with an organizational structure or to clarify the name because additional files or folders have been created.

Function	Directions
Rename: toolbar or menu	**Select** the **file or folder** to rename. **Select Organize** from the toolbar, **Rename** from the menu, or **File**, **Rename** from the menu bar. **Type** the **new name** and **press Enter**.
Rename: shortcut	**Right-click** the file or folder to rename. **Click Rename** on the shortcut menu. **Type** the **new name** and **press Enter**.
Rename: click–pause–click	**Click** the file or folder **name**. Pause, and **click again**. **Type** the **new name** and **press Enter**.

Organizing Folders

Most users store files on removable storage media (USB storage devices or CDs), on hard drives, and on network file servers. Files must be organized to make it easier to locate and retrieve them—and electronic files must be organized for the same reason that filing cabinets need to be organized. Electronic files are organized on the storage media in folders and subfolders.

Root Level	The "root" is the top level on which the folders reside. This level stores files the computer needs to access at startup. A general rule is that a folder or file listing of the root level should not occupy more than one screen's worth of information.
Folders	Folders organize programs and data files. Before creating them, think about the nature of the work and the programs it requires. Most software programs automatically make a directory for their program files when they are installed. Be careful to ensure that these directories "fit" the organizational structure of the work world. Customize them during installation if needed.
Subfolders	Subfolders are contained within other folders. They provide further division or structure to the organization of files.

Some rules for creating and using the folder and subfolder structure are summarized here:

1. Place each application suite in its own folder, with subfolders holding each application program. This structure makes installation of new versions, deletions of old versions, and maintenance of files easier. Some suites also create subfolders for shared suite files and create the necessary structure automatically during the software installation process.

2. Place programs not belonging to application suites in the Program Files folder in their own subfolder, with an appropriate name representing the application. For example, Adobe Acrobat Reader should have its own subfolder. Some users create a folder called Downloads and then create subfolders within it for each program downloaded. These subfolders are then backed up and used whenever needed. Other users also create a Utility folder off the root, and then place each utility program in its own subfolder within the Utility folder. For example, Norton Anti-Virus, Norton Utilities, and WinZip would each have a subfolder in the Utility folder.

3. Create folders for storing data files. Never store data files on the root, as this structure means that they will get mixed up with essential computer files. Instead, create a Data folder off the root. In the Data folder, create subfolders for each user on the system. Let each user then create the appropriate subfolders in his or her Data folder. While the hard drive contains Documents, Pictures, Music, and Games folders under your user account,

most people prefer to create their own structure. (A different scheme may be enforced in computer labs or public spaces.)

4. Create a Graphic Library folder off the root or in the Data folder for storing graphic images. The Graphic Library folder could contain subfolders representing graphic file formats or categories. For example, you might create subfolders to hold JPG and GIF graphic files or subfolders called Pets, Cities, and Computers. Some users also create a subfolder to hold photographs, as many users exchange pictures of family and friends.

5. Use appropriate folder names. No two folders in the same level can have the same name, but subfolders within different folders can have the same name. It is probably better not to name any folder on the computer with the same name as another folder. When folders have the same name it is very easy to forget which folder you are working in and to edit or delete the wrong file.

Disk Management Concepts

This section covers a few disk management concepts that are critical to working with the computer and the operating system.

Copying a USB Storage Device

Once the user creates and organizes his or her files and folders, it is a good idea to make a copy of the disk. The simplest way to do so is to copy all files and folders on the disk to another USB storage device, to a CD, to your network file server space, or to your second hard drive or external hard drive. Note here that this guidance applies to the user's personal data; the rules may be different for confidential data in a hospital setting where no removable storage devices may be allowed.

To copy a USB storage device:

1. **Double-click** the storage device in the Computer window.
2. **Select** all files and folders on the device (**Ctrl+A**), or select only those files and folder to which changes were made.
3. Either **right-click** the selection, **select Copy**, go to the backup location, and **right-click** to select **Paste** *or* **drag** the selection to the backup location.
4. Repeat Step 3 as needed to back up the files. When backing up files and folders to the same place the second time, you will be prompted to replace the existing files on the backup storage device. **Select** the **Copy and replace** option.

NOTE: If you are copying files and folders to a new CD, insert the CD into the writeable drive, select the **Burn files to disk** option, and type a title for the disc. The computer will then format the disc to prepare it to receive the files. You can then drag and drop the files onto the CD window.

Backing Up a Disk

Because of the size of hard drives today, most people no longer back them up. However, that practice will eventually cause the user problems because of hardware or software failures. The key question to ask is this: How important are the data? Although applications for the most part can be reinstalled, data may be lost forever if a failure occurs and no backup exists. At the very least, users should back up all data files, including documents, images, pictures, and, in some cases, downloaded freeware. Back up anything that cannot be quickly reinstalled or re-created. Data stored on the local drive of a networked computer are not routinely backed up when the network is backed up; instead, only data on the file server are backed up during this process.

Chapter 2 covered hardware, including storage devices such as tape drives, optical drives, and removable hard drives that people can use for backing up data. The user needs to seek answers to questions such as the following:

- What type of data do I have that cannot be replaced easily? How much data can I afford to lose?
- What capacity do I need for the backup device?
- How often do I need to back up my data?
- How reliable is the backup medium?
- How easy is it to use?
- What will it cost?

Ideally, backup systems for large operations should be done automatically and regularly. This backup does not include the data found on local hard drives on users' personal computers, however. For this reason, many organizations require users to store critical data on the network file sever itself so that the data are routinely backed up as part of the full system backup. Some organizations permit no critical data to reside on local hard drives. Those users who do store some data on the local hard drive can regularly back up the data to their personal space on the file server or copy that data to a removable hard drive, CD, or USB removable storage device.

For a home computer or a small business, this kind of backup is more difficult to do without a managed network. Solutions to this dilemma might include use of a second hard drive installed internally or use of second hard drive that is connected to the computer via a USB or FireWire port. With this approach, the user must remember to perform regular backups, set the timing for automated backups through the Backup Wizard, or use software such as SmartSync Pro to automate the backup process. Automating the backup process requires the computer to be left on. This approach, however, does not solve the issue unless the backup files are stored in a different place from the originals. Some experts suggest having a third backup that is stored in a safety deposit box or off site in a secured place and whose contents are recycled regularly.

Another solution is to use an online backup service. Several companies (e.g., HP Upline and SOS Online Backup) now offer backup services for a small monthly fee. Although this approach might sound like a great solution, it has some drawbacks. Some services discourage users from backing up certain types of files, such as MP3 files (music), and others limit how frequently the backups can occur. Some do not have easy-to-use interfaces. This approach requires a high-speed Internet connection, trust in the security of the servers used for backup, and trust that the company will not go out of business or not secure your data. Each user must find a solution for backing up critical data that works for him or her.

To back up the hard drive of your PC:

1. **Right-click** the **hard drive** in the Computer window.
2. **Select Properties** from the shortcut menu.
3. **Click** the **Tools** tab.
4. **Click** the **Backup now** button.
5. Follow the directions given by the Backup Wizard to set up the backup.

NOTE: Make sure the backup medium has enough space to hold the files you want to back up. After creating or updating the backup, store this medium in a different location from the hard drive.

Creating Shortcuts

Shortcuts can save time when users are working in the Windows environment. Instead of forcing users to work with the Computer feature to try to find files, folders, or programs, shortcuts provide access to frequently used items on the desktop. Files, folders, application programs, and storage devices can all have shortcuts. Recall that a shortcut is a pointer to an object; it tells the computer where to find the object but is not the actual object. Double-clicking the shortcut opens the object that the shortcut "points to."

The general rule for using shortcuts is to create them for frequently used objects. Many people create shortcuts to their data files, the printer, Internet Explorer, and selected applications. Do not create shortcuts to infrequently used items, or your desktop will rapidly become overly cluttered.

A small curved arrow in the lower-left corner of an icon denotes that the icon is a shortcut. See Figure 3-2. Because it is simply a pointer to an actual object, deleting the shortcut deletes just the shortcut, not the actual object to which it is pointing.

To create a shortcut on the desktop:

1. **Find** the object that the shortcut will point to.
2. **Resize** the windows to make the desktop visible.

3. **Right-drag** the object to the **desktop**.
4. **Select Create Shortcut(s) Here** from the shortcut menu.

In addition, shortcuts can be created for objects on the left side of the Start button menu by right-clicking the object, clicking **Send to**, and then selecting **Desktop (Create Shortcut)**. The objects Documents, Computer, and Network Places from the right side of the Start button menu can be placed on the desktop by right-clicking the object and selecting the **Show on Desktop** option from the shortcut menu.

Some people also place shortcuts to frequently used applications on the Quick Launch area of the taskbar to keep their desktop from too much clutter.

Managing Files with Scan Disk and Defragmenter

Before running any of these programs, use the Disk Cleanup program to remove any unwanted files. This utility is available only for cleaning the hard drive on your system; it is not applicable to removable storage devices. The unwanted files include things such as temporary Internet files and downloaded program files; these files simply take up space and slow down the computer. Empty the Recycle Bin to free up even more disk space. This step should be done on a weekly basis. See Chapter 9 for more on temporary Internet files and cleanup.

Access the Disk Cleanup program by selecting **Start, All Programs, Accessories, System Tools,** and **Disk Cleanup**. Select just your files or all files on the computer, and then run the program.

Next, use an error-checking tool (Scan Disk) to check the file system for errors and bad sectors. Some technicians recommend using this tool once a week; others recommend using it once a month. In reality, many users perform a Scan Disk check once or twice a year. Close all programs including any program running in the background before running Scan Disk. If a program is running, Scan Disk will restart itself over and over. On networked computers, this tool may not be accessible unless the user is logged on as the administrator. **Figure 3-18** shows the Properties, Tools tab.

To access this error-checking tool:

1. **Close** all files.
2. **Open** the **Computer** window.
3. **Right-click** the storage device.
4. **Select Properties** and the **Tools** tab.
5. **Click** the **Check now** button [Check Now...] in the error-checking part of the screen (see Figure 3-18).
6. Place a check in the **Automatically fix file system errors** and **Scan for and automatically repair bad sectors** squares, and then click the **Start** button.

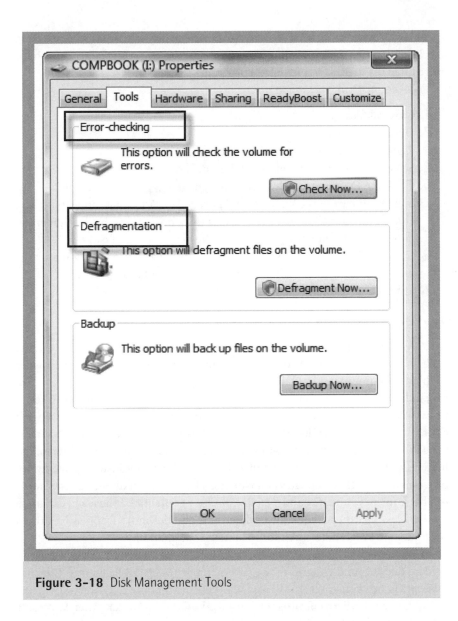

Figure 3-18 Disk Management Tools

This program takes a while to do its job, depending on the size of the device being checked. Once the work is complete, Scan Disk produces a status report for the check. Click **Close** when the program is finished.

The last file management program discussed here is the Defragmentation utility. This program consolidates fragmented files and folders on the storage device so that each one is stored in a contiguous space. This neater organization provides for performance improvements in accessing files and folders. Once again, all programs must be closed before this utility is run, as this program checks and moves data. This tool should be run about two times per month, or more often if a user loads and deletes programs frequently.

To access the Defragmentation utility:

1. **Close** all files.
2. **Open Computer.**
3. **Right-click** the storage device.
4. **Select Properties,** and then select the **Tools** tab.
5. **Click** the **Defragment Now** button [Defragment Now...] in the Defragmentation part of the screen (see Figure 3-18). A message appears stating either that your file system is fine and does not need to be defragmented now or that it is not okay and needs to be defragmented now.
6. **Click OK** if the system doesn't need attention. **Click** the **Defragment Now** button [Defragment now...] to begin the defragmentation process.
7. **Select** the **drives to defragment** and **click OK.**

Applying Updates and Patches

All software programs—whether programs such as Word, operating systems such as Windows, or device drivers for printers, monitor and other hardware such as the computer itself—issue periodic upgrades or patches. Updates are generally enhancements to the software that provide additional features or functions, whereas patches are generally fixes for problems discovered in the software after its original release. Many of these patches focus on fixing security problems inherent in the software that might make the user's computer vulnerable to hackers and viruses. The first thing that should be done after installing a software program is to check for updates and patches. Then, every so often, the user needs to check for new updates and patches. Some people make these checks once a month, while others check for updates and patches more frequently; others configure the program to check for such items automatically.

In Windows Vista and XP, the Start menu contains an option called Windows Update that is found either on the main menu or under All Programs. Clicking this option takes the user to Microsoft's Web site. Follow the directions given for updating the Microsoft programs installed on the computer. After Microsoft scans the computer, it presents a list of updates or patches. These items are generally divided into Critical Updates, Windows Vista and Driver Updates, and so forth. Select the desired updates and download them to the computer. (The computer must have an active Internet connection to complete this step.) Note the size of the files before downloading them; some of them are quite large and may take substantial time to download, especially over dial-up connections. In addition, a message appears periodically on the right side of the taskbar reminding the user to check for updates.

In the Microsoft Office suite, access the updates option by clicking the Office button, the Options button, the Resources option, and the Check for updates button [Check for Updates]. Follow the directions on the screen for obtaining the updates.

Summary

This chapter oriented the user to the operating system and the Windows interface, including the common objects found on the desktop. Desktop management skills include setting screen savers, changing desktop colors, moving objects, and managing windows. File and folder management concepts are also essential knowledge for today's users, who need to know which commands create, rename, move, copy, and delete files and folders. This chapter also presented some basic ideas about organizing files and folders and introduced a few utilities for managing the software.

Whether the operating system is proprietary, such as Windows, or open source, such Linux, one thing is certain: A system for managing the hardware and interfacing with the end user is always needed. That system is not static, however, but rather will evolve to reflect changes in technology and in user needs.

EXERCISE 1 Managing a Desktop and Windows[1]

■ **Objectives**
1. Identify and describe the desktop.
2. Apply a screen saver.
3. Arrange the desktop to work efficiently and effectively.
4. Change the colors of the desktop.
5. Open, close, minimize, maximize, size, and arrange windows.
6. Switch between windows.

■ **Activity**
If necessary, make sure to turn on the computer and log on. You may also need to turn on the monitor.

1. Identify the following desktop objects using their *generic* group names, not the specific name of the object the icon represents. Complete these statements:

   a. An object like [icon] is called a(n) _____. Use it to _____.

   b. An object like [icon] is called a(n) _____. It represents _____.

   c. An object like [icon] is called a(n) _____. It is used for _____.

   d. An object like [icon] is called a(n)_____. Use it for _____.

   e. The following bar is called the _____. It is used for _____.

   [taskbar image]

   f. The sidebar is used to _____.

2. Apply a screen saver.
   a. **Right-click** a **blank area** of the desktop.
   b. Choose **Personalize** from the shortcut menu.
   c. **Click** the **Screen Saver** option.
   d. **Click** the **screen saver down arrow**, and select **Bubbles**.
   e. **Set** the amount of time to wait before activating the screen saver to **10** minutes.
   f. **Click Apply** and then **OK**. **Figure 3-19** shows the screen saver dialog box.

3. Move and arrange objects on the desktop.
   a. **Drag** the **Internet Explorer** icon [icon] to the lower-right side of the desktop.
   b. **Drag** the **Recycle Bin** icon [icon] to the lower-right side of the desktop.
   c. **Right-click** a **blank area** of the desktop. Click **Sort by**, and then select **Name**.

---

[1]This exercise is available electronically from the textbook Web site.

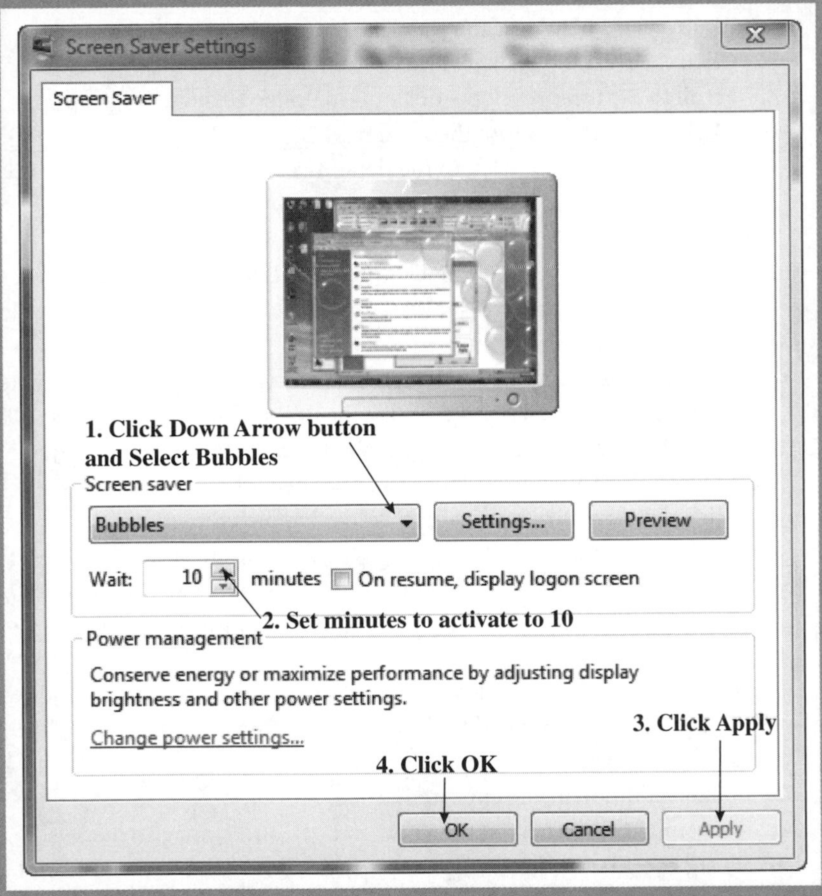

Figure 3-19 Steps to Activate or Change a Screen Saver

    d. What happened to the icons? _____
    e. **Drag** the **Internet Explorer** icon 🔵 to the upper-right side of the desktop.
    f. **Drag** the **Recycle Bin** icon 🗑 to the upper-right side of the desktop.
    g. **Right-click** a **blank area** of the desktop. Select **View, Align to Grid**.
    h. What happened? _____
    i. **Drag** the **taskbar** to the top of the screen.

HINT: If the icons snap back into place, right-click a **blank area** of the desktop, select **View**, and then select **Auto Arrange**. This series of actions removes the check mark next to the Auto Arrange feature and permits you to move the icons. If the taskbar doesn't move, **right click** the taskbar and select **Lock the Taskbar** to remove the check mark.

4. Change the desktop background.
   a. **Right-click** a **blank area** of the desktop and click **Personalize**.
   b. **Click** the **Desktop background** option.
   c. **Scroll to Textures** (click the first option under Textures **Img5 options**).
   d. **Click OK** and then **close** the window.
   e. To change the setup back to the default colors, repeat Steps a–d except choose **Img42** under Vistas.

5. Open, browse, and manage windows.
   a. Open the Computer window by **double-clicking** the **Computer** icon . If this icon is not on the desktop, **click** the **Start** button and select **Computer** from the menu.
   b. Using the title bar, **drag** the Computer window to the right approximately 3 inches. If it is set to fill the screen, use the **Restore** button to make it smaller.
   c. **Click** the **Maximize** button . What happened to the window?
   d. **Click** the **Restore** button . What happened?
   e. **Click** the **Minimize** button . What happened?
   f. **Click** the **Computer** button on the taskbar.
   g. Place the pointer on the **right border** of the **Computer** window.
   h. With the double-headed arrow, **drag** the **window border** to the right 2 inches.
   i. Place the pointer on the lower-right corner of the **Computer** window.
   j. **Drag** the **window border** up and to the left, making the window approximately 3 inches square.
   k. Which additional bars appeared?
   l. Why might you need to know how to open and manage windows?
   m. **Drag** to enlarge the **Computer** window, making it approximately 6 inches square.
   n. **Double-click** the **Local Hard Drive** icon (usually C). **Double-click** the **Windows** folder. Notice that the default in Windows is to open each new folder in the same window.
   o. **Click** the **Back** button until the Computer window is open.

6. Change the default folder option and switch between windows.
   a. In the Computer window, select **Organize** from the toolbar, **Folder and Search Options** from the menu, or **Tools, Folder options**. See **Figure 3-20**.
   b. **Click** the **Open each folder in its own window option** under the **Browse Folders** section of the dialog box.
   c. **Click Apply** and **OK**. Now each folder will open in its own window.

HINT: If the menu bar isn't displayed, press the **Alt** key to display it or select **Organize** from the toolbar, **Folder and Search Options** from the menu, click the **General** tab, and select the **Open each folder in its own window** option.

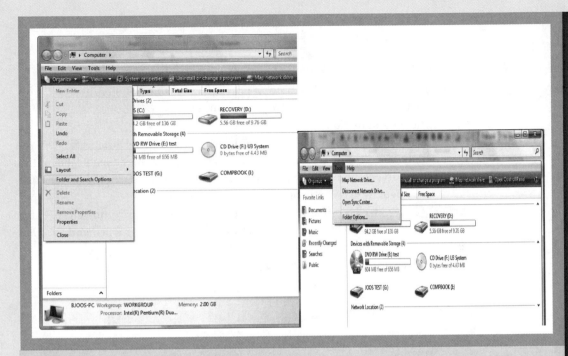

Figure 3-20 Changing Folder Options

d. To try out the new setting, **click Start**, **Control Panel**, and **Appearance and Personalization**.

e. What happened?

f. **Click** the **Computer** button on the taskbar.

g. What happened?

h. **Move** the Computer window so that the Control Panel window is visible.

i. **Click** anywhere in the **Control Panel** window.

j. Hold down the **Alt** key and press the **Tab** key. This brings up a window for switching between open applications. Use this feature to toggle between open windows.

k. **Press** the **Tab** key again while still holding down the **Alt** key.

l. Release the **Tab** and **Alt** keys. What happened?

m. Why might you want to switch between windows?

n. **Click** the **Close** buttons to close all open windows.

EXERCISE 2 Managing Folders and Files

■ **Objectives**

1. Create folders and files.
2. Move, copy, and rename folders and files.

3. Delete files and folders.

4. Empty the Recycle Bin.

■ **Activity**

In this exercise, the term "USB storage device" refers to the flash drive.

1. Create a folder and subfolders on a removable storage device.

a. **Open** the **Computer** window.

b. **Double-click** the **USB storage device** icon. It should be labeled "Removable Disk" or USB Disk or some other label if you added a label to the drive, plus a letter such as G, H, I, and so forth depending on the configuration of your computer.

c. **Right-click** a **blank area** of the device window. This command may also be accessed by clicking the **Organize** button on the toolbar and selecting **New Folder**.

d. **Select New, Folder**. See **Figure 3-21**.

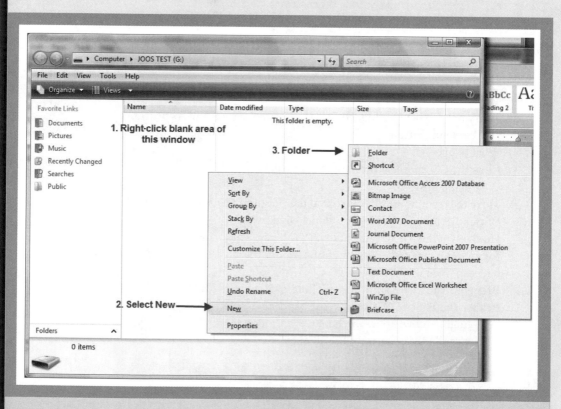

Figure 3-21 Creating a Folder

e. **Type Computer Class** in the text box that appears and then **press Enter**.

f. **Double-click** the **Computer Class** folder.

g. **Right-click** a **blank area** of the Computer Class window.

h. **Select New, Folder**.

i. **Type Class Notes** and then **press Enter**. A new folder can be created either by using the right-click method or by selecting the command from the toolbar.

j. Repeat the process twice, making two more subfolders in the Computer Class Folder. Call these folders **Exam Review** and **Homework Submitted**.

k. If the professor wants to see your work, submit the removable storage device or open the **Computer Class** folder displaying the subfolders, **click Print Screen**, open **Word**, **type** your name, and **press Ctrl+V** to paste the print screen image into the Word document. Print the Word file and submit it. The results should look like **Figure 3-22**.

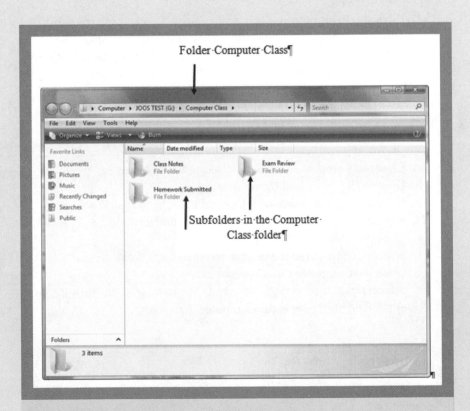

Figure 3-22 Printout of Word with Subfolders Displayed

2. Create files.
   a. **Double-click** the **Class Notes** folder.
   b. **Right-click** a **blank area** of the Class Notes folder. **Select New**, **Word Document**.
   c. **Type Internet Notes** and then **press Enter**.
   d. **Right-click** a **blank area** of the **Class Notes** folder. **Select New**, **Word Document**.
   e. **Type Security Notes** and then **press Enter**. (Steps b–d result in the creation of two blank Word documents.)
   f. Create one more **blank Word** document with your name on it.
   g. **Expand** the Class Notes window to fill the screen and click the **Print Screen** button.
   h. **Open** the Word file that has your name as the file name.
   i. **Press Ctrl+V** to paste the print screen file in the Word file.
   j. **Click** the **Save** button on the Quick Access toolbar to save the file. If the Save button is not on the Quick Access toolbar, click the **Office** button and then **Save**.
   k. **Click** the **Print** button if it is in the Quick Access toolbar *or* **click** the **Office** button and then **Print**. The Print dialog box appears.
   l. Send one copy of the current document to the default printer by clicking **OK**. Submit the printout to your professor. Note that some professors may require the submission of the files on your USB storage device. The Word document should look like the document in **Figure 3-23**.

3. Copy, move, and rename folders and files.

Clipboard Method
   a. **Close** all open windows except the Computer window.
   b. **Double-click** the **Local Drive** (usually C) icon 🖾.
   c. **Double-click** the **Windows** folder and then the **System32** folder.
   d. Scroll down in the System32 folder window until the **Calc** file 🖩 is visible.
   e. **Click** the **Calc** file to select it.
   f. **Select Organize** from the toolbar and then **Copy** from the menu.
   g. **Open** the **Computer Class** folder.
   h. **Select Organize** from the toolbar and then **Paste** from the menu. A copy of the Calc file is now in the Computer Class folder.

HINT: This task can be accomplished by dragging the Calc file to the USB storage device if both windows are visible. Recall that the default action when you drag and drop files and folders from one storage device to another is to copy the item. The calculator icon is now in both windows.

   i. Close the **local hard drive** window.

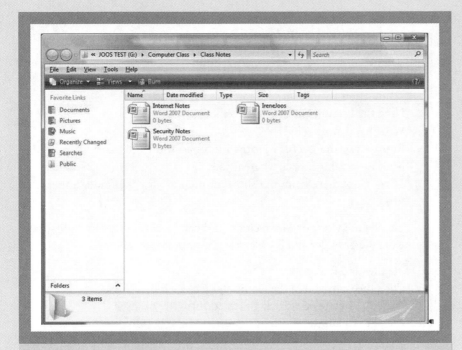

UNFIG 52

Figure 3-23 Printout of Files in the Class Notes Folder

Drag and Drop Method
a. Open the **USB storage device** window if necessary.
b. **Right-drag** the **Calc** icon file onto the **Class Notes** folder.
c. **Select Copy here** from the shortcut menu. Notice that the calculator now exists in both folders.
d. Why do you need to right-drag the icon when copying from a file in USB storage device to the same USB storage device?

There are two ways to rename files and folders, and each process is the same for both files and folders. The first technique uses the command from the shortcut menu; the second uses the click–pause–click method.

Rename a File Using the Menu
a. Right-click the **Calc** icon in the Computer Class folder.
b. **Select Rename**.
c. **Type Calculator** and then **press Enter**. The icon now has a new name.

Rename a File Using the Click–Pause–Click Method
a. **Click** on the **text** of the Class Notes folder in the Computer Class window once, and then **click again**. The text in the folder icon should be highlighted, but not the icon. FIG 24
b. Type **Lecture Notes** and then press **Enter**.

For the next task, the Computer window setting must be set to **Show each folder in its own window** (click **Organize**, **Folder and Search options**; check **Open each folder in its own window**; and click **OK**). See **Figure 3-24** for how the two windows should look.

Drag and Drop

a. **Drag** the **Lecture Notes** folder to the USB Device window.

b. What happened? Why?

c. **Right-drag** the **Lecture Notes** folder to the Computer Class folder window, putting it back where it was.

d. **Select Copy here** from the shortcut menu. Now the folder appears in two places.

The default Copy or Move command can be overridden by right-dragging the file or folder and by selecting the appropriate command.

4. Delete files and folders.

a. **Click** the **Calc** icon in the Computer Class window.

b. **Press** the **Delete** key. **Click Yes** to confirm the deletion.

c. **Close** the **Computer Class** window. If the window is set to open all folders in the same window, click the USB device letter in the address bar instead of closing the Computer Class folder.

d. Change the view of the icons in the USB device window to **List**.

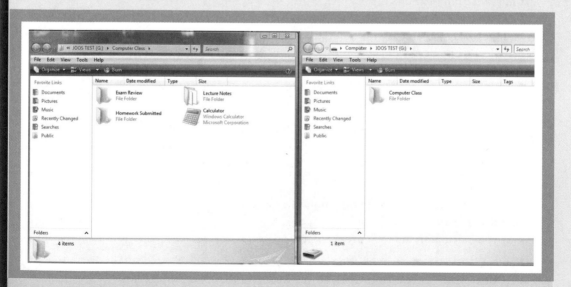

Figure 3-24 Dragging Between Two Open Windows

e. If necessary, move the USD device drive window so that the Recycle Bin is visible.

f. **Click** the **first icon** in the row or column. Hold down the **Shift** key, and click the last icon. All of the icons are now selected.

g. **Drag** the **selected folders** onto the Recycle Bin.

h. When the Recycle Bin turns greenish-blue, **release** the mouse button.

i. **Click Yes** to confirm the permanent deletion of files and folders.

j. **Close** all windows.

> HINT: Files that are deleted from a USB storage device do not go to the Recycle Bin, which is why the question asking to confirm permanent deletion appears. Files from the desktop go to the Recycle Bin when they are deleted, so the question doesn't appear.

5. Empty the Recycle Bin. When you delete files from internal storage devices such as the C drive or desktop, you should empty the Recycle Bin periodically. In Windows Vista, you can "see" trash building up in the icon.

a. Create **two blank Word documents** on the desktop. Call one **test** and the other **test2**.

b. **Drag** and **drop** the new files on top of the Recycle Bin.

c. **Double-click** the **Recycle Bin** icon. A list of contents appears.

d. **Click** the **Empty the Recycle Bin** button on the toolbar or select **File, Empty Recycle Bin** from the menu bar.

e. **Click Yes** to confirm the deletion.

f. **Close** the Recycle Bin window.

g. How often should the recycle bin be emptied?

EXERCISE 3 Software Decisions and Organization Skills

■ Objectives

1. Begin to select appropriate software and justify its purchase.
2. Organize a hard drive or removable device with folders and subfolders.
3. Identify appropriate file names for given documents.

■ Activity A

1. You are the manager on Unit 93, a 40-bed general medical–surgical unit. You received approval for a new computer for managing the unit's information needs, but now need to specify which software the computer will need. List the necessary software and explain why the unit will need it (see Chapter 2 for brief descriptions of software categories or look in computer advertisements for specific software programs). Make sure the software complies with the facility's default standards. For example, does

your facility require everyone to use Word for word processing or Excel for spreadsheets? Does it let users determine whether OpenOffice or Microsoft Word better meets their word processing needs? Include an operating system in your request. Some examples of common categories are listed here:

Word processing

Spreadsheet

Database

Presentation graphics

Browsers and HTML editors

Utilities such as antivirus programs, Norton Utilities, WinZip, and Acrobat Reader

Specific software such as medical dictionaries, lab tests, and drug calculation programs

2. You must organize the hard drive so that things are orderly and easy to maintain. Describe the organization of the hard drive. Remember that each program should have its own folder, and that similar programs and data should reside in the same folders or subfolders. Most applications are located in the Program Files folder.

3. Use your removable storage device to create the previously mentioned folders and subfolders on that device.

4. It will take the information systems staff 3 weeks before they can install your software. If you decide to do it yourself, how will you go about installing the software?

■ **Activity B**

This chapter suggested ways to organize your work for easy retrieval and provided you with the skills to create these folders.

1. You are storing data files on the hard drive, so you will not have to deal with removable devices. This means that the path to these folders will be **C:\ DATA**. In that data folder (**DATA**), you will create a series of subfolders. As an example, the structure should begin to look like **Figure 3-25**.

   a. Place an appropriate file name in the blank column.

	Document File Name
Memos Folder	
Request for more staff	
Request for communication software	
Response to a procedure change	
Response to vacation request	

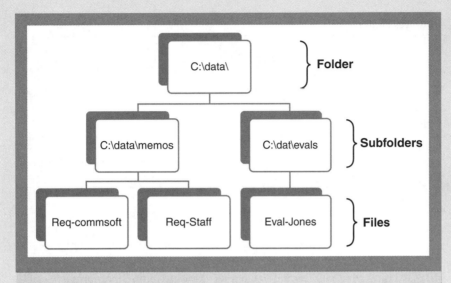

Figure 3-25 Organization of Folders and Files

Committee Folder

Subfolder for policics and procedures

Subfolder for accreditation

Sample template for policies and procedures

Minutes of the policies and procedures meeting
held September 15, 2009

Teaching Materials Folder

AIDS: What you should know

Orientation to our unit

So you are going to have surgery

Evaluations Folder

One subfolder each for RN–Jones, LPN–Smith, and
Unit Clerk–White

Evaluation template

Evaluation for Jones–2009

Evaluation for Smith–2009

Budget Folder
Unit budget for 2008
Unit budget for 2009
Unit budget for 2010
Web Pages Folder
Introducing our staff
Services provided on our unit
Contact information

   b. Create these folders on the hard drive or your removable storage device.
   c. Create the files in the appropriate folders.
   d. Using what you learned in Chapter 1 about zipping (compressing) a file, zip (compress) the data folder.
   e. Send the compressed folder to the faculty member as directed by the faculty member or email it to a classmate. Can you and your classmates unzip the folders that were emailed?

EXERCISE 4 Customizing the Start Menu and the Taskbar

■ **Objectives**
   1. Alter the taskbar.
   2. Alter the Start menu.
   3. Work with and alter the sidebar.
   4. Download and add other gadgets to the sidebar.

Some of these tasks may not be available in computer laboratories or in the work environment unless you are logged on as the administrator.

■ **Directions**
   1. Change the taskbar.
      a. **Right-click** on a **blank area** of the taskbar and select **Properties**. The Taskbar and Start Menu Properties dialog box appear.
      b. **Click** the **square** to the left of the Show Quick Launch text to place a check in the square. This will display programs that enable you to show desktop, switch between windows, and so forth in the Quick Launch area of the taskbar. Clicking on these programs will start them.
      c. **Click** the **Apply** and **OK** buttons.

d. Add a few Microsoft Office icons to the Quick Launch area of the toolbar. Click the **Start** button, and select **All Programs, MS Office**. Right-click **MS Office Word 2007** and select **Add to quick launch**. The Word icon appears in the Quick Launch area, ready for you to start the program.

e. Repeat Step d to add icons for other frequently used Microsoft Office programs to the Quick Launch area. If more icons are added than can easily fit a right pointing chevron appears indicating more icons are there.

2. Alter the Start menu.

   a. **Right-click** the **Start** button and click **Properties**.

   b. **Click** the **Start** menu tab in the **Taskbar and Start Menu Properties** dialog box. If you do not like the new look, you can change it to an old look.

   c. **Click** the **Customize** button next to the Start menu option.

   d. **Click** to increase the number shown on the Start menu to **10.**

   e. **Scroll down** until you see **Use large icons**. Click to remove the check mark next to this option.

   f. **Click OK** and then **Apply.**

   g. **Click OK** to apply the changes. Look at the changes to the Start menu: You should see small icons and a list of 10 applications.

> HINT: Notice the Privacy area in the Taskbar and Start Menu Properties dialog box. If you do not want someone to see which programs were recently accessed on the computer or which files were recently opened, remove the check marks next to these options. Also notice the Notification area, which can be customized to change what it hides or what it shows.

Pin an Item to the Start Menu

   a. Find **MS Office OneNote** in the **All Programs** menu. If you do not have this program, use another one.

   b. Right-click the text and select **Pin to the start menu**. The program now appears in the top-left pane of the Start menu; it can be accessed more easily from this location than by going through several layers. Use this feature for programs used regularly but not daily.

Some users like to control the All Programs menu so that it does not become too unwieldy. Doing so requires thinking about how to organize the programs into appropriate categories and having administration rights on the computer. Here is one suggestion: Place all like programs together. For example, create a folder called Multimedia, and place all multimedia programs in that folder. Create a Utilities folder, and place all utilities in that folder.

Organize the All Programs Menu on the Start Menu

   a. **Right-click** the **Start** button and then **click Explore.**

   b. **Select** the **Start** menu on the left side of the window if it is not highlighted.

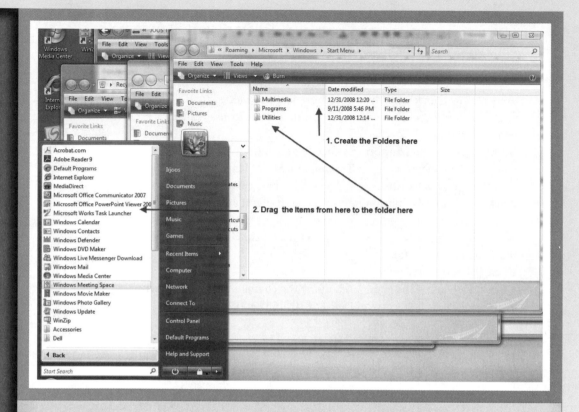

Figure 3-26 Altering the Start Menu, All Programs

    c. **Right-click** a **blank area** of the right window. See **Figure 3-26**.
    d. **Select New, Folder**, and type **Utilities**.
    e. Repeat the process to create a **Multimedia** folder.
    f. **Drag** the appropriate programs into the folders. For example, move QuickTime and Real Player into the multimedia folder and Norton Anti-virus and WinZip into the Utilities folder.
    g. If a message appears saying you need administration permission, **click Continue** and then **click Continue** again. The program will now move to the new location if you have administrative permissions.
    h. **Close** all open windows, and look at the Start menu.
3. Work with and alter the sidebar.

Close a Gadget on the Sidebar
    a. **Point** at the gadget, then click the gadget's **Close** button. For example, point to the **clock** and click the **Close** button.

Add a Gadget to the Sidebar

a. **Click** the **plus** sign at the top of the sidebar. The Gadgets dialog box appears.

b. **Double-click** the **calendar** gadget. The calendar gadget appears on the sidebar.

Use a Gadget on the Sidebar

a. Place the **mouse over** the calendar and **click**. The whole calendar for the month appears.

b. **Click** a **date**, and that date appears. You can move from month to month or date to date.

Close the Sidebar

a. **Right-click** the **sidebar** and select **Close**. The sidebar now disappears from the desktop.

Open the Sidebar

a. **Right-click** the **Windows sidebar** in the notification area of the taskbar.

b. Select **Open**.

4. Download additional gadgets for the sidebar. This part of the exercise can be completed only if you have permission to download and install objects to the computer.

Obtain an Additional Gadget

a. Open your Web browser.

b. Type **desktop.google.com** in the URL address box.

c. **Click** the **gadget** hyperlink at the bottom of the screen.

d. **Click** the **technology** hyperlink on the left-side panel.

e. **Click** the **Download** button under the temperature convertor icon ???.

f. **Click** the **Open** button on the dialog box. The gadget now appears on the sidebar.

Use the New Gadget

a. Place the mouse **over the temperature** conversion gadget, and click the **chevron**. The size of the gadget increases. See **Figure 3-27**.

b. Type **98** in the °F Fahrenheit text box, and click the **temperature gauge** to the right of the text box. The values all change.

Many gadgets are available on the Internet. Make sure you obtain ones from trusted sites.

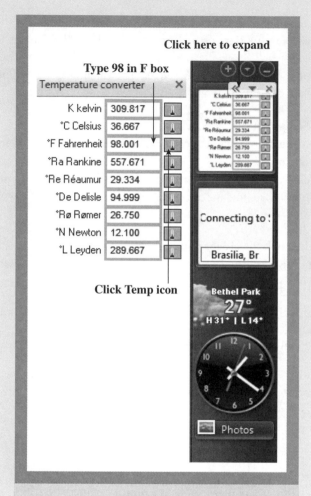

Figure 3–27 Using a Gadget

■ **Directions**

1. Create the following objects on the desktop. Refer to the appropriate chapter discussions if you cannot remember how to create these objects.
   a. Shortcuts to the printer and to the **Documents** folder
   b. A folder for your downloaded graphics files
   c. A **Word** file named **All About Viruses**
   d. **Computer** on the desktop
   e. A new gadget of your choice on the sidebar

2. Define the following terms:
   a. icon
   b. folder
   c. file
   d. shortcut
   e. taskbar
   f. sidebar
   g. gadget
   h. shortcut menu
3. Rearrange the desktop.
   a. **Place** the shortcuts to the printer and to the **Documents** folder on the upper-right side of the desktop.
   b. **Place** the **Graphics** folder on the lower-right side of the desktop.
   c. **Place** the **All About Viruses** file centered at the top of the desktop.
   d. Keep all of the other objects except the taskbar on the left side of the desktop.
4. Change the theme of the desktop to **Nunavut-Nature-Animals**.
5. Move the taskbar to the left side of the desktop.
6. **Click** the **Print Screen** button to place the desktop image on the clipboard.
   a. **Start WordPad** or a word processing program.
   b. **Click** the **Paste** button on the **Home** tab, the clipboard group, or the Paste icon on the toolbar.
   c. Print the file with the new desktop image.
7. Restore the desktop.
   a. **Close** all windows.
   b. **Reset** the default to the **Windows Vista** theme.
   c. **Place** the taskbar at the bottom edge of the desktop.
   d. **Delete** the objects created in Step 1.
   e. Turn in the Print Screen copy showing the restored settings.

ASSIGNMENT 2 Working with Files and Folders

■ Directions
1. **Create** folders.
   a. **Create** a folder on your **USB storage device** named **Learning 1**.
   b. In the Learning 1 folder, create a **Graphics** folder, a **Word** folder, an **Excel** folder, and a **PowerPoint** folder.
2. Find and copy files.
   a. Find a **PNG** file on the hard drive. **Click** the **Start** button. **Type** *.png in the search box and **press Enter**.

    b. **Copy** any of the files found to have a .png extension to the folder Learning 1 on the **USB storage device**.

3. Create data files in the **Learning 1** folder.
    a. Create a **Word file** named **Word Review Guide**.
    b. Create an **Excel file** named **Unit 5 Budget-2010**.
    c. Create a **PowerPoint** file named **Health Habits**.

4. Move files to the correct folders.
    a. Move the **PNG** file into the **Graphics** folder.
    b. Move the **Word Review Guide** file into the **Word** folder.
    c. Move the **Unit 5 Budget-2010** file into the **Excel** folder.
    d. Move the **Health Habits** file into the **PowerPoint** folder.

5. Rename a file.
    a. Rename the **Health Habits** file to **My Nutrition100 Presentation**.
    b. Place your name on the **USB storage device** and turn it in to the professor.

ASSIGNMENT 3 Additional File and Folder Work

■ **Directions**

1. Develop an appropriate structure for storing your work this semester. Include folders representing the courses you are taking this semester as well as a few subfolders representing the work of each course. You may also complete this exercise using your personal or work environment.

    Sample structure (these are all folders). You do not need to include the label "folder" or "subfolder"; that status can be easily determined from the structure. Your main folder should be **YOURNAME**.

    YOURNAME (folder)
      IST105 (subfolder)
        Exams (subfolder)
        Exercises
        Grades
      NUR208 (folder)
      CHEM111 (folder)

2. Create your structure based on the preceding example on your USB storage device under a folder with your last name.

3. Find three files created this semester and place them in the appropriate folders. List the files and their related folders here: _____ _____.

4. Create a folder called **Downloads**. Go to www.adobe.com and **click** the Get **Adobe Reader** button. **Download** the **Adobe Reader** file to the **Download** folder on your USB storage device.

5. Compress the main folder (**right-click** the folder, select **Send To**, and then **select Compressed folder**). Submit this work as directed by the professor.

ASSIGNMENT 4 File and Hard Drive Management

■ **Directions**
1. Use the file provided to you by the professor to answer these questions. Save it as Chap3–Assign 4–Your last name.
2. Use the system and maintenance dialog box to identify the following information:
   a. Operating system
   b. Operating system version and service pack last applied
   c. Processor running the computer
   d. Processor speed
   e. Amount of RAM on this computer
3. List and describe the three main tools available to maintain the files on your storage medium.
4. Use the help system to determine how you would make a file or folder have read-only status; with a read-only file, others can read the file, but not change it unless they rename it.
5. Make a backup folder on your USB storage device and copy all of your current files and folders into the backup folder. Rename the original files and folders (not the ones in the backup folder).
6. List two ways to delete files and folders. Where do the files go once you delete them from a removable storage device?
7. **Print** this file and turn it to your professor.

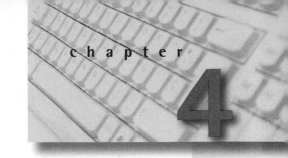

Software Applications: Common Tasks

Objectives

1. Identify standards common to applications running in the Windows environment.
2. Describe and use the online help that the applications provide.
3. Use the MS Office ribbon and its tabs, groups, and commands.
4. Perform common tasks such as creating, opening, closing, saving, finding, and printing files.
5. Use cut/copy/paste functions to move or copy data from within the same file, from one file to another, or from one application to another.

This chapter describes common tasks that are performed when working with application programs regardless of the application. In the Windows environment, certain standards exist so that many applications share a common desktop environment with menus and toolbars to access commands. For example, menus provide the paths to action. Commands on a menu that are followed by an arrow result in the appearance of a submenu of commands; those followed by an ellipsis (. . .) produce a dialog box. Many applications display a title bar, menu bar, one or more toolbars, status bar, and graphical buttons.

Microsoft Office 2007 uses a new interface that is designed to provide the appropriate tools at the time they are needed. This chapter uses Microsoft (MS) Office Word 2007 to explain and demonstrate this new interface. There is also an exercise using WordPad to demonstrate the traditional title, menu, and toolbars.

Common Layout

MS Office 2007 uses a "fluent user interface" that is presented as a "ribbon." Although the ribbon looks different than the command layout for Office 2003, once you become familiar with it, the tasks and commands are very similar. The tab names resemble menu names, and the ribbon resembles a toolbar, as in previous versions of Word. **Figure 4-1a** shows the ribbons for Word, Excel, and

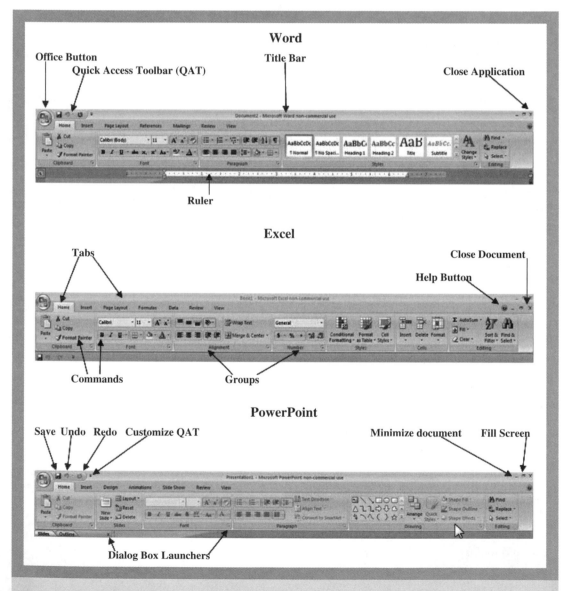

Figure 4–1a Sample Ribbons from MS Office 2007

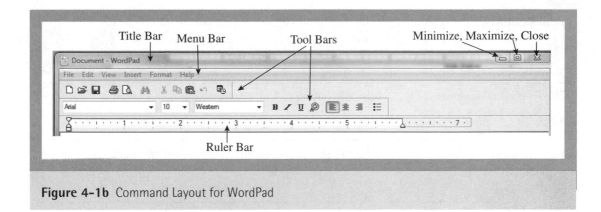

Figure 4–1b Command Layout for WordPad

PowerPoint with common features identified. **Figure 4-1b** shows the command layout for WordPad; a similar interface is also used by several other applications such as Office 2008 for the Mac and Office OneNote.

Office Button	Click on the Office button in Word and a list of commands appears: New, Open, Save, Save As, Print, Prepare, Send, Publish, and Close.
Quick Access Toolbar	The default items on the toolbar are Save, Undo, Redo, and Quick Print. Other commonly used items can be added for fast and easy access by right-clicking on the command/tab and choosing **Add to Quick Access Toolbar.** They can also be added by first clicking the **Office** button, then clicking **Word Options** at the bottom of the window, and finally choosing **Customize** from the list. A window appears with many icons that can be added to the toolbar. You can also change the position of the toolbar on the screen to the top or bottom of the ribbon. On public computers, however, you may not be allowed to alter this toolbar.
Title Bar	The title bar shows the program and document titles.
Ribbon	The ribbon is composed of task-oriented tabs, groups, and commands.
Tabs	Tabs vary among applications, but all share the Home, Insert, Review, and View features. Some tabs, such as Home and View, are always available. Contextual tabs come and go depending upon what you are doing. Tabs function much like menu bars.
Groups	Each tab has several groups that show related items together. Groups function much like toolbars.

Help Button	The Help button opens a dialog box for Word, Excel, or PowerPoint Help. Type the keyword or topic in the search text box and click Search *or* browse the topics listed in the dialog box.
Fill Screen or Maximize	Use this button to fill the screen with the document.
Restore Down	Use this button to resize the document to its original size before it was maximized.
Minimize	Use this button to minimize the document so that the desktop or other documents are visible.
Close Application	Use this button to close the current document or when you are finished with the application and have saved your work.
Dialog Launcher	This button opens a dialog box with related commands and options.
Save	Use the Save button to keep the file on the storage device for future reference.

Microsoft Office Button Functions

Figure 4-2 shows the menu and related commands that appear when you click the Office button. These items are described in more detail below, using Word as an example. The commands are the same in PowerPoint and Excel, with one exception: Instead of Word Options, for PowerPoint and Excel, Options is used. Note the list of Recent Documents that appears to the right of the menu. Each file name has a pushpin icon next to it. To "pin" a file to the Recent Documents list so that it always stays there, click the pushpin icon. To unpin the file, click the green pushpin icon.

New	This item opens a new blank document or Blog Post. Many choices for the type of document are available, such as calendars, envelopes, letters, memos, minutes, résumés, schedules, timesheets, and templates. More options are available from Microsoft's Web site.

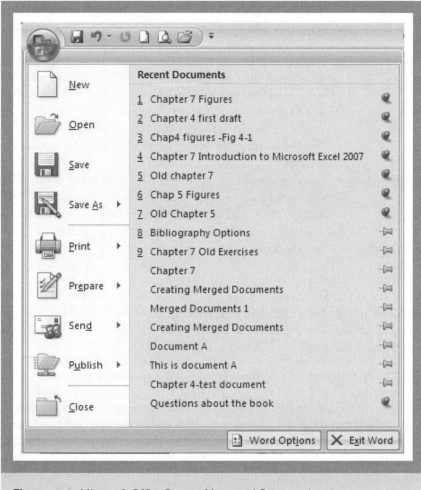

Figure 4-2 Microsoft Office Button Menu and Commands

Open	Choose from the list of Recent Documents that appears next to the commands under the Office button, or click Open and look in other areas of the storage devices.
Save	Save the file. If you are saving the file for the first time, the file will need a name and location in which to save it.
Save As	Holding the cursor on the Save As command without clicking brings up a menu of file formats in which to save the document. Click a file format and the Save As dialog box appears. Here the file is named (or renamed) and a place to save the file is selected. Click the command Save As to go straight to the Save As dialog box.

Print	Using the same point but don't click approach you can choose Print, Quick Print, or Print Preview, which then provides a dialog box for choosing where, how, and what to print.
Prepare	This item allows you to check the properties of the document, add a digital signature, inspect or encrypt the document, and check for compatibility with earlier versions of the application.
Send	Use this option to email or fax a copy of the document.
Publish	Use this command to publish to a blog or to a server.
Close	Close the document. You will be reminded to save any changes if necessary.
Word Options	Choosing Word Options opens a list with many choices that include popular options for Word; display options; ways to proof, save, customize, and secure a document; and resources. Some of the same options appear in the other Office applications.
Exit Word	Close the application.

Some of these commands are followed by an arrow ▶. It leads to a dialog box that offers additional choices, such as those described for the Save As and Print commands. These commands are similar to the commands obtained from the File menu for software that does not use the ribbon interface. Other commands are followed by ellipses (. . .) that lead to a dialog box.

Tabs and Groups

Basic task-oriented **tabs** appear across the top of the ribbon in Word (see **Figure 4-3**), Excel, and PowerPoint. Four of them are the same in each application: Home, Insert, Review, and View. Tabs are broken into subsections called **Groups** (see Figure 4-3) that further define the tasks associated with that group. Clicking a tab shows tasks associated with that tab. For example, the Page Layout tab allows you to define themes, set margins, add page breaks, and define indent and spacing parameters in

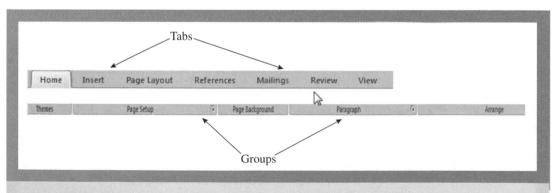

Figure 4-3 Tabs and Groups in Word

Word. Clicking the **Dialog Box Launcher** [⬚] in a group opens a dialog box where further options are available. When a down arrow [▾] appears in a ribbon button, it means more choices are available. When the mouse arrow is held over an option in the ribbon, a ScreenTip appears that describes its function. A task pane is a small window that displays additional options and commands for certain features. A con textual tab occurs in a window that is available only in a certain context or situation.

Status Bar

Figure 4-4 shows the status bar in Word. It shows the page number, number of words in the document (the document pictured is a new one), some view buttons, and the Zoom slider. Zoom allows you to examine a part of the document more closely or to see a complete page of the document. Setting the Zoom level to "page width" can be helpful when working with a document in landscape mode. Right-click the status bar, and a menu opens that allows you to customize it.

Keyboard Commands

Keyboard commands (access keys) make it easy to choose tasks in a ribbon. Press the **Alt** key to activate access keys, and **KeyTip** badges (letters and numbers) appear. **Figure** 4-5 shows what happens when the Alt key is pressed. Simultaneously

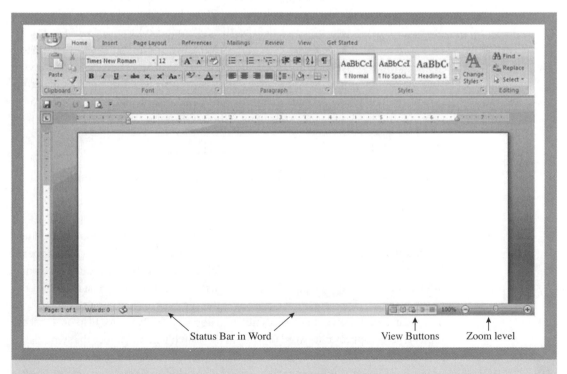

Figure 4-4 Status Bar in Word

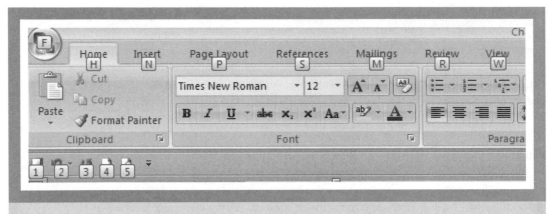

Figure 4-5 KeyTips (Shortcut Symbols) for Accessing Commands from the Keyboard

pressing the Alt key and one of the letters shown causes shortcut letters and numbers to appear for the groups in that tab. For example, press **Alt+H** and you will see the KeyTip for bold; press **Alt+1** and the next thing typed will appear in bold. If the cursor is inside a word, that word will be changed to bold. To cancel KeyTips, press Alt again. Pressing the **F10** key will also show KeyTips.

In other applications such as Publisher 2007, browsers, or Office 2008 for the Mac, shortcut keys are shown next to the command on the drop-down menu. If you press **Alt+F** in Word 2007, the drop-down menu for the Office button appears. Next to each command is the keyboard shortcut. For example, to save the current document, press **S**. These letters work only when this particular drop-down menu is present. Otherwise, **Ctrl+S** is the keyboard shortcut for the Save command. These shortcuts work in all Office 2007 applications.

Common Tasks

This section describes common tasks that one does in most applications.

Obtaining Help

Access the Help feature through the blue question mark 🔵 on the ribbon or the Help option on a menu bar. Click the question mark, and a Word Help screen appears (**Figure 4-6a**). Topics describe what is available in online help; if you are working offline, the symbol 🔵 Offline is shown. To use online help, you must be connected to the Internet. If you hold the cursor over the symbols at the top of the window, a ScreenTip description of the object's function appears. To search for help on a specific topic, type the appropriate word or topic in the search text box under the symbols.

Note the dialog box in the lower-right corner of Figure 4-6a. Clicking the green ball 🟢 at the lower-right corner of the dialog box causes the menu for

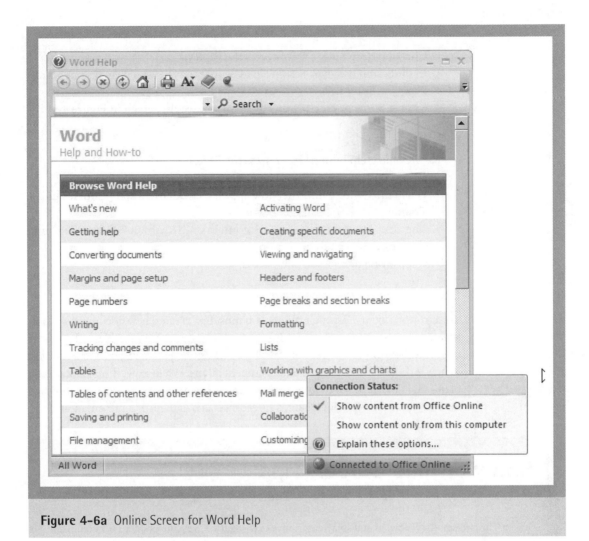

Figure 4-6a Online Screen for Word Help

choosing either online or offline help to appear. If you are online, you will find
more options for assistance at the end of the Help window. For example, you can
choose More on Office Online Downloads | Training | Templates Downloads, Training, or Templates.

To select a help topic:

1. **Click** the **Help** button or press the F1 key.
2. **Click Lists** in the Table of Contents section of the window.
3. **Click Create a bulleted or numbered list**.
4. Review the article.
5. **Click** the **Home** symbol at the top of the Word Help window. It returns
   you to the original list of topics.

To find help using a keyword:

1. **Click** the **Help** button 🔘 or press the **F1** key.
2. In the Search box, type **ScreenTips**. (Be sure to type ScreenTips as one word.)
3. **Press** the **Enter** key.
4. Choose **Show or hide ScreenTips**. You will see the screen in **Figure 4-6b**.

To access Microsoft Office Training online:

1. **Click** the **Help** button 🔘 or **press** the **F1** key.
2. **Click Training** under "More on Office Online."
3. When the Office Online window appears, **click Office 2007 Courses** under Training.
4. The next window that appears contains a list of 2007 Office Training Courses, as shown in **Figure 4-6c**.
5. Choose one to review if you have time!

Creating a New File (Document)

To start working in most applications, you must first create a new document, spreadsheet, database, or presentation. Most applications open to a new, blank document or spreadsheet or present a series of dialog boxes asking you to respond to questions. When Word is started, a new blank document opens. When PowerPoint is started, a blank title slide appears. In Excel, a worksheet is opened. A Word document is used here to represent a text document, a spreadsheet, a database, or a presentation.

Show or hide Screen Tips

Screen Tips are small windows that display descriptive text when you rest the pointer on a command or control.

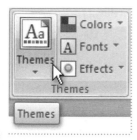

Figure 4-6b Show or Hide ScreenTips Screen

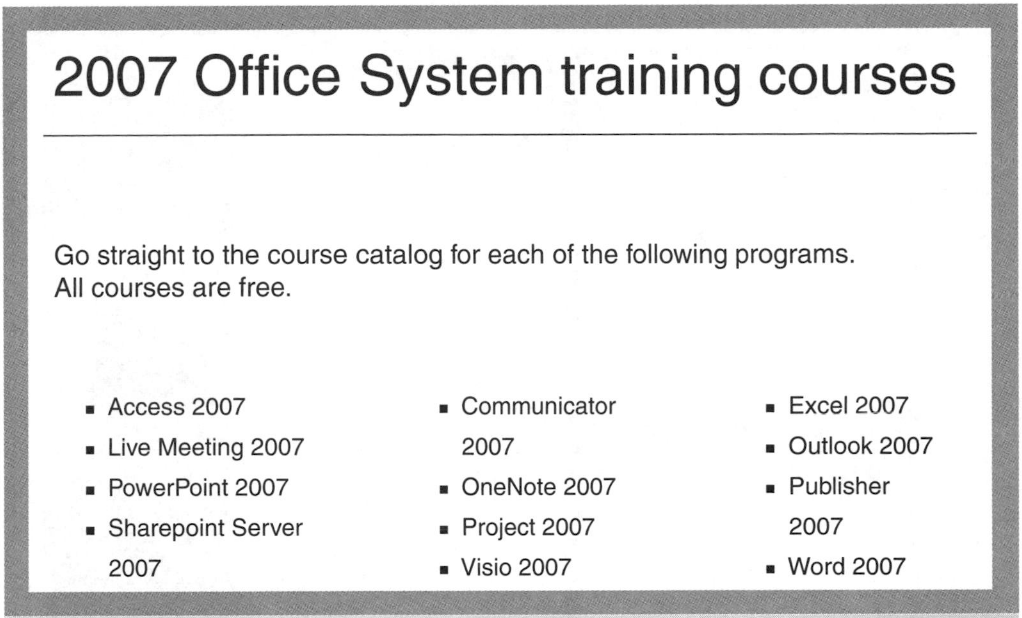

2007 Office System training courses

Go straight to the course catalog for each of the following programs.
All courses are free.

- Access 2007
- Live Meeting 2007
- PowerPoint 2007
- Sharepoint Server 2007

- Communicator 2007
- OneNote 2007
- Project 2007
- Visio 2007

- Excel 2007
- Outlook 2007
- Publisher 2007
- Word 2007

Figure 4-6c 2007 Office System Training Courses Screen

When the computer is on and you have a task to complete, an application must be selected. For Microsoft Office, click **Start**, select **All Programs**, and then select **Microsoft Office** in the next menu that appears; next select the correct application. **Figure 4-7b** shows the screen in Vista; **Figure 4-7a** shows Windows XP. A new document will open such as the one shown in Figure 4-4.

You can also go to the Start button ▨ and open a Microsoft Office application from the Start menu if it appears above the Start button, as shown in **Figure 4-8**. Microsoft Office icons may also be placed on the Quick Launch area of the taskbar or on the desktop. Using this approach, the user clicks the correct button on the taskbar or double-clicks the shortcut icon on the desktop to launch the program.

To start another document once the application is open:

1. **Click** the **Microsoft Office** button ▨ and choose **New. Figure 4-9** shows the dialog box that appears.
2. **Click** the **Create** button on the lower-right side of the screen to select a new blank document.
3. Alternatively, **press Ctrl+N** and a new blank document opens.

There are also several templates you can use to minimize formatting time. Templates are either installed on the computer, made from previously constructed documents, or available online.

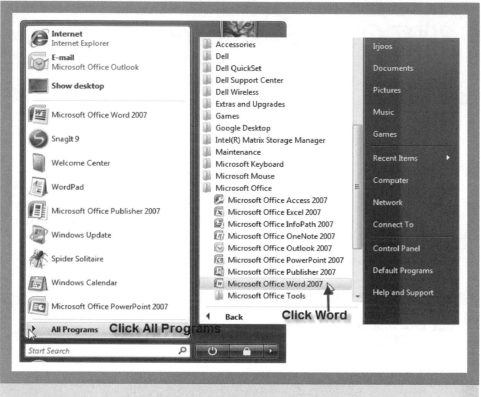

Figure 4–7a Menu for Opening Microsoft Office Word 2007 in Vista from Start and All Programs

To create another document using a template:

1. **Click** the **Microsoft Office** button and choose **New.**
2. **Click Installed Templates** in the left column.
3. **Select** a template from the **choices that appear.**
4. When a choice is made, **click Create.**

Now two documents are open. All documents remain open and accessible through the Word menu box—   Document1 - Micro...   (Vista) or   2 Mi... ▾   (XP)— found at the bottom of the screen until you close them.

Opening, Minimizing, and Closing a File

All applications require you to open and close files. Once a document has been created, it may be saved and often is reopened later for additions and/or corrections.

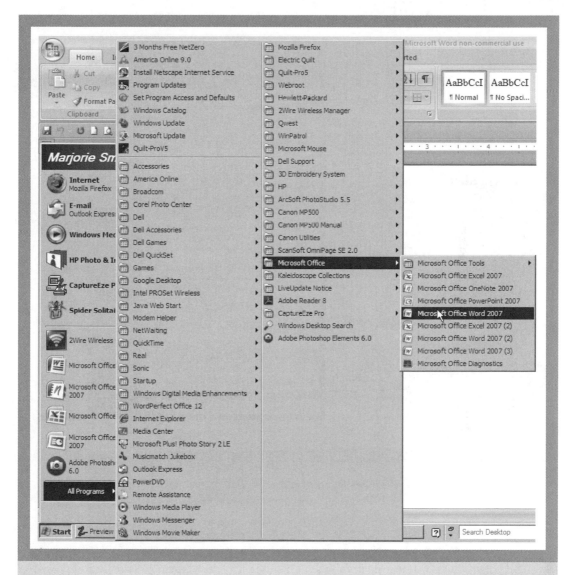

Figure 4–7b Menu for Opening Microsoft Office Word 2007 in Windows XP from Start and All Programs

Open Files

In the Windows world, a file can be opened in many ways. In some applications, you select File, Open on the menu to do so. Because the focus here is on Office 2007, this section demonstrates the use of the Microsoft Office button.

1. **Click** the **Office** button, and move the mouse pointer to **Open**. A list of recent documents appears on the right.

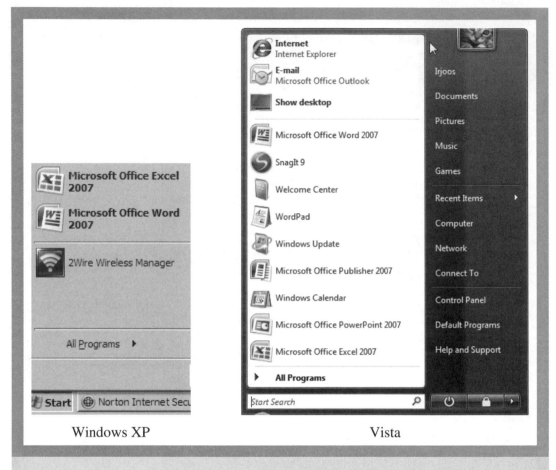

Figure 4-8 Start Menus for Windows XP and Vista

2. Choose a document from that list, if it is the one desired.
3. If the file doesn't appear in the list, **click Open**; a dialog box appears like that shown in **Figure 4-10**. Several choices are available. In Figure 4-10, Vista shows **Documents** under the Favorites link. Select the correct location from the left pane and then the correct file from the right panel. For Windows XP, **My Documents** is selected from the Look in list, and the Navigation Pane with its list of Folders/Files is shown on the right.
4. **Click** to choose the appropriate document. If the document is located on an external storage device or a network file server, select **Computer** or My **Computer** to see those devices.

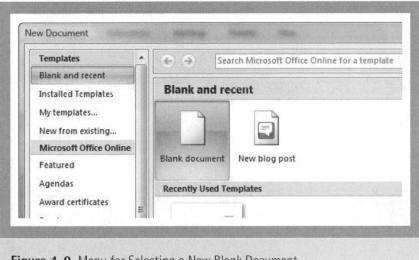

Figure 4-9 Menu for Selecting a New Blank Document

Files can be opened in many ways. Examples include:

- In a window or on the desktop, double-click the **file**.
- **Click** the **Start** button on the taskbar. **Select Recent Items** (Vista) or **My Recent Documents** (Windows XP), and **click** the one desired. The last 15 files that were opened appear on the menu list, regardless of file type.
- In an application, press **Ctrl+O**.

Minimize Files

Click the Minimize button – in the upper-right corner of the window, and the document will disappear. It can be accessed again by clicking in the Word button 2 Mi.. ▾ on the taskbar. Choose the document you desire.

Close Files

To close a file:

1. **Click** the **Office** button, and then move the mouse pointer to the **Close** command   *Close*.
2. **Click** the **Close** command. If changes were made to the file and it was not saved, a prompt appears to remind you to save the file before closing it.

Other options for closing files:

- **Click** the   in the upper-right corner of the window.
- **Press Ctrl+F4** on a traditional keyboard.
- On some newer keyboards, **click** the **Close** button (F6) found at the top of the keyboard.

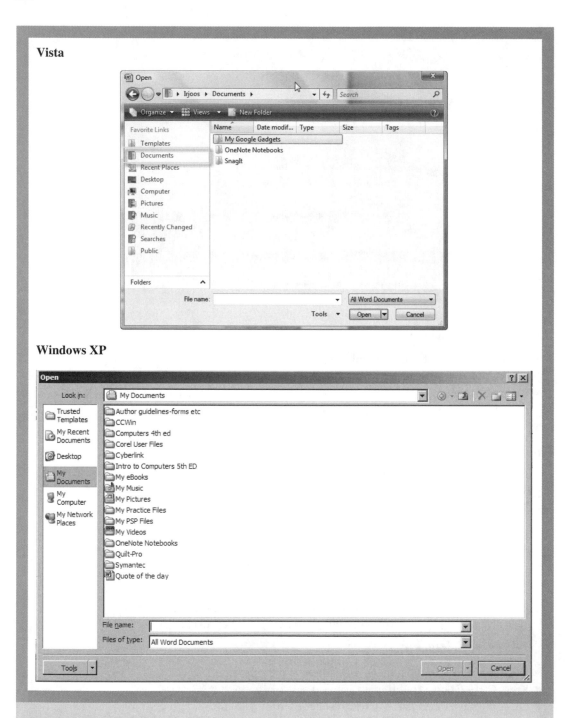

Figure 4-10 Open Dialog Boxes for Vista and Windows XP

Saving Files

Once work begins on a file or document, it will need to be saved for future reference or revision. It is safest to name and save the document when it is first opened. You can then simply press **Ctrl+S** (or the **Save** button on newer keyboards) periodically to save your work and prevent loss of data. The first time that a file is saved, you must specify a location and name for the file (see Chapter 3 for a discussion of file naming conventions). If a location is not specified, the file is saved in the default location. In Microsoft Office, the default location is the Documents (Vista) or My Documents (Windows XP) folder on the hard drive (C). Once the file has a name and location, use the **Save** command to update the file and save any changes to it. The Save As dialog box does not appear after the file has been saved the first time.

To access the Save command:

1. **Click** the **Save** button 🖫 on the Quick Access toolbar. Alternatively, click the **Office** button and **select Save** from the **menu**.
2. If the file has not been saved before, the **Save As** dialog box appears. Name the file and select the location in which to save it. See **Figure 4-11**.

When the cursor is *hovered over* the **Save As** command 🖫 Save As ▸ , a menu appears asking you to choose the format in which to save the file. The file can be saved in the default format (Word 2007), as a template, in a Word 97-2003 format, or in another format such as a PDF (if the free Microsoft plug-in has been obtained). Other choices are also available. Once the choice of format is made (click it), the **Save As** dialog box appears (see Figure 4-11). This dialog box works like the Open dialog box. Select the location from the **Favorite Links** section or **Save in** column, then either choose an appropriate folder or choose **Create New Folder** 🗀 if desired; name the new folder and then type the file name in the **File name** text box and click **Save**. Although you have the option to place the file on the storage device without placing it in a folder, this is not a good practice.

When the Save As command is *clicked*, a dialog box appears, bypassing the format type menu. From that dialog box, you choose the format in which to save the file, the location for the file, and the file name.

Use the Save As command to change the name or location of a document or to save a copy of the revised document while keeping the original document as is. To use the keyboard to save a file, press **Ctrl+S** or the **Save** function key.

The computer can be set to automatically save information every 1 to 120 minutes; this information can then be recovered if a power failure or other problem with the computer occurs. To set the automatic save feature:

1. **Click Word Options** on the Office Button menu.
2. Choose **Save**.

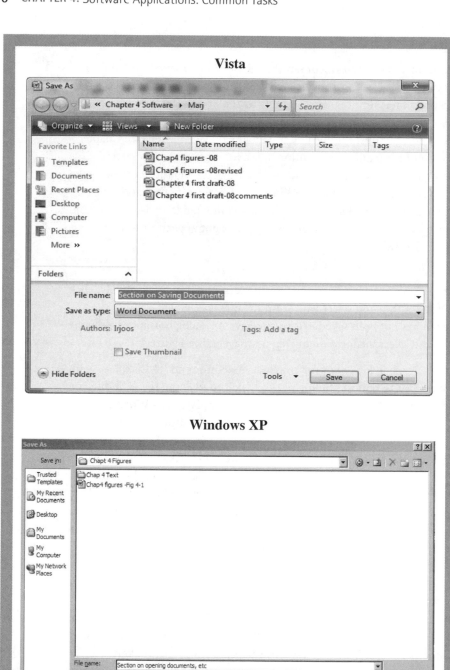

Figure 4-11 Save As Dialog Boxes for Vista and Windows XP

3. **Place** a **check** in the square to the left of **Save AutoRecover information every** and then set the time to 10 minutes or whatever time is appropriate (**Figure 4-12**). The default location for saving files can be noted here or changed as desired. Note that automatic recovery should not be used as a replacement for saving your document (**Ctrl+S**) on a regular basis (every 10 minutes or so). On public computers, you will not be able to alter the recovery time settings.

Printing Files

To print a file:

1. **Click** the **Office** button. Hold the arrow over **Print** 🖨 Print ›, and a list of Print choices appears.
2. **Click** the **Print option** desired. The Print dialog box appears, as shown in **Figure 4-13**.
3. Choices available in the Print dialog box include changing the printer; choosing the number of copies to print; printing the total document, the current page, the selection, or selected pages; or collating multiple-page documents. Adjust the options as needed.
4. **Click OK.**

Two other options for printing documents are Quick Print and Print Preview. Quick Print skips the dialog box and prints the document directly. Print Preview shows the document as it will look when printed. In addition, pressing **Ctrl+P** or clicking the printer icon 🖨 on the Quick Access Toolbar (if present) will open the Print dialog box. Some keyboards have a Print function key located on the F12 key as well.

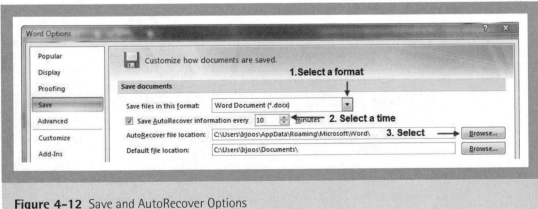

Figure 4-12 Save and AutoRecover Options

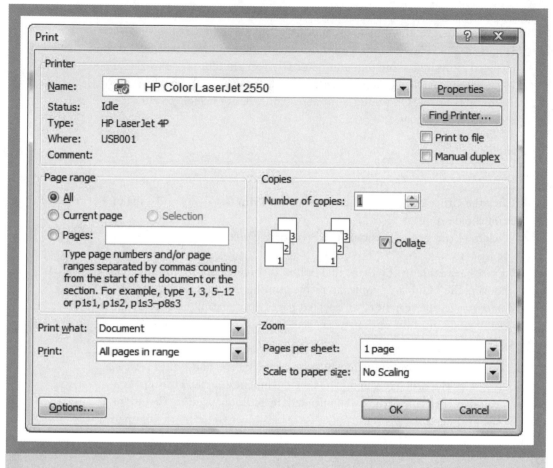

Figure 4-13 Print Dialog Box

Finding Files or Words

Another common task performed in many applications is to find, or find and replace, specific files or words within a folder or document. Suppose it is necessary to use a document that was previously created and now must be altered to fit the current situation. Or perhaps a file or email must be forwarded to someone else. Instead of manually searching for these files or replacing these words, let the computer do it.

To access this feature:

1. In some applications, you can select **Edit, Find or Replace**.
2. In Office 2007, select the **Home** tab, and choose **Find** or **Replace** from the Editing group.

Figure 4-14 shows the Find and Replace dialog boxes that will appear in Vista and Windows XP.

Once the dialog box is open, to find a word:

1. **Type** the word in the **Find what** text box and click **Find Next**. This choice will find the next occurrence of the word and highlight it.
2. Continue clicking **Find Next** until all instances of the word or file are found.

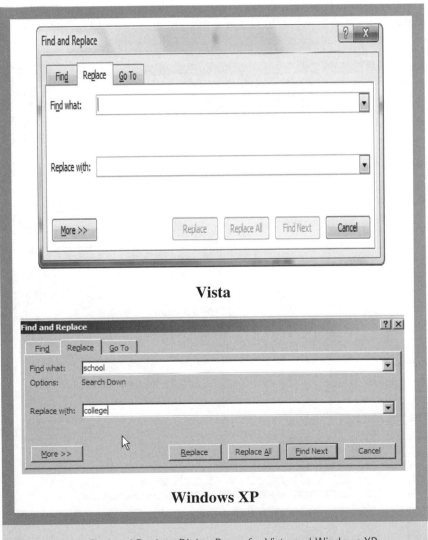

Figure 4-14 Find and Replace Dialog Boxes for Vista and Windows XP

To find and replace text using the Find and Replace dialog box:

1. Click the **Replace** command in the Editing group. If already in the dialog box, click the **Replace** tab.
2. **Type** the text or word in the **Find what** text box.
3. Click the **Replace with** text box.
4. Type the replacement text or word, and then **click Find Next**.
5. **Continue clicking Find Next** until all of the instances of the word are either left alone or replaced.

Figure 4-15 shows the options available when **More** ⟨More >>⟩ is clicked and **Match case** is also selected. In this example, the word to find is "school", and

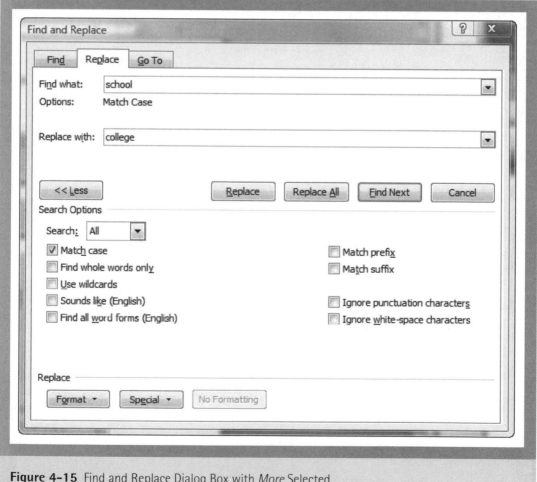

Figure 4-15 Find and Replace Dialog Box with *More* Selected

the replacement word is "college". Be careful when using the Replace All button. This button results in the program automatically finding all incidents of the text "school" and replacing it with "college": It also means that "schoolbook" will be replaced with "collegebook". The find feature is not case sensitive, although the option to match case was selected here.

Selecting Text or Objects

Selecting text or an object means to highlight the text or object, such as a word or a cell in a worksheet. This task is often necessary when editing documents. Although the Delete and Backspace keys are acceptable for completing minor editing tasks, using these keys is not efficient when you are editing or copying whole lines, sentences, paragraphs, columns, rows, cells, or the entire document. The selection feature is also used when you are formatting documents (word processing, spreadsheets, and so forth). Although each item can certainly be formatted separately, this technique is very time-consuming.

Each application has some minor variations in how you select or highlight text and cells. Described here are some of the most common techniques for selecting items. Additional methods are presented in each application chapter as appropriate.

Select	Mouse Action
A word	**Double-click** the word.
Several words	**Click** and **drag** the mouse over the words. Or select the **first** word, hold down the **Shift** key, and click the **last** word.
A sentence	**Hold down** the **Ctrl** key and click on the **sentence**.
A line	**Click** in the **Quick Select area** (the cursor turns into a right-slanted arrow when placed in the margin on the left side of the line).
Entire document	**Triple-click** the Quick Select area. Press **Ctrl+A**.
A cell	**Click** the **cell**.
Multiple cells	**Drag over** the cells.

In addition to working with the mouse, the keyboard can be used to select text. This technique is especially helpful when the item that must be selected spans greater distances or is located on the edge of the document. For example, to select text that spans several pages, place the cursor at the beginning of the text to be selected, hold down the Shift key, and use the arrow keys to move down the document. As the cursor is moved, all of the text will be highlighted. This technique also works in worksheets to select multiple cells.

If the entire document must be selected, press **Ctrl+A**. The entire document is now selected. You can also use the **Editing** group on the **Home** tab to select text. Click **Select** and these options appear:

Editing Text

Three basic editing features are used in applications: inserting, deleting, and replacing items.

Insert means to add new text, slides, rows, columns, and so forth. In word processing programs, the insert mode is the default. When you start typing, the characters are placed at the insertion point. In applications for spreadsheets and graphics, commands must be used to insert rows, columns, or new slides. These commands are covered in each application chapter of this book.

Delete means to remove some text, row, column, or slide from the document. Select what must be deleted and press the **Delete** key. If a mistake is made, go to the Quick Access toolbar and click the **Undo** button. In some applications, you would go to the **Edit** menu and choose **Undo Typing** to reverse the last action. If the Undo button was clicked in error, click the **Redo** button (or select **Repeat Typing**). Additional features available for deleting are covered later in the appropriate application chapters. Be aware that the Delete key and the Backspace key both delete text, but have an important difference: the Delete key deletes text to the **right** of the insertion point, whereas the Backspace key deletes text to the **left** of the insertion point.

Replace means to substitute one thing for another. In most cases, it is not necessary to first delete the text and then type the new text in its place. Instead, highlighting or selecting the text puts the application into the replace mode. Typing the replacement will then automatically delete what was highlighted. Thus it is not necessary to delete the text before typing.

Copying or Moving Text

The last of the common tasks presented in this chapter deals with copying or moving text from one place to another in the same document, from one document to another, or from one application to another. The most common method for carrying out this task is to use the cut/copy/paste commands. These commands rely on the concept of a clipboard that serves as a temporary holding place for the cut or copied material. In Excel, PowerPoint, and Word, the tools for cutting and copying can be found in the same place on the ribbon—under the Office button on the far left of the Home tab.

Another method for copying and moving text is the drag and drop method. In this method, you select the desired text and use the mouse to drag it to the new spot.

Which technique is best? The general rule for selecting a copying/moving method is based on how far you want to move or copy the material and how many times you want to paste the item. For short distances in the same document, use drag and drop. To copy or move data over longer distances (to another page, to another document, or to another application), use the clipboard strategy. To paste items multiple times, use the clipboard.

The Format Painter 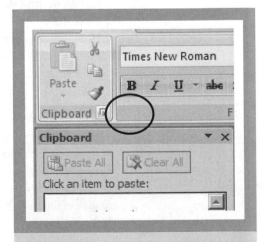 is used to copy formatting from one place to another.

Cut/Copy/Paste With The Clipboard

To copy data using the clipboard:

1. **Select** the **data** to be copied.
2. **Click** the **Copy** button .
3. **Place** the **insertion point** (cursor) where the data are to be copied.
4. **Click** the **Paste** button .

To move data using the clipboard:

1. **Select** the **data** to be moved.
2. **Click** the **Cut** button .
3. **Place** the **insertion point** where the data are to be moved.
4. **Click** the **Paste** button .

It is important to know where the insertion point is located because that is where the Paste command will place the data. The mouse pointer (I-beam) does not reflect where the data will go. If data are to be moved to another document or application, either use the Office button and then the file name to access the other document in the application or click the application button from the Start menu to get to the other application (refer to Chapter 3 if you are unsure about how to do this).

To collect items in the Office clipboard, the Office clipboard must be displayed.

To display the Office Clipboard task pane:

1. **Click** the **Dialog Launcher** in the Clipboard group.
2. The Clipboard task pane appears, as shown in **Figure 4-16**. Items that are cut or copied will appear there.

Multiple data may be placed on the Office clipboard at one time and may be used in any other documents. The Clipboard task pane will show how many items are

Figure 4–16 Clipboard Dialog Launcher and Task Pane

on the clipboard, with the last item copied appearing at the top of the list. You have the choice of pasting one or more of these items into a new document or clearing the clipboard. The clipboard can hold 24 items at one time. When the 25th item is added, the first one added to the clipboard is deleted. The last item added to the Office clipboard is also sent to the system clipboard.

To paste the contents of the Office clipboard into a new document:

1. **Open** a new document.
2. Display the **Office Clipboard** task pane.
3. **Click** the **items** to add to the new document. A new document can be created from multiple items on the Office clipboard. When using the paste function, the system clipboard is used, not the Office clipboard.

Data stay in the Office clipboard until the user exits Microsoft Office or clicks the Clear All button ⬚ Clear All in the Clipboard task pane. When the Office clipboard is cleared, the system clipboard is simultaneously cleared as well. If you have stored a large amount of data on the clipboard, you will be asked if you want those data to be available for another application when you quit Word.

Drag and Drop

The Cut/Copy/Paste commands can also be accessed through the keyboard. After selecting the text, press **Ctrl+X** for cut or **Ctrl+C** for copy; press **Ctrl+V** to paste the text in a new location. On some keyboards the X, C, and V keys are labeled as "Cut," "Copy," and "Paste."

To move data using the drag and drop method:

1. **Highlight** the **data** to be moved.
2. **Place** the **pointer** on the selected area.
3. **Hold down** the **left mouse** button.
4. **Move** the mouse so that the insertion point (broken vertical bar) is in the place where the text should be moved.
5. **Release** the mouse button.

Notice how the look of the mouse pointer changes when you use the drag and drop technique. The mouse pointer turns into a left-slanted arrow with a box below it, and the insertion point turns into a broken vertical bar.

Move is the default option for the drag and drop method when editing text. Do not confuse this technique with the drag and drop method of moving files, where the default option depends on the storage device.

To copy data using the drag and drop method:

1. **Select** the **data** to be moved.
2. **Place** the **pointer** on the selected area.
3. **Hold down** the **Ctrl** key.

4. **Hold down** the **left mouse** button.

5. **Move** the mouse so that the insertion point (broken vertical bar) is in the place where the text should be copied.

6. **Release** the mouse button and then the **Ctrl** key.

It is important not to release the Ctrl key until after you release the mouse button or else the selected data will be moved, not copied. When you are copying text, the pointer has the same appearance as when you are cutting text, except that a plus sign appears in the box below the pointer.

Keyboard Shortcuts

Some keyboard shortcuts were introduced in earlier parts of this chapter. **Table 4-1** lists the shortcut keys commonly found in Office 2007; they will work in most Office applications.

TABLE 4-1   SHORTCUT KEYS FOR OFFICE 2007

Command	Shortcut
Select All	Ctrl+A
Bold	Ctrl+B
Copy	Ctrl+C
Delete	Ctrl+D
Center	Ctrl+E
Find	Ctrl+F
Go To	Ctrl+G
Replace	Ctrl+H
Italics	Ctrl+I
Justify (Full Justify)	Ctrl+J
Insert Hyperlink	Ctrl+K
Left Align (Left Justify)	Ctrl+L
Indent	Ctrl+M

(continues)

TABLE 4-1   SHORTCUT KEYS FOR OFFICE 2007 *(continued)*

Command	Shortcut
New Page	Ctrl+N
Open a Document	Ctrl+O
Print	Ctrl+P
Right Align (Right Justify)	Ctrl+R
Save	Ctrl+S
Tab	Ctrl+T
Underline—Underscore	Ctrl+U
Paste (Velcro)	Ctrl+V
"Do You Want to Save Changes?"	Ctrl+W
Cut	Ctrl+X
Redo	Ctrl+Y
Undo	Ctrl+Z

Summary

This chapter presented some standard commands that are used in applications in the Windows Vista/Windows XP/Office 2007 environment. It described the online help provided in applications. Common tab and group commands for performing such tasks as creating, opening, closing, saving, finding, and printing files were introduced as well. In addition, the cut/copy/paste and drag and drop functions, which allow users to move or copy data from one file to another in the same or different applications, were presented. These commands and tasks cross applications and provide some consistency when working with the various Windows applications.

EXERCISE 1 Using Online Help in an Application

■ **Objectives**

1. Use the various forms of Help available in application programs.
2. Navigate through the Help screens.
3. Compare different ways of using online Help.

■ **Activity**

1. Find help in Microsoft Office Word 2007.
   a. Start **Word**.
   b. **Click** the **Help** button 🔘 on the tabs bar on the far right. The Word Help window appears.
   c. **Click Creating specific documents** under Browse Word Help.
   d. Look for the option **Set up a document; click** it.
   e. Read the beginning paragraphs and list under "What do you want to do?"
   f. **Click** the **Home** button 🏠 on the toolbar. The original window appears.
   g. **Type open document** in the Search text box.
   h. **Click Search** 🔍 Search ▾. A list of topics appears.
   i. **Click Open a file.** The Help screen opens.
   j. Move down to **Open a file** and click it. Review the information if necessary.
   k. **Click** the **Home** button 🏠 on the toolbar.
   l. **Click** the **arrow** ▾ in the Search box. Review the list of past searches there.
   m. Close the **Help** screen.
   n. Did you prefer looking at a list of topics or did you prefer using the search bar for the information needed? Why?
2. Find help in Excel 2007.
   a. Start **Excel**.
   b. **Click** the **Help** button 🔘 on the far right of the tabs bar.
   c. **Click** the **Table of Contents** button 🔖 on the toolbar. A table of contents appears. Note that if the book icon is open the table of contents pane should already be present on the left side of the screen.
   d. **Click What's New** 📖 What's new in the Table of Contents task pane. More options appear.
   e. **Click Use the Ribbon** in the options that appear in the Table of Contents task pane.
   f. Review the Ribbon help screen.
   g. Close the Table of Contents task pane by **clicking** ✖ in the Table of Contents task pane. Leave the help screen open.

h. **Type create a workbook** in the Search text box and click the **Search** button.

i. **Click** <kbd>Get to know Excel 2007: Create your first workbook Training</kbd> . Make sure there is an active Internet connection. A video starts once you are connected to Microsoft's Web site.

j. Listen to the Introduction.

k. **Click** 📋 **Quick Reference Card** on the list on the left side of the screen displaying the video.

l. Review the Information. **Click** the **Close** button 🗙 .

m. Close the Overview-Training window by clicking the **Close** button 🗙 .

n. Close the **Help screen** window and then close **Excel**.

o. What were the similarities between this Help command and the one from Activity 1 with Word?

3. Obtain additional help without using the Help button.

a. Open Word.

b. Place the mouse pointer over the **Line spacing** button 📑 in the **Paragraph** group in the **Home** tab. Do *not* click.

c. What happens after a few seconds?

d. What is this called? When would you use this feature?

4. Have more practice in finding additional help in Word.

a. Open Word if necessary.

b. **Click** the **Help** button ❓ on the far right of the tabs bar. Make sure there is an active Internet connection. The Help window appears.

c. **Type format a document** in the Search text box and **click Search**. Your results are displayed.

d. **Click** ❓ Insert the date and time a document was created, last printed, or last saved
   Help > Automation and programmability . The Help screen appears.

e. How would you insert a date and time?

f. Why might this information be helpful to know?

5. Use Office Online for Training (Figure 4-6a).

a. Make sure Word is open.

b. **Click** the **Table of Contents** button 📖 .

c. **Click Training** 📖 Training in the Table of Contents. You will need to scroll down to find it.

d. **Click Bullets, numbers and lists**.

e. **Click Create lists as you type** under Overview. You may need to click the + sign next to Simple Lists to see this option.

f. Listen to that section.

g. **Click** the **Quick Reference Card** on the left task pane in the MS Office Online Help window.

h. Review the contents.

i. **Close** all open windows.

EXERCISE 2 Common Tasks: Create, Open, Close, Find, Print, Save

■ Objectives

1. Create a new document using the Office button, New option or the New button on the Quick Access toolbar.
2. Use the commands from the Office button menu and the Quick Access toolbar to open, close, print, and save a file.
3. Use the Find and Replace command to replace text and the Find command to locate a file.

■ Activity

1. Start an application.
   a. **Click Start, All Programs, Microsoft Office**, and **Microsoft Office Word 2007**. Other methods may be used to start Word. Use the technique that is appropriate for the computer being used.
   b. Type **I'm learning how to create a new word processing document using Word 2007.**
   c. **Click** the **Office** button .
   d. **Click** the **Save** command button .
   e. Select **Documents** (Vista), **My Documents** (XP), or whatever folder and storage device are used for this class. (This could be a folder created in Chapter 3 with the name of your course.)
   f. In the File name text box, type **Learning Word**.
   g. **Click Save**.
2. Open and save another document.
   a. **Click** the **New** button in the Quick Access toolbar. (If the button is not there, **click** the **Office** button, **right-click New,** and then choose **Add to Quick Access Toolbar**.)
   b. Type **I'm creating this second document to tell you about why I entered the healthcare field.**
   c. **Press Ctrl+S.**
   d. Select the appropriate folder and storage device as directed by the professor.
   e. In the File name text box, type **Choosing a Healthcare Profession.**
   f. **Click Save** or **press Enter.**
3. Open, edit, and save an existing document.
   a. **Click** the **Office** button.
   b. **Click Learning Word** under Recent Documents. (If this file is not visible, make sure that the correct storage device and folder are selected.)
   c. Edit the document by adding a sentence or two stating what you want to learn about Word.

    d. **Click Save** under the **Office** button or **press Ctrl+S**. Notice the Save As dialog box did not appear because the file already has a name and location. The file was just updated.

    e. The file remains open.

4. Print the document.

    a. **Click** the **Office** button and move the cursor to **Print**. What are your choices?

    b. **Select Quick Print** from the menu.

    c. What happened?

5. Open and edit the second document.

    a. **Click** the **Office** button.

    b. **Click Choosing a Healthcare Profession** under Recent Documents. (If this file is not visible, make sure the correct storage device and folder are selected.)

    c. **Click** the **Office** button, and point to **Save As** 🔳 Save As ▸. The file format type menu appears.

    d. **Click Word Document**. The Save As dialog box appears.

    e. **Type Nursing** or your healthcare major in the File name text box and **press Enter** or click **Save**. The file now has a new name.

6. Find and replace text.

    a. Make sure the **Choosing a Healthcare Profession** file is open.

    b. **Click Replace** 🔍 Find ▾ / Replace in the **Editing** group on the **Home** tab.

    c. **Type** the words **healthcare field** in the Find what text box.

    d. Tab to the **Replace with** box.

    e. **Type** the lowercase word **nursing** or your **healthcare major** in the Replace with text box.

    f. **Click Find next** in the dialog box.

    g. **Click Replace.** (Be very careful when using Replace All. Undesired things can happen to the document.) A Word message appears stating that Word has finished searching the document.

    h. **Click OK** and then click **Close** ✕ in the dialog box.

    i. Notice what happened to the Word document.

    j. **Click Save** to save the file.

7. To close a document.

    a. **Click** the **Office** button, then **click Close** 📁 Close or **click** the **Close** button ✖ at the top of the window to close the document. You will also exit Word if this is the only Word document that is open.

8. Find a file using the Windows search feature.[1]

---

[1]A version of this activity for Windows XP is available on the textbook Web site.

■ **On the Hard Drive**
   a. **Click** the **Start** button. The Start menu opens.
   b. **Type Learning Word** in the Search text box. As you type, files appear above the Search text box.
   c. **Click** the **Learning Word** document. The document opens provided it was stored on the hard drive during Activity 1e.

■ **On a Removable Storage Device**
   a. **Double click Computer**, which should be located on the desktop or from the Start button, Computer option.
   b. **Click** the **removable storage device** where you are storing your files.
   c. **Type Learning Word** in the Search text box. A screen like that shown in **Figure 4-17** appears.
   d. **Click** the **Date modified down arrow** key on the contextual toolbar and select today's date. Note the other options available.
   e. **Double-click** the **Learning Word** document. The document opens provided it was stored on the removable storage devices during Activity 1e.
   f. Close all open windows.

EXERCISE 3 Copy and Move Data Using Cut/Copy/Paste and Drag and Drop

■ **Objectives**
1. Copy and move text from one place in the document to another using the clipboard.
2. Copy and move text from one place in the document to another using drag and drop.
3. Copy text from one document to another.

■ **Activity**
1. Start the program and enter data or retrieve a data file.
   a. Start Microsoft Office Word 2007. Select **Start**, **Programs**, **Microsoft Office**, and then **Microsoft Office Word**. Use the default Word setting for font (Calibri, 11 points).
   b. *If you are not using the copy-move file from the textbook Web site use the following to create your document:*
      If using the Copy-Move file, go to 1e. Type **Understanding how to copy and move data is an important skill that can save the user time**.
   c. **Press** the **Enter** key twice.
   d. **Type** the following text, pressing the **Tab** key between items and the **Enter** key at the end of the row.

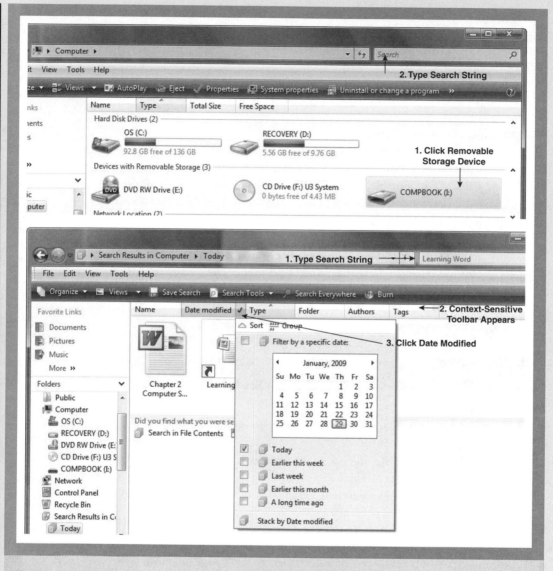

Figure 4-17 Windows Search Screen for a Removable Storage Device

Below is a list of physicians and their associated specialty. Please use the beeper number to access these physicians during off-hours.

Dr. M. Smith	Orthopedics	*4567	Monday/Wednesday/Friday
Dr. K. Bones	Orthopedics	*4512	Tuesday/Thursday/Saturday
Dr. P. Roberts	Oncology	*5678	Sunday
Dr. Z. White	Internal Med	*3489	All week

e. If you created the file, **click** the **Save** icon 💾 and name the file **Practice-CMwith Drag** or if you opened the Copy-Move file from the textbook Web site, rename the file Practice-CMwithDrag using the **Save As** command.

2. Move text using drag and drop.

   a. **Select** the **Dr. Smith** line. (The quickest way to do this is to place the pointer in the Quick Select area. Place the pointer out at the margin across from Dr. M. Smith; when the pointer is a right-slanted arrow, **click**.)

   b. **Place** the pointer on the **highlighted** area. Hold down the left mouse button, and drag the selection to the blank line below the "D" in "Dr. Z. White." Release the mouse button. If the Enter key was not pressed after the last line, you will not be able to go to the line below "Dr. White." Go to the right of "k" in "week" and place text there. **Click** to the left of the "D" in "Dr. M. Smith," and press **Enter**.

   c. "Dr. M. Smith" is now at the end of the list.

3. Move text using the clipboard.

   a. **Select** the **second line** of text in the list. It begins with Dr. P. Roberts.

   b. **Click** the **Cut** button ✂.

   c. **Click** to the left of "Dr. M. Smith" so the blinking vertical line is to the left of the "D". Do not select the entire line.

   d. With the insertion point to the left of the "D" in "Dr. M. Smith," **click** the **Paste** button 📋. The list should now look like the one shown in **Figure 4-18**.

4. Copy text using drag and drop.

   a. Go to the **end** of the document.

   b. **Press** the **Enter** key twice to create two blank lines.

   c. **Type** the following information, remembering to use the Tab key between items and the Enter key to go to the next line.

Chris Walker	**Nursing Assistant**
Mary Robb	**Registered Nurse**
Lee Dock	**Nurse Practitioner**

   d. **Click** the **Save** button 💾.

Dr. K. Bones	Orthopedics	*4512	Tuesday/Thursday/Saturday
Dr. Z. White	Internal Med	*3489	All week
Dr. P. Roberts	Oncology	*5678	Sunday
Dr. M. Smith	Orthopedics	*4567	Monday/Wednesday/Friday

Figure 4-18 Results of Moving Text with Drag and Drop

    e. **Select** the first line of text in this list ("Chris Walker" through "Assistant").

    f. **Place** the pointer over the selected text.

    g. **Hold down** the **Ctrl** key and the **left mouse button**, and drag the text so that the broken vertical bar is to the left of "Mary."

    h. **Release** the **mouse button** and then the **Ctrl** key. The text is copied.

    i. **Highlight Chris** in the second row, and type **Brian**.

5. Copy text using the clipboard.

    a. **Select** the text from "Mary Robb" through "Registered Nurse."

    b. **Click** the **Copy** button.

    c. Move the pointer to the left of the "L" in "Lee Dock" and click. Do not highlight the text.

    d. **Click** the **Paste** button.

    e. **Highlight** the second **Mary** and type **Nancy**.

    f. **Click** the **Save** button to save the document.

6. Copy text from one document to another.

    a. **Select** all the **text** from "Chris" through "Practitioner."

    b. **Click** the **Copy** button.

    c. **Click** the **New Document** button on the Quick Access toolbar or the Office button menu.

    d. **Click** the **Paste** button. The text is now inserted into a new Word document.

    e. Save the document as **Practice-CMwithClipboard2**.

7. Copy text from one application to another.

    a. **Click Start**, **All Programs**, **Microsoft Office**, **Excel** (or use one of the shortcut techniques to open Excel).

    b. **Click** the **Paste** button. The contents of the clipboard are now inserted into an Excel worksheet. Columns will need to be enlarged to see all the data. Names should be in column A and Job title in column B unless you added two tabs between items forcing the Job title to column C. More on tabs and their settings in the Word chapter.

8. Close all files and programs. There is no need to save anything again unless requested to do so by your professor.

ASSIGNMENT 1 Using Help

■ **Directions**

1. Use the Excel online Help feature to learn about "What's new" in Excel. Click "Use the ribbon" and review the material. Review any other feature you are interested in.

2. Print one or two appropriate Help screens for future reference.

3. Using Word, Excel, or PowerPoint, find out how to insert a SmartArt diagram in a Word document, Excel spreadsheet, or PowerPoint presentation. Use the online Help feature to learn how to complete this task in each application.
4. Open WordPad (Start, All Programs, Accessories, and WordPad). Copy and paste the directions for inserting SmartArt from the Help screen into the WordPad document. Make a note regarding the source of this material. Save the document as Insert SmartArt.
5. Submit the prints from Steps 2 and 4.

ASSIGNMENT 2 Copy and Move Text

■ **Directions**
1. Create a one-page document describing how to perform the following tasks. Each description should take the form of its own paragraph. Place your name on the document.
   Save a document.
   Print a document.
   Create a new document.
   Move text in a document.
2. Print the original **document** and save it as **Assign-CM-Yourlastname**.
3. Using the "move text" feature of the program, rearrange the text as follows:
   Create a new document.
   Move text in a document.
   Save a document.
   Print a document.
4. Save the **document** as **Assign-CMRev-Yourlastname**. Print the revised document. Submit both documents in either print or electronic form.

Introduction to Word Processing

Objectives

1. Define common terms related to word processing.
2. Create, format, edit, save, and print Microsoft Word documents.

Word processing applications are used to create text—letters, memos, reports, proposals, newsletters, and even books! They make any job easier once a few of the possibilities are revealed. This chapter provides the basics of word processing using Microsoft Word 2007.

Common Terms in Word Processing and Office Applications

Block   A block is a selected (highlighted) section of text that is treated as a unit. Most individual formatting functions, such as bold and underline, can be applied to blocks of text, thereby making formatting and editing functions much more efficient.

Clipboard   A clipboard is a holding area or buffer for copied or cut data for later use. You can place data onto a clipboard and can then paste it into another document, another application, or another location within the original document. In the 2007 version of Office, the Office Clipboard can hold as many as 24 items at a time (see Chapter 4 for details).

Font	A font defines a descriptive look or shape (font face or typeface), size, style, and weight of a group of characters or symbols. For example, one font is Times Roman, 12 point, bold, italic. Another font is Calibri, 10 point, italic. The default font for Word 2007 is Calibri. Several other terms are important to understanding fonts:

Pitch	Number of characters printed in 1 inch (cpi).
Point size	Height of the font given in printing language, measured as 72 points per inch of height. The default point size in Word is 11 points.
Spacing	Proportional or fixed pitch. "Proportional" means a variable amount of space is allotted for each character depending on the character width. "Fixed space" or "monospace" means a set space is provided for each character regardless of the character width. For example, an "I" is allowed the same amount of space as a "W".
Style	The vertical slant of the character—normal (upright), condensed, or italic (oblique). Many word processing programs also include bold and other effects.
Symbol set	The characters and symbols that make up the font.
Typeface	The specific design of a character or symbol, commonly referred to as the font face. For example, Helvetica, Courier, Times Roman, Times Roman Bold, and Times Roman Italic are all different typefaces.

Footer	The footer is an information area that is placed consistently at the bottom of each page of a document. It can hold the name of the document, the page number, the date, or any information that is helpful.
Format	Formatting is the process of editing the appearance of a document by using indentations, margins, tabs, justification, and pagination; format conditions affect the document appearance. In Word, format features vary depending on whether you are formatting characters (font, size, emphasis, and special effects such as highlight or superscript/subscript), paragraphs (alignment, indentation, line spacing, and line breaks), or pages (margins, paper size, and orientation).
Grammar Checker	A grammar checker (an add-in that often comes with word processing programs) provides feedback to the user about errors in grammar. For example, using "there" when "their" is appropriate

or using subjects and verbs that do not agree will cause a wavy green line to appear under the offending sentence or phrase. Within the grammar checker, several settings and styles can be selected. In Word 2007, spelling and grammar appear together under the Review tab. This feature shows the errors as the user types; it is turned on by choosing **Office Button**, **Word Options**, **Proofing**, and **Mark grammar errors as you type**.

Hard Return The hard return is a code inserted in the document by pressing the Enter key. It is usually placed at the end of a paragraph. In Word, the paragraph mark is ¶. Users may toggle the paragraph markers on to show marks in the document when typing or toggle them off by **clicking** the **paragraph button** ¶ in the Paragraph group of the Home tab or by **clicking** the **Office** button, choosing **Word Options**, **Display**, and placing a check in **Paragraph marks**.

Header The header is an information area that is placed consistently at the top of each page of a document. It can hold the name of the document, page number, date, or other identifying information.

Indent To "indent" text means to establish tab settings that place subsequent lines of text the same number of spaces from the margin until the next hard return.

Insert To "insert" means to add characters in the text at the point of the cursor, thereby moving all other text to the right. Insert mode is the opposite of overtype mode and is the default in most word processing programs. In Office 2007, the Insert tab is next to the Home tab on the ribbon and is used to insert pages, illustrations, links, and so forth.

Justified Justified text is aligned relative to the left and right margins.

Center Centering places the text line equidistant from both margins.

Full Full justification is alignment of text flush against both the left and right margins.

Left Left justification is alignment of text flush against the left margin and staggered on the right.

Right Right justification is alignment of text flush against the right margin and staggered on the left.

Move Move is a function in word processing programs that permits the user to relocate text or graphics to another place in the document or to another document.

Outliner Outliner is a feature of many word processing programs that enables the user to plan and rearrange large documents in an outline form.

Overtype	Overtype means to replace the character under the cursor by the character typed. To turn it off, **click** the **Office** button, **click Word Options**, **click Advanced**, and then clear the **Use the Insert Key . . .** and **Use overtype mode** check boxes.
Page Break	A page break is the place where Word ends the text on one page before it continues text on the next page. Insert a page break by going to the **Insert** tab and selecting **Page Break** from the Pages Group or by pressing **Ctrl + Enter**. The software then places the break at the point where the cursor is located. It is a good idea to review the document when it is finished to determine where page breaks are needed. Use this feature cautiously until all revisions of the document have been completed. A page break can also be inserted from the Page Layout tab in Word: **Choose Page Layout** and then **click Breaks**. A list of choices appears. You may also select column, text wrapping around objects, and section breaks here.
Pagination	Pagination consists of the numbers or marks that are used to indicate the sequence of the pages. It is a process of determining when a sufficient amount of text appears on one page and then starting the next page. Word processing programs automatically perform pagination if this feature is turned on. Most programs permit the variation of placement and style of the page number. Add page numbers by going to the **Insert** tab and **choosing Page Number** from the Header and Footer Group. A list of options for page number placement appears. Select the option preferred.
ScreenTips	ScreenTips are small windows that display descriptive text when you rest the pointer on a command or control. Screen-Tips are enhanced in Office 2007 with larger windows and more text.
Scrolling	Scrolling is the process of moving around a document to view a specific portion of a page of text. (All of the document may not fit on the screen.) This navigation process does not change the location of the insertion point until the user clicks elsewhere in the document.
Section Breaks	Section breaks permit you to create layout or formatting changes in the document and apply them only to that section.
SmartArt	SmartArt is a new feature in Office 2007 that permits you to easily create a visual representation of your information.
Smart Tags	A Smart Tag is a popup that appears when you place the insertion point over certain text. Marks (purple dotted underlines)

appear when Word recognizes certain types of data and places a mark in the document.

When a Smart Tag appears, move the insertion point over the underlined text until the Smart Tag Actions button appears. Click the button to see the menu of actions that you can take. Data such as addresses, dates and times, names, and telephone numbers can have smart tags assigned . If Smart Tags don't display, **click** the **Office button**, **Word Options**, **Proofing**, **AutoCorrect Options** button, and then **Smart Tags** tabs. Adjust the settings as desired.

Soft Return A soft return is the code inserted in the document automatically when the typed line reaches the right margin.

Spell Checker Most programs come with an embedded spell checker, which is a program that checks words for correct spelling. Word combines the spelling and grammar checker. A wavy red line under a word means that it is misspelled or that it is not in Word's dictionary. If you right-click the mouse button, Word brings up a menu where you can choose the correct spelling if you so desire.

Tab A tab is a setting that places the subsequent text on that line a certain number of spaces or inches in from the left margin. Tab settings by default are five spaces (0.5 inch). These settings can be changed, however. Five styles of tabs are available—left, right, center, decimal, and bar. All deal with the alignment of the text around the tab mark.

Thesaurus A thesaurus is a built-in feature that helps you search for alternative words. In Word 2007, the Thesaurus appears in the Proofing Group under the Review tab.

Toggle Toggling switches from one mode of operation to another mode: on or off. For example, a user might toggle from insert mode to replace/overtype mode.

Word Wrap This feature automatically carries words over to the next line if they extend beyond the margin.

Data Exchange

Word processing software saves documents in file formats that are unique to that software program. Many word processing programs allow the option of saving documents under another file format by using the Save As feature. For example, a Microsoft Word 2007 document can be saved in several ways, such as in Word 2007, Word template, rich text, Word 97–2003, PDF, or XML. This feature permits you to exchange a file with others who are working with different word processing programs, versions, or systems. It also permits you to save a word processing file as a Web page. Other file formats are also available. Word 2007 files cannot be read by earlier versions of Word unless a viewer is downloaded from Microsoft. Word 2007 uses the .docx extension (not the .doc extension).

Saving Work

Every person probably has at least one horror story that he or she can tell about lost data or documents. To avoid accidental loss of data, follow these tips:

1. Periodically save your work. When typing a document, the computer holds that document temporarily in random access memory (RAM). Once the program is instructed to save the document on a storage device, the document exists both in RAM and on the storage device. If power is lost (even temporarily), all of the data in RAM are lost; conversely, data stored on the removable storage device, in temporary backup files, or on the hard disk are maintained.

2. Pay attention to warnings that the software gives. These warnings are hints to remind you that doing certain things will have a certain result. For example, saving a document with the same name as another one results in a message asking whether the file is to be replaced (**Figure 5-1**). Do not respond with "Replace existing file" unless you have no need for the original document.

3. Always keep a backup or duplicate copy of a document. That backup could consist of a CD, USB storage device, or another hard drive. Store the backup in a different place. If something happens to the original document or the computer, the backup copy will then be available for restoring the data. A particularly valuable document, such as a thesis or research paper, should have a backup that is kept in a different location from the primary

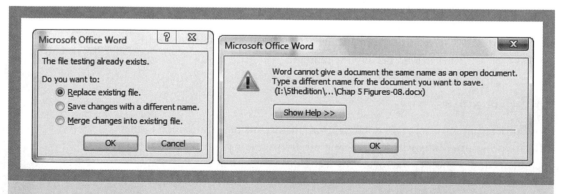

Figure 5-1 Warnings That a File Exists with the Same Name

document. Many options for automatic backup are available today from places like Mozy Home or Unlimited. If you select an online backup service, do your homework first.

Introduction to Microsoft Word 2007

Examples in this text use Microsoft Office Word 2007 for Windows Vista or Windows XP. Using Microsoft Office Word 2008 for the Macintosh, however, is essentially the same; the menu and toolbars include most of the same headings and icons. Therefore, both Macintosh and Windows users can use the chapters in this book on word processing, spreadsheets, and graphics presentation with very few changes between operating systems. Office 2008 for the Mac, however, continues to use the type of menu and toolbar system found in former editions of Office (File, Edit, View, Insert, Font, Tools, and so forth). See **Figure 5-2a**.

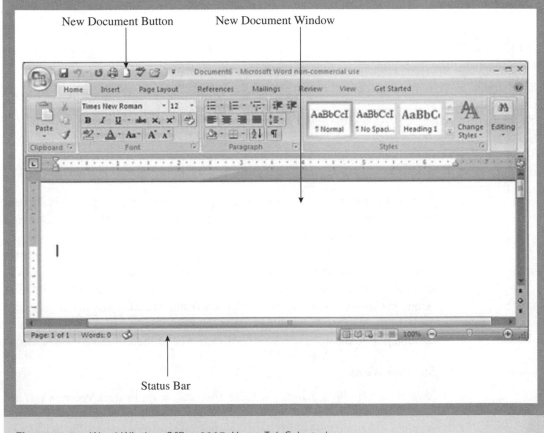

Figure 5-2a Word Window Office 2007, Home Tab Selected

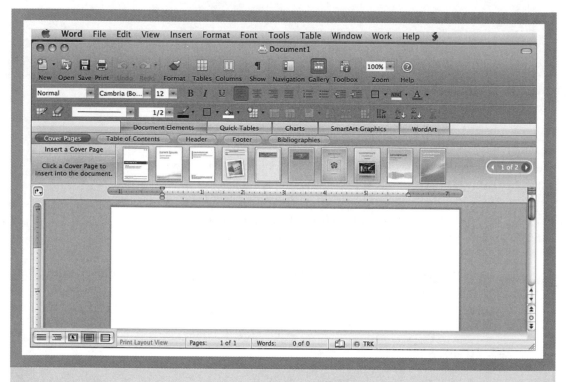

Figure 5-2b Word Window Office 2008 for the Mac, Cover Pages Selected

Ribbons, Menus, and Keyboard Commands

Most word processing programs are menu driven, meaning that you can carry out commands by selecting icons or choosing from a menu of options. Menu-driven programs provide you with two options—to select items from the ribbon (menus) and icons by using the mouse or to use keystroke combinations to issue the command. Some programs are faster when you issue commands through a series of keystroke combinations. Keystroke options were described for the Microsoft Office ribbon in Chapter 4. For example, **Ctrl + Enter** inserts a hard page break in a document. In the Macintosh operating system, the Apple key (or command key), which is found next to the space bar, acts like the Ctrl key on the Windows system.

Starting Word

As with all Windows programs, there are many ways to start Word; a few are presented here. Several ways of opening a new or existing Word document were also described in Chapter 4 (see the sections on creating, opening, closing, and saving files).

1. **Click Start**, **All Programs**. **Select Microsoft Office**, and then **choose MS Office Word** from the available options (Figure 4-7).
2. **Double-click** the **MS Office Word icon** if it appears on the Start button menu or on the desktop (Figure 4-8).
3. **Click** the **Word** 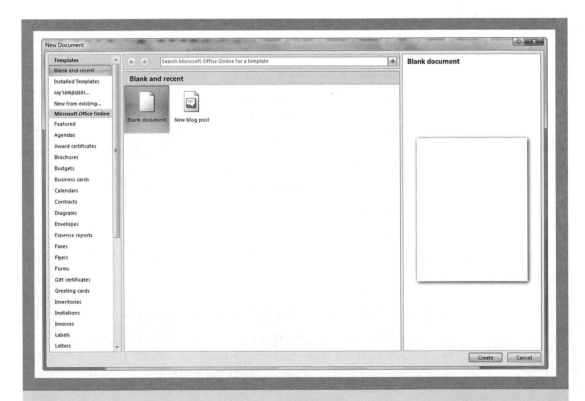 icon on the Quick Launch area of the taskbar if it appears there.

Creating a New Document

After starting Word, a new blank document is opened by default. At this point, you can simply type and format the text as desired.

Two methods to create a new document once the Word application is open are described here:

1. **Click** the **Office Button** and then **New**. A window appears (**Figure 5-3**). **Click Blank document**, and a new document appears that is formatted using the normal template. Note the choices available for a new document under Templates.

Figure 5-3 New Document Dialog Window

2. Add the New Document symbol to the Quick Access toolbar. **Click** the **Office** button, **choose Word Options, Customize, New, Add** Add >> , and **OK**. Now the New Document button ⬜ has been added to the toolbar. **Click** it and the new document window appears. See Figure 5-2a.

NOTE: You can also click the **Office** button, right-click **New** from the menu, and then select **Add to Quick Access Toolbar.**

For each document, Word presents a screen with the ribbon at the top, a blank window or workplace in the center, and scroll bars on the right side and bottom-right corner. A blinking vertical bar, or insertion point marker, represents the position of the cursor in the document. In Figure 5-2a, the cursor appears at the beginning of the document.

Opening a Previously Saved Document in Word

When changes or additions are necessary in a document, several options are available for opening the document again after it is saved (see Chapter 4 for additional ways to open existing documents).

If the application is not running:

1. Start **Word** and **click** the **Office** button. A list of Recent Documents appears on the right. **Click** the desired document.
2. Start **Word**, **click** the **Office** button, and **choose Open**. The Open dialog box appears (Figure 4-10) with a list of documents. Note that you can also choose Recently Changed; this choice brings up a complete list that includes the name of each document as well as its size, type, and date modified.

To open an existing document once the application is running:

1. **Click** the **Office** button. A list of Recent Documents appears.
2. If the file is not in the list of Recent Documents, **click** the **Open** button. The Open dialog box appears, allowing you to search for the needed file (Figure 4-10).

The Ribbon in Word: Microsoft's "Fluent User Interface"

The menu bar in any Office 2007 program for Windows (Excel, PowerPoint, Access, and so on) has been replaced by a ribbon, as described in Chapter 4. The ribbon comprises a series of task-oriented tabs and groups that are organized to keep like tasks together (Figure 4-3). Each tab contains a different group of commands or tasks that help you to use Word. No matter which tab is chosen, the Office button and Quick Access toolbar are always available.

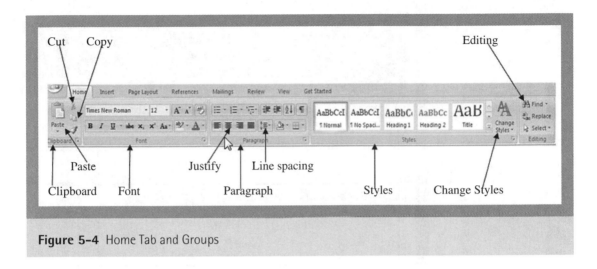

Figure 5-4 Home Tab and Groups

Following is a brief description of each tab and its groups in Word 2007.

Home   **Figure 5-4** shows the Home tab and its groups: Clipboard, Font, Paragraph, Styles, and Editing. These groups allow you to format the document by (1) cutting, copying, or pasting items to the clipboard; (2) selecting a font style, size, and color; (3) setting margins, indents, spacing, and text alignment; (4) adding bullets or numbers to a list; and (5) selecting a document style.

Insert   The Insert tab (**Figure 5-5a**) has groups such as Pages, Tables, Illustrations, Links, Header and Footer, Text, and Symbols. You

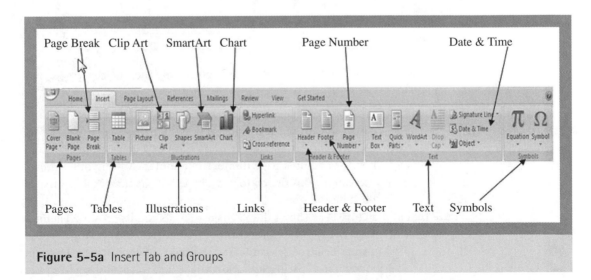

Figure 5-5a Insert Tab and Groups

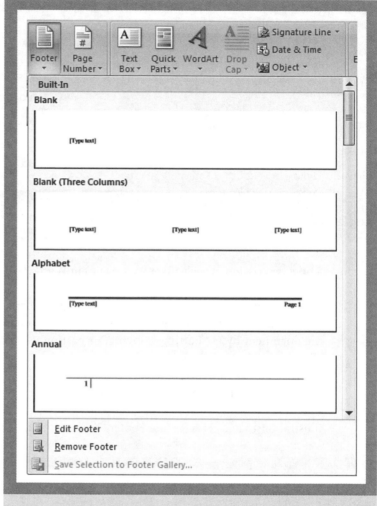

Figure 5–5b Dialog Box for Adding a Footer and Page Number

can add a cover page or insert a blank page, page break, table, chart, SmartArt, or clip art using this tab. **Figure 5-5b** shows the box for adding a page number in a footer. Among other things you can use this ribbon to add a hyperlink, bookmark, text box, or the date and time.

Page Layout **Figure 5-6a** shows the Page Layout tab and its groups: Themes, Page Setup, Page Background, Paragraph, and Arrange. These groups help you select the font style and color, margins, paragraph indents and spacing, and allow you to add watermarks, add a page

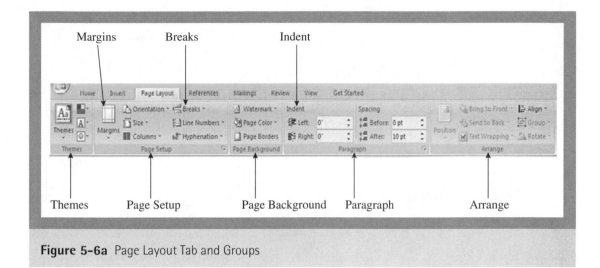

Figure 5-6a Page Layout Tab and Groups

border, or change the page color or arrangement. **Figure 5-6b** shows the Page Setup group when the document fills the screen (that is, when it is "maximized").

References   Groups found under the References tab (**Figure 5-7**) include Table of Contents, Footnotes, Citations and Bibliography, Captions, Index, and Table of Authorities (cases, statutes). These groups help you add endnotes, footnotes, citations, index, and tables, and then update these items as necessary. For example, you can cite a book or journal, insert the citation in the document, and choose the style for the source such as APA or MLA. In addition, a longer paper can be set up to automatically generate a table of contents.

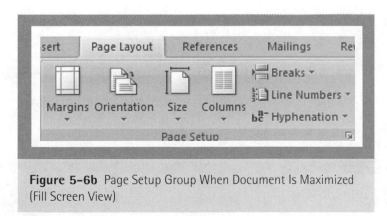

Figure 5-6b Page Setup Group When Document Is Maximized (Fill Screen View)

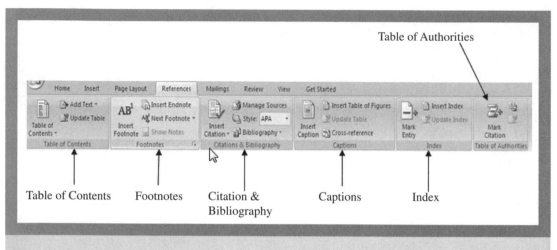

Figure 5-7 References Tab and Groups

Mailings   The Mailings groups (**Figure 5-8**) help you prepare envelopes, labels, mail merge letters, and recipient lists.

Review   You can use the Review groups for proofing a document; for example, these groups help you check spelling and grammar, do a word count, track changes, insert comments, enable ScreenTips for showing a word in another language, or protect a document

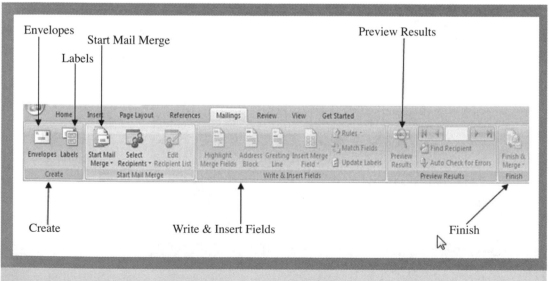

Figure 5-8 Mailings Tab and Groups

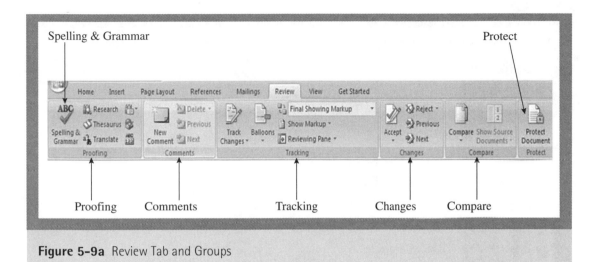

Figure 5-9a Review Tab and Groups

from changes by someone else (see **Figure 5-9a**). **Figure 5-9b** shows the Proofing group when the screen is maximized.

A readability index may also be used to test the readability level of the document. To set this option, **click** the **Microsoft Office** button; **click Word options, Proofing**; make sure there is a check next to **Check grammar with spelling**; and **click** in the square next to **Show readability statistics**. Now, when you check the spelling and grammar of the document, a readability index will also appear. This consideration is very important when developing patient educational materials. However, this approach is not effective for measuring the health literacy level needed to understand the document being reviewed. Health literacy is further explained in Chapter 14.

View   The View tab includes commands that allow you to view the document in print layout, full screen reading, Web layout, outline, or

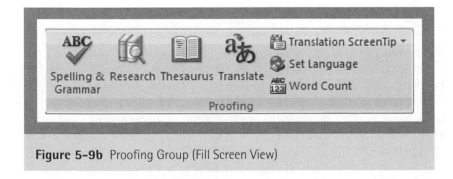

Figure 5-9b Proofing Group (Fill Screen View)

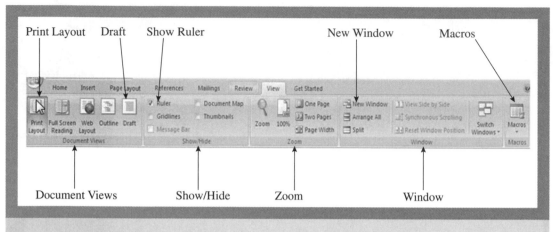

Figure 5-10 View Tab and Groups

draft form (**Figure 5-10**). The next group has commands to show or hide various items in Word, such as the ruler, gridlines, the message bar, the document map, and thumbnails. Zoom controls can be found in the Zoom group or on the status bar at the bottom of the window. Options also allow you to view one or two pages of the document. The next group focuses on the window and provides ways to view a document or to switch between windows. The last group is Macros; a macro is a sequence of operations that has been automated and can prove useful for repetitive tasks.

Get Started This group, which is found in the Home and Student versions of MS Office, helps the new user get started with Word 2007 (**Figure 5-11**). To access the training guides and videos, you must have access to the Internet.

Moving Around the Document

There are several ways to move around a document.

Arrow keys	Move the insertion point or cursor one line or letter at a time.
Ctrl + arrow keys	Move one word, section, or paragraph at a time.
Home key	Move the cursor to the beginning of the line.
End key	Move the cursor to the end of the line.
Ctrl + Home	Move the cursor to the beginning of the document.
Ctrl + End	Move the cursor to the end of the document.
Page Up and Page Down	Move the cursor quickly through the document one screen at a time.
Ctrl + Page Up	Move the cursor to the previous printed page.
Ctrl + Page Down	Move the cursor to the next printed page.

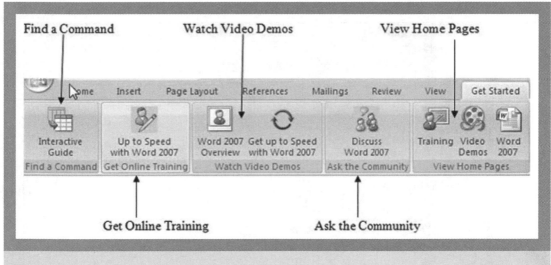

Figure 5-11 Get Started Tab and Groups

A scroll bar is located at the right side of the screen (Figure 5-2a). The View Ruler icon ⌨, which is located at the top of the right scroll bar, toggles the ruler bar off and on. Placing the mouse pointer in the open box in the scroll line ⬚ allows you to click or drag the box, thereby moving up or down the scroll line as quickly as desired. The single arrow in the scroll bar is used to move up ▲ or down ▼ one line at a time, but does not alter the location of the insertion point. The double arrows (chevrons) are used to move up ⯅ or down ⯆ a page. Clicking and dragging the dotted triangle on the lower-right corner ⋰ of the window (when it is doesn't fill the screen) allows you to change the dimensions of the window. If you click (and hold) on the top of the window, you can then move the window around the screen. When the window does not fill the screen, a horizontal scroll bar appears in the status bar.

NOTE: A scroll wheel on a mouse will also let you scroll through a document by moving the wheel back and forth.

Formatting the Document

Page Formatting

Described here are the options for changing page formats:

1. Open a new document and choose the **Page Layout** tab. **Click** the dialog launcher ⬓ at the lower-right corner of the Page Setup group; the Page Setup dialog box appears (**Figure 5-12**). Use it to adjust the document's margins and decide on paper orientation (portrait or landscape), paper size, and layout. Usually margins are set 1 inch at the top and bottom of the page and

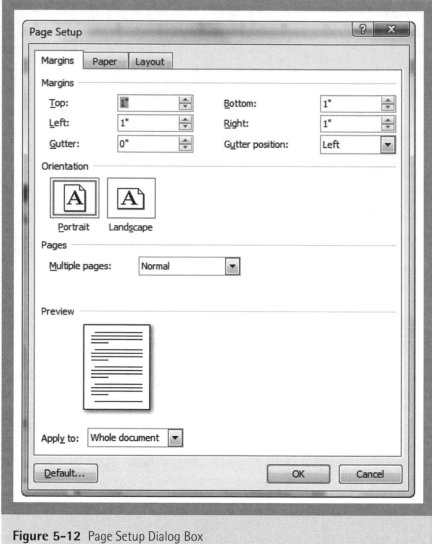

Figure 5-12 Page Setup Dialog Box

1.25 inches at the left and right sides of the page. Vertical centering of the text is also set in this dialog box; use this feature to center a title page.

2. Set a page break by pressing the **Ctrl + Enter** keys or by selecting the **Insert** tab and then **Page Break** from the **Pages** group (Figure 5-5a). If other page, section, or column breaks are needed, use the **Page Layout** tab and **click** the **Breaks** option in the **Page Setup** group.

3. Use the **Header & Footer** tool to have text appear on each page of the document.

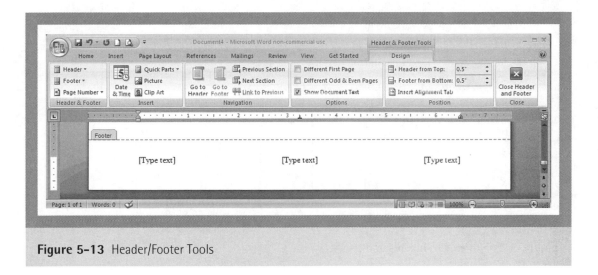

Figure 5-13 Header/Footer Tools

To add a header or footer to a document:

1. **Choose** the **Insert** tab and **select Header or Footer** from the **Header & Footer** group (Figure 5-5a).
2. Select either header or footer. See Figure 5-5b for choices for a footer.
3. Select one of the style options. **Figure 5-13** shows the document window that appears after the footer **Footer ▾** was selected. Note the addition on the ribbon of the Header/Footer Design tab.
4. Type the text wanted in the footer (or header) box by highlighting [**Type Text**]. The tab key moves the cursor from the left side to the middle of the page, and then to the right side. Choose the appropriate spot for inserting the name of the document, the date, or page number. You can also select options from the groups such as Page number, Date and Time, Options, or Position.
5. **Click** the **Close** button when finished (Figure 5-13).

Paragraph Formatting: Indents

Word has four indents: first line, left, right, and hanging (**Figure 5-14**). These indent markers are displayed on the ruler bar. Dragging the top indent marker to the right (first line indent) indents the first line of a paragraph; pressing the Tab key does the same thing. The middle marker is the left indent marker; use it to indent all lines of the paragraph except the first one. The top and middle markers will move together with the bottom marker when it is selected and moved. The middle marker is the hanging indent when it is placed to the right of the first line indent marker. To apply a hanging indent (to the right of the first line),

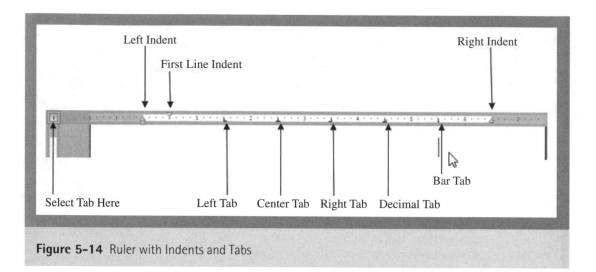

Figure 5-14 Ruler with Indents and Tabs

drag the middle marker ⌂ to the right of the first-line indent marker. A hanging indent will indent all lines of a paragraph except the first line.

To set the indents:

1. Place the insertion point at the beginning of the document, in the paragraph that will be indented. Alternatively, highlight multiple paragraphs.
2. Drag the appropriate marker to the chosen tick mark on the ruler bar. The indents may also be accessed under the **Page Layout** tab, **Paragraph** group or by clicking the dialog launcher ◰ in that group.

Paragraph Formatting: Tabs

Word sets tabs every 0.5 inch along the ruler, although they are not visible to you. It also offers five standard tab types (from left to right): left tab ⌞L⌟, center tab ⌞⊥⌟, decimal tab ⌞⊥⌟, right tab ⌞⌐⌟, and bar tab ⌞¡⌟ (Figure 5-14). The tabs can be placed and adjusted on the ruler using the mouse.

To set the tabs:

1. **Click** the **Left Corner Tab** button ⌞L⌟ on the ruler bar until the correct tab mark appears.
2. **Click** the ruler setting where the tab should be. (The ruler bar must be showing to use this option.) The tab settings may also be adjusted and additional features applied through the **Page Layout** tab by **selecting** the **Paragraph** group and then **Tabs** ⌞Tabs...⌟ at the bottom of the dialog box.

To remove a tab:

1. **Click** a tab and drag it off the ruler into the document.
2. To clear all the tab settings at once, use the **Tabs** dialog box that appears when you double-click a tab spot on the ruler.

Paragraph Formatting: Alignment, Numbering, Bullets, and Borders

The icons for justification, numbering, and adding bullets or borders are found under the Home tab in the Paragraph group. **Figure 5-15** shows the icons for text alignment or justification: left ≣ , centered ≣ , right ≣ , and full ≣ (both right and left, respectively). Above them are the icons for bulleted ⊟ ▾ or numbered ⊟ ▾ text or for a multilevel list ⊞ ▾ . Other icons relate to line spacing ⊟ ▾ , shading, borders (allows for a partial or complete border around selected text), indents, sorting, or showing/hiding paragraph marks.

Character Formatting: Font Size and Style

As in previous examples, you can choose the font size and style in several different ways.

1. **Click** the **Home** tab. Choose a font style and size from the **Font** group (**Figure 5-16**).
2. **Click** the dialog launcher ▫ in the **Font** group and the Font dialog box appears (**Figure 5-17**). You can select a font, font style, size, effects, color, and character spacing in this dialog box. You can also choose a font style and size that will then be used as the default style for all documents. By default,

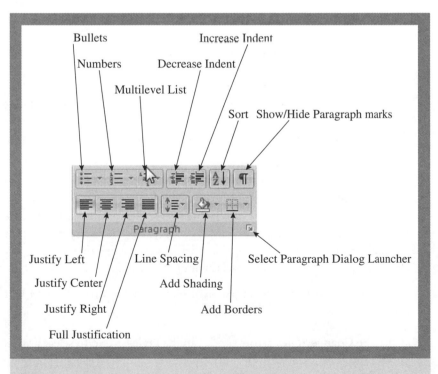

Figure 5-15 Paragraph Group in Home Tab

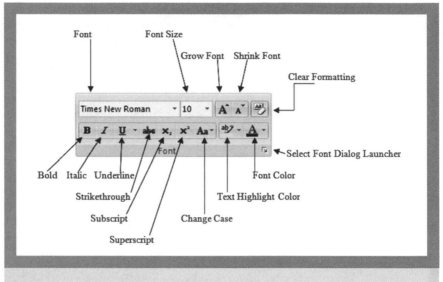

Figure 5-16 Font Style Group in Home Tab

the font size for business documents is 10 to 12 points, but you may also choose a larger size that can be read easily on the screen if you like. Later, you can change the font if necessary. For example, you can highlight the entire document by **choosing Select** in the **Editing** group and then **Select All** (or press **Ctrl + A**) and reduce the print size before printing by choosing another font size or print style or both.

3. Style buttons are available in the Font group for bold, italic, and underline (Figure 5-16).
   To use the Style buttons for bold, italic, and underline:

   - **Highlight** a word or section of text.
   - Click the desired Style button that appears. You can use the **Style** button in the **Font** group to change style attributes. Alternatively, when you highlight a word, a small toolbar will appear as you hold the mouse arrow over the highlighted word; you can then choose bold, italic, or another font size from among the other choices on the toolbar.
   - Clicking a Style button again will change the style back to its previous style.

   These attributes can also be turned on or off by pressing **Ctrl+B**, **Ctrl+I**, or **Ctrl+U**.

4. Click the **Change Styles** arrow in the **Styles** group to select a style, color, and font for text. Even more styles and choices are available when you click the dialog launcher in the **Styles** group. See **Figure 15-18**.

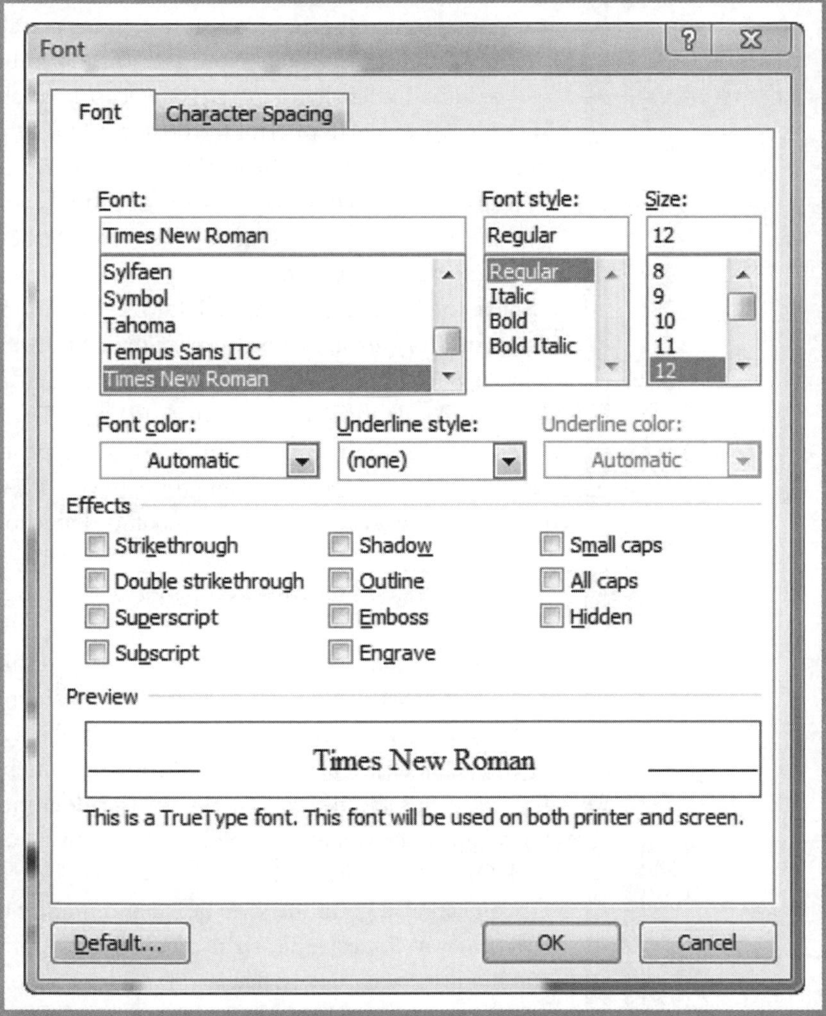

Figure 5-17 Font Dialog Box

Preparing a Document

You can prepare the formatting for a document in two ways: (1) by setting the formatting before you begin to type the text or (2) by typing the text and then formatting the document. The decision as to how to proceed is based on personal preference; remember, however, that the idea is to create and format the document efficiently and effectively. The process described here focuses on setting the formats before the document is created.

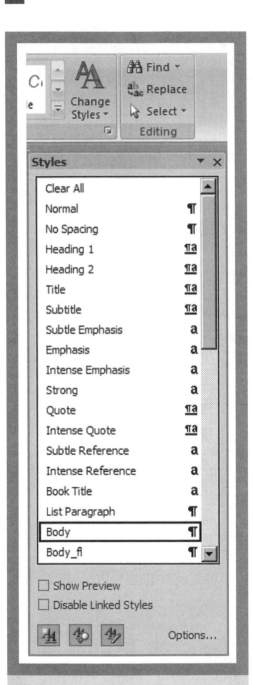

Figure 5-18 Styles Menu

Although the formatting features can be accessed from the Home tab, many of these settings are also available under the Page Layout tab. If the product will be bound, a left-hand margin of at least 1.5 inches is needed. If you plan to print the document on letterhead, measure the letterhead's height. A margin of as much as 2.4 inches may be needed to make sure that the body of the letter begins below the letterhead. To change the margins of a section of the document, **choose** the **Page Layout** tab; **click Margins**; **choose Custom Margins** at the bottom of the box and do what is needed; and then **select this point forward** from the **Apply to** options (Figure 5-12).

Go back to the **Home** tab and select the type and size of font desired from the Font group. In Word 2007, the default font and size is Calibri, 11 points. This choice can be changed by (1) clicking the dialog launcher in the **Font** group, (2) selecting the desired font and size in the dialog boxes, (3) clicking the **Default** button in the lower-left corner of the window, and (3) responding **Yes** when asked if you want to change the Normal template. The last step ensures that Word will always open to this font and size for any future documents. If the settings should be changed for this document only, ignore the Default box, change the settings, and click **OK**. (See Figure 15-17.)

You can also go to the style boxes and modify the style that way. For example, right-click on a style option and modify it accordingly. The arrows move the boxes up or down or bring up the complete style list.

Next choose the **Paragraph** group and click the dialog launcher. The Paragraph dialog box appears as shown in **Figure 5-19**. Besides selecting an alignment option, you can choose single, 1.5, or double-spacing options under Line Spacing in this dialog box. You can also choose the line spacing by clicking on the arrow next to the line spacing box in the Paragraph group.

On a computer screen, it may be easier to work on a document using 1.5 or single spacing. Later, you can change this option to whatever spacing is required or

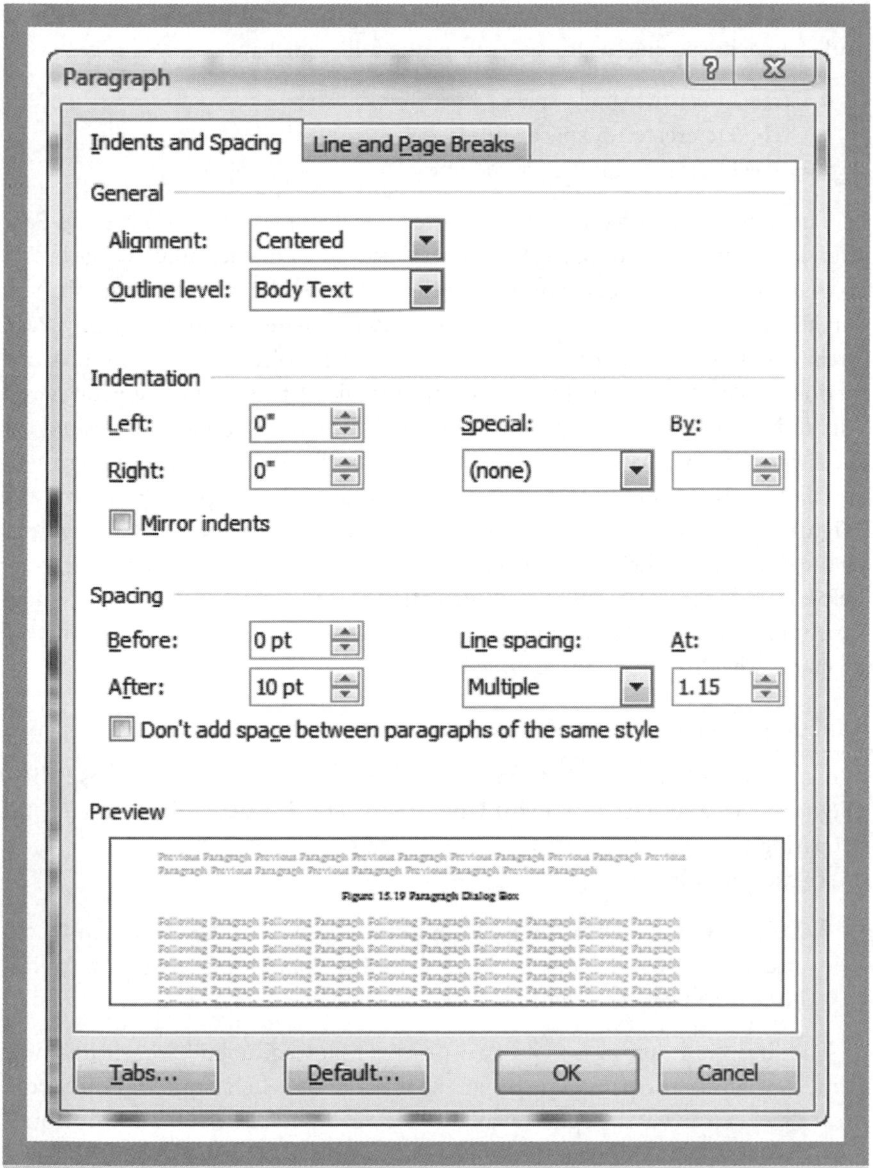

Figure 5-19 Paragraph Dialog Box

preferred in the final product. You can also highlight the entire document (**Ctrl+A**) and change its spacing by pressing one of the following key combinations:

- **Ctrl+1** to create single-spaced lines
- **Ctrl+5** to create 1.5-spaced lines
- **Ctrl+2** to create double-spaced lines

The same Paragraph dialog box (Figure 5-19) includes a tab for Line and Page Breaks. Clicking the Widow/Orphan Control box under that tab adjusts page breaks so that a page always begins or ends with at least two lines of a paragraph. You can also insert a page break by going to the **Page Layout** tab and choosing **Page Breaks**. A dialog box appears containing additional choices for text, columns, and section breaks. Be careful with inserting page breaks as they are problematic as you edit and revise a document. To force lines and paragraphs to move as desired use the appropriate pagination options of keep lines with next and keep lines together.

Clicking the paragraph sign (¶) in the Paragraph group of the Home tab (Figure 5-15) will add formatting marks for spaces, tabs, and ends of paragraphs to the document. **Click** this sign again, and the marks disappear. The marks are helpful if a document needs to be reformatted or if you are not sure why the document looks the way it does. Remember that it is always better to use tabs instead of spaces when formatting a document.

Viewing a Document

Word provides several ways to view a document on the screen. Choose **View** (Figure 5-10) and select the **Print Layout** tab. This is usually the best view for preparing a document.

To change a view:

1. **Select View** and **click** the **View Option** desired from the choices in **Document Views** or click one of the icons in the Zoom group that corresponds to the view desired (Figure 5-10).

The first View option is Print Layout; it is followed by Full Screen Reading. Print Layout ▤ shows the document as it will look when printed. Full Screen view ▥ maximizes the space available for reading. The next View option is Web Layout ▤ —a view that shows how the document would look when displayed in a browser.

The next View option is Outline, which provides an outline view of the document. **Click Outline** and the outlining ribbon appears (see **Figure 5-20**). You can also access the Outline view by clicking the **Outline View** button ▤ in the status bar of the Word window. An outline provides a map to guide the writing process for a document. It can also help when you want to arrange pictures or columns and so on. Word uses its built-in heading styles for outlines (Heading 1, Heading 2, and so forth) by default.

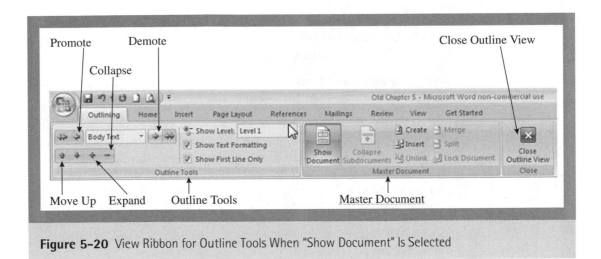

Figure 5-20 View Ribbon for Outline Tools When "Show Document" Is Selected

Draft ≣ view consists of text only with very large print. Other groups in the View tab are Show/Hide (as in ruler or gridlines); Zoom, which allows for viewing the document as one page or two pages; Window; and Macros.

Using Numbered and Bulleted Lists

Automatic bulleting and numbering can be helpful—and frustrating! For example, you might want to stop the list and then start another list later in the document. Word will pick up the previous number and continue numbering from it until you adjust the settings.

To create a numbered list:

1. **Select** the **Home** tab.
2. Put the cursor in the document where the list will begin.
3. **Click** the **Numbering** button ≣ ▾ in the **Paragraph** group (Figure 5-15).
4. Type the list, **pressing** the **Enter** key at the end of each item.
5. When you are finished, **press** the **Enter** key twice or **click** the **Numbering** button to turn off the numbers.

Alternatively, you can type the first number and press the **Enter** key; for the next item, Word will add the 2. If the list is ended, simply backspace to get rid of the next number or press the **Enter** key twice.

To create a bulleted list:

1. Type the list.
2. **Highlight** the list.
3. **Click** the **Bullets** button ≣ ▾ in the **Paragraph** group (Figure 5-15).

You may also click the bullet button and start typing the list as you did with the numbered list above. To modify the appearance of numbers and bullets, click the arrow in the button and choose an appropriate style.

Checking Spelling and Grammar

Spelling and grammar checks, translation, and a thesaurus are tools included in Word 2007 under the Review tab (Figure 5-9b). Word automatically checks spelling and grammar as you type. If a word is misspelled, a wavy red line appears under the word. If a grammar error is detected, the wavy line is green. Because some people are distracted by the wavy lines, Word provides an option to turn this feature off.

To correct the error:

1. **Right-click** the error.
2. **Select** a correction, choose to ignore it, or add the word to the spelling dictionary.

Figure 5-21 shows the menu that appears when "error" is misspelled.

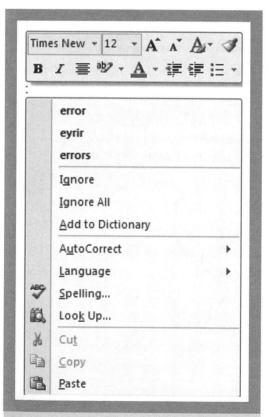

Figure 5-21 Spelling Assistance Menu

When adding a word to the dictionary, be sure that it is correct. The spelling dictionary is stored on the hard drive, so it is available only on the computer to which it was added. Some computer labs may refresh the computer image each time a new user logs in; in such a case, any words added to the dictionary will not be permanent.

To turn the spelling and grammar checker off:

1. **Click** the **Spelling & Grammar** button in the **Review** tab. You must have some text in the document for this to work; otherwise it will just run the spell checker.
2. **Click Options** in the dialog box that appears.
3. **Uncheck** the boxes **Check spelling as you type** and **Check grammar as you type**.
4. **Click OK**.

After this is done, to check spelling and grammar:

5. **Click** the **Spelling & Grammar button** under the **Review** tab.

The spelling and grammar checks are typically turned on while the document is typed. When text is entered into the document, the Spelling & Grammar icon appears in the status bar. When a red X appears on the icon 🔏, Word has detected a possible spelling or grammar error.

Analyzing Readability Statistics

Readability statistics are possible by choosing **Word Options** under the **Office** button, **Proofing**, and then selecting both **Check grammar with spelling** and **Show readability statistics**. The readability level of the document should match the reading ability of the audience for whom the document is intended. It is best to perform grammar, spelling, and readability checks after the document is finished, and with the cursor placed at the beginning of the document. It will still be necessary to proofread the document, however, as Word will not find all of the misspellings or grammar problems that might exist.

Creating Word Counts

Also found under the Review tab is the Word Count button , which appears in the Proofing group (Figure 5-9b). Performing a word count is very helpful when you are writing an abstract or paper that is limited to a certain number of words. You can also determine the number of lines, paragraphs, or characters in a document by using this option. Note also that Word lists the number of words in the document in the left part of the status bar.

Using Word Templates

Word provides several templates that can be applied to a new document, as shown in the New Document box (Figure 5-3). The first section shows templates available in the program; many other choices are available from Microsoft Office Online.

　　If a certain style is modified and needs to be saved as a template, choose **Save As** under the **Office** button. When Save As is highlighted, choose **Word Template** from the column on the right. Name the document template and choose the appropriate template folder in which to save it.

Creating a Table

The Tables group under the Insert tab is used in many ways. For example, it helps you set columns for recording minutes of a meeting or for organizing any kind of information. Tables are also essential to research reports. It is a good idea to plot out the kind of table needed in terms of number of rows and columns required before selecting them. Among the choices for a new table in the Tables group are Insert Table, Draw Table, or (built-in) Quick Tables. **Figure 5-22** shows the dialog boxes that appear when Table and Quick Tables are selected under the Insert tab. **Figure 5-23** shows the dialog box that appears when Insert Table (under the grid) is selected.

　　To draw a table, **click** the **Table** button. Place the mouse over the grid and highlight the number of rows and columns needed. Keep dragging until the correct size is reached. The Table Tools Design Ribbon appears (**Figure 5-24**) once the table is in place.

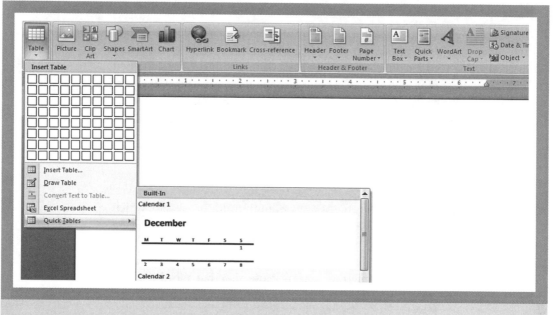

Figure 5-22 Table Menu Plus a Quick Table Example

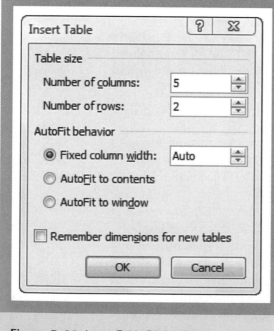

Figure 5-23 Insert Table Dialog Box

To create a table:

1. Place the insertion point where the table should appear in the document.
2. **Click** the **Insert** tab, the **Table** button, and **Insert Table**.
3. Select the number of rows and columns and click **OK** or, if using the mouse, drag over the cells for the number of rows and columns desired.

Remember that a row is needed for headers. Additional rows or columns can be inserted if necessary.

To insert a row:

1. **Right-click** in a row.
2. From the menu, **select Insert . . .** and **choose Insert rows** either above or below the row selected.

You may also insert multiple rows at one time by selecting the number of rows to be inserted

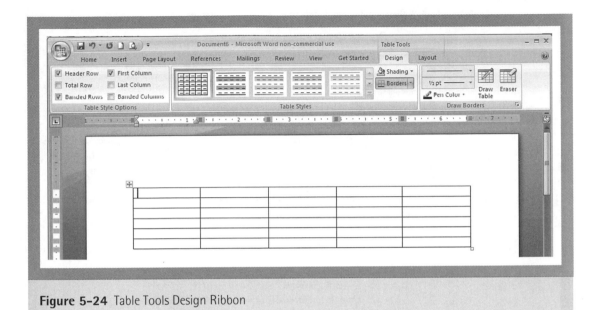

Figure 5-24 Table Tools Design Ribbon

using the quick select area in the left margin, and right-clicking the selection. Follow the directions from the shortcut menu. Columns are inserted the same way.

Many more commands are also available under the Table menu to change the width or height of a row or column, alter the style of the table, or delete grid lines. To delete the table, highlight it, and then either backspace or **choose Cut.**

Creating an Outline

To create an outline before you start the document, choose **View**, then **Outline**. Outlines are based on heading styles; they can include a maximum of nine levels of headings. **Figure 5-25** shows a multilevel outline of Chapter 4. While shown in this figure, the title of the chapter is not generally included in the outline levels. It is better to use the heading styles for major content areas of the document, not the document title.

To make an outline:

1. In Outline View, type the first line in the Outline, Heading 1.
2. Press **Enter**. Another line of the same level appears.
3. Type the next line or press the **Tab** key. The Tab key demotes the next line to the Heading 2 level. Note that a plus symbol ⊕ appears in front of the first line; this symbol indicates that there is a heading below it. If the minus symbol ⊖ appears, then there are no subordinates.

If you want to create an outline after you write a document, be sure to apply the appropriate heading styles to the headings in your document. If you don't want to use Word's preset styles (**Figure 5-26**), you can redefine the formula for

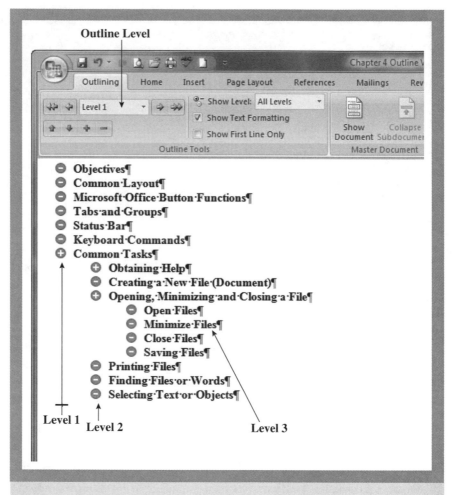

Figure 5-25 Outline View of Chapter 4 with Outlining Ribbon

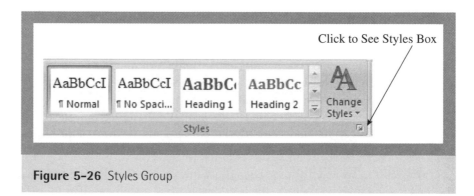

Figure 5-26 Styles Group

the default heading styles or apply a different style by choosing the **Styles** group dialog launcher ▣, selecting the level to change, right-clicking, and making the desired changes (see **Figure 5-27**).

Creating a Table of Contents

A table of contents (TOC) usually appears at the beginning of a document after the title page and provides a list of headings from a certain level along with their page numbers. **Figure 5-28** shows a partial table of contents for Chapter 4. Each heading in the document had to have a heading level assigned to it. Each heading was highlighted and a heading level assigned to it by clicking on an appropriate level in the **Add Text** command in the Reference tab, **Table of Contents** group. See **Figure 5-29**.

You can make your own custom table of contents, if you like. Choose **References**, **Table of Contents**, and then click **Insert Table of Contents**. A dialog box appears (**Figure 5-30**) in which you can choose options for showing and aligning page numbers, formats, and other options. If you choose **Modify** in this box, another dialog box appears (**Figure 5-31**). The style for each heading is described and can be changed, if you wish, by choosing **Modify** in the **Style** dialog box. You can then change the font type and size as well as its appearance (bold, italic, color, and so forth).

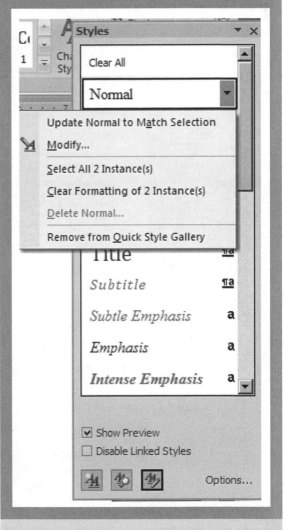

Figure 5-27 Styles Pane After Right-Clicking to Modify a Style

Creating Merged Documents

Word has features that will help you create envelopes and form letters and print personalized copies of both for each person on a list. Word replaces merge fields from a main document with information from a data source. As with many other Word functions, there is more than one way to send a form letter to a list of people. The Step by Step Mail Merge Wizard will be used to prepare the documents in the example in this section.

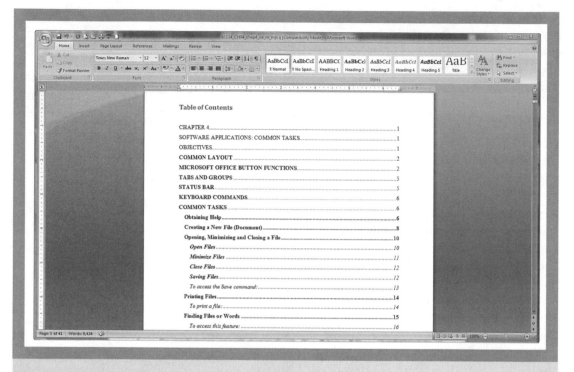

Figure 5-28 Table of Contents for Chapter 4

Two documents will be created:

- A data source contains the name, address, and whatever else must be individualized for each letter. A series of subdocuments can also be set up that Word will merge into a main document. The data source can be an Outlook address book, an Access database, an Excel spreadsheet with column headings, or a Word table. In this example, the data source is a Word table. Every data source consists of three parts: records, fields, and field headers. Each paragraph in a data source is a record, and each column is a field. You must plan the data source carefully so that it does what you want it to do.

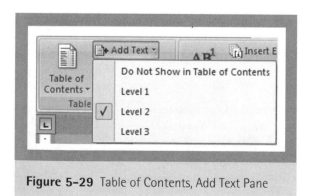

Figure 5-29 Table of Contents, Add Text Pane

- A main document contains the same text that will appear in each letter and the field code from which to insert the personalized data from the data source.

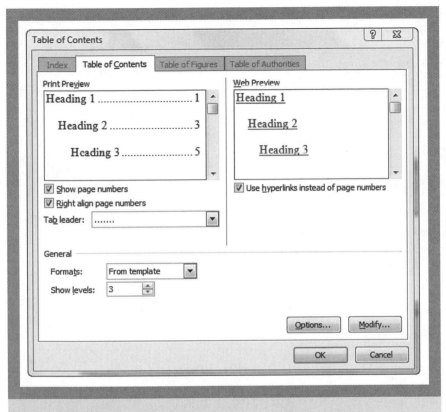

Figure 5–30 Table of Contents Dialog Box

To perform a step-by-step mail merge:

1. **Open** a new Word document.
2. **Select** the **Mailings** group, then **click Start Mail Merge** (**Figure 5-32**).
3. **Click Step by Step Mail Merge Wizard**. The next screen that appears shows Step 1 of 6 (**Figure 5-33**).
4. **Choose** tab **Letters** ⦿ Letters .
5. **Click Next: Starting Document**.
6. **Choose Start from a template**, and then **click Select Template** [Select template...] .
7. **Click Letters** tab in the Select Template window and **select Origin Letter** (**Figure 5-34**).
8. **Click OK. Figure 5-35** shows part of the letter that appears. Because the computer used to prepare this example belongs to Marjorie Smith, that name appears automatically at the top of the letter.
9. **Click Next: Select Recipients**.

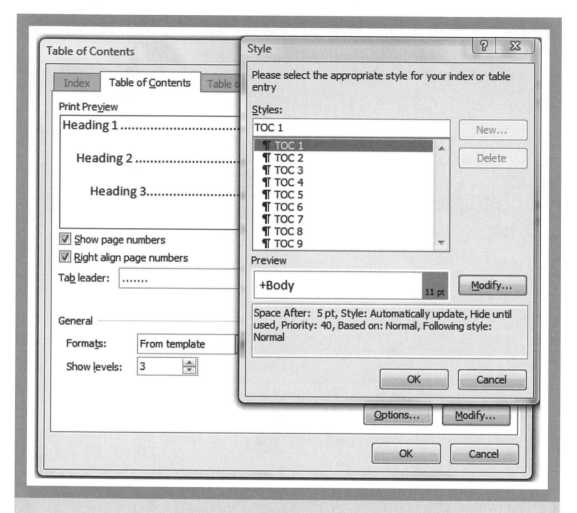

Figure 5–31 Style Dialog Box That Appears When "Modify" Is Selected from the Table of Contents Dialog Box

10. Select **Type a new list** and then **click Create**.

11. Type the **title**, **first name**, **last name**, **address** (usually one), **city**, **state**, and **ZIP** code for the first recipient. (Use the Tab key to move between the address fields.) Some fields may be hidden, and the table must be enlarged left to right.

12. **Click New Entry** and add a second recipient. **Figure 5-36** shows the New Address List window that appears after street names were added. Add two or three more recipients.

13. **Click OK** at the bottom of the window. You will be asked to name your list and save it in "My Data Sources." **Type** a **name**, click **Save** and then **OK**. Figure 5-37 shows the Select Data Source window that appears when lists already exist. In this case you would select the correct data source and **click Open. Click OK**.

    Figure 5-38 shows the Mail Merge Recipient List that appears after the list.

14. **Click Next: Write your letter** in Step 3.

15. Step 4, "Write your letter," appears. See **Figure 5-39** for Steps 4–6.

16. Type a name in the upper-right-hand space if it isn't there. Add an address and a phone number.

17. Place the cursor at the red arrow. **Click Address block . . .**

18. Delete the lines below the address block ("Type recipient name, address and phone").

19. **Click [Type the Salutation]**. Click **Greeting line . . . Figure 5-40** shows the dialog box for choosing the type of greeting line you desire. **Click OK** when you are finished.

20. Highlight the body of the letter and type a message.

21. **Click [Type the closing]** and type **Sincerely.**

22. Add your name and appropriate information at the bottom of the letter. Choose a date by clicking the arrow that appears when you click [Pick the date].

23. **Click Next: Preview your letters** in Step 4 (Figure 5-39).

24. Preview the letters by **clicking** on **Recipient 1**, **Recipient 2**, and so forth.

25. When you are satisfied with the way the letters look, **click Next: Complete the Merge** in Step 5.

26. In Step 6, **choose Print**. A dialog box appears (**Figure 5-41**).

27. Choose to print all of the letters, the current record, or just those records between selected numbers.

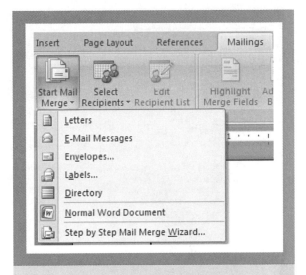

Figure 5–32 Start Mail Merge Drop-Down Menu

Using Bibliography Options

One of the new features in Word 2007 is the ability to automatically generate bibliographies in several formats. The Citations and Bibliography tools in Word

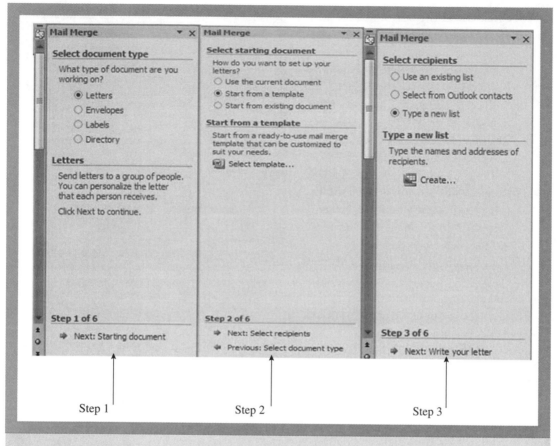

Figure 5-33 Steps 1–3 of the Mail Merge Wizard

work well if you set the style before you enter the source. Even if you change your mind later, you won't have to reenter all your source information. You are most likely to use one of two specific styles:

NOTE: If you are using this function for a course assignment, be sure you use the specific format and version of that format that is acceptable to the faculty who will grade your paper.

- APA—American Psychological Association
- MLA—Modern Language Association

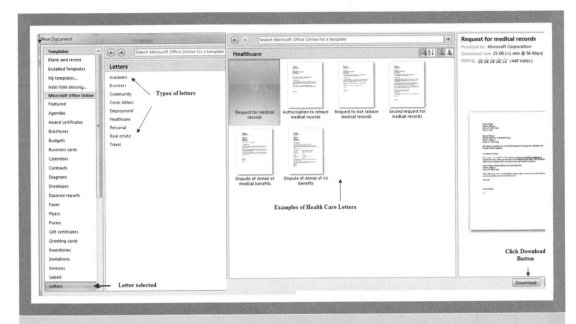

Figure 5-34 Dialog Window for Selecting a Letter from Templates

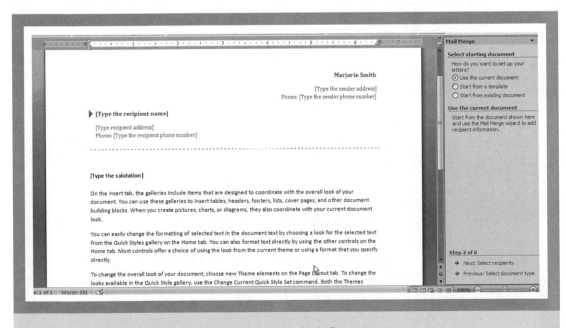

Figure 5-35 Template for the "Origin Letter" for the Main Document

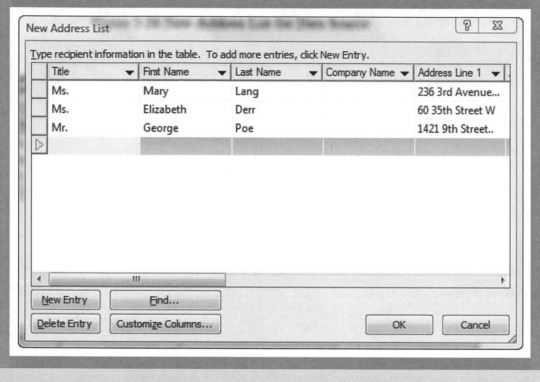

Figure 5-36 New Address List for Data Source

To add a source:

1. Choose an appropriate style. For this example, APA is used.
2. **Click** the **References** tab.
3. **Choose Manage Sources**. The Source Manager dialog box opens (**Figure 5-42**).
4. **Click** the **New** button. The Create Source dialog box opens (**Figure 5-43**).
5. Choose **Book**.
6. **Type** the author's name, the book title, year of publication, city where published, and publisher. If the book has more than one author, **click Edit**. Type the information for the first author, **click Add**, repeat until all authors are added. **Click OK**. Use **Add** if the source has more than one author. The citation is listed in both the Master and Current lists. Additional citations can be added at this time or later.

NOTE: Also available from Microsoft's Web site are APA templates for formatting the document using that style manual.

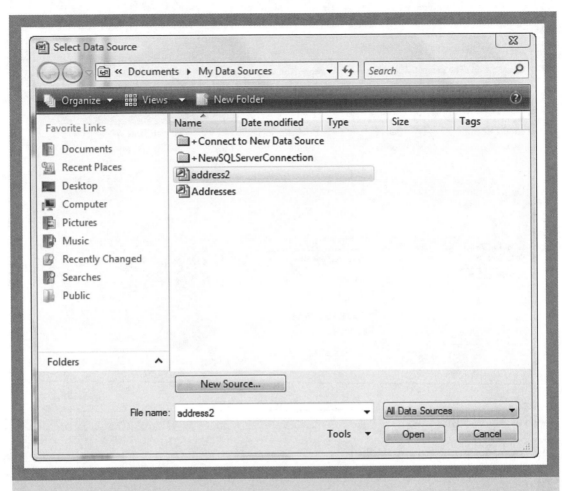

Figure 5-37 Select Data Source Dialog Box

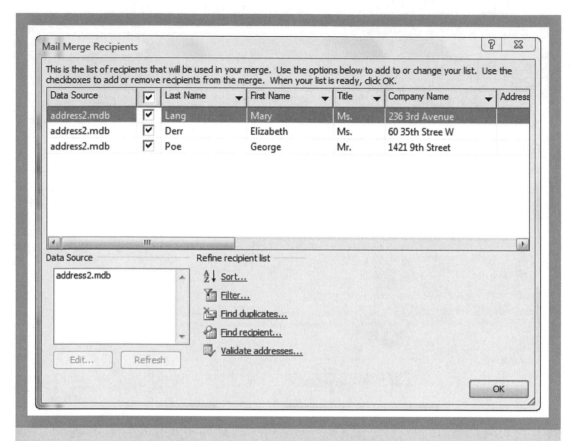

Figure 5-38 Mail Merge Recipients List

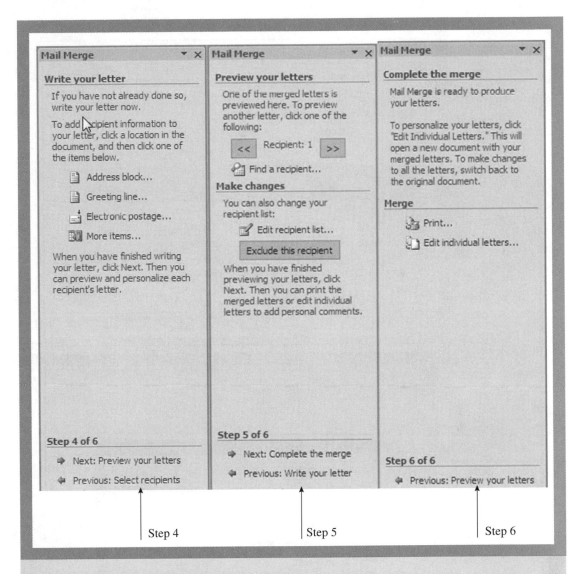

Figure 5-39 Steps 4–6 of the Mail Merge Wizard

Insert Greeting Line

Greeting line format:

| Dear ▼ | Joshua ▼ | , ▼ |

Greeting line for invalid recipient names:

Dear Sir or Madam, ▼

Preview

Here is a preview from your recipient list:

◁◁ ◁ | 1 | ▷ ▷▷

Dear Mary,

Correct Problems

If items in your greeting line are missing or out of order, use Match Fields to identify the correct address elements from your mailing list.

Match Fields...

OK   Cancel

Figure 5-40 Insert Greeting Line Dialog Box

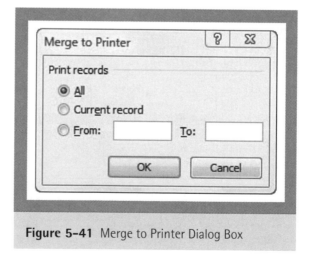

Merge to Printer

Print records

◉ All

○ Current record

○ From: [   ] To: [   ]

OK   Cancel

Figure 5-41 Merge to Printer Dialog Box

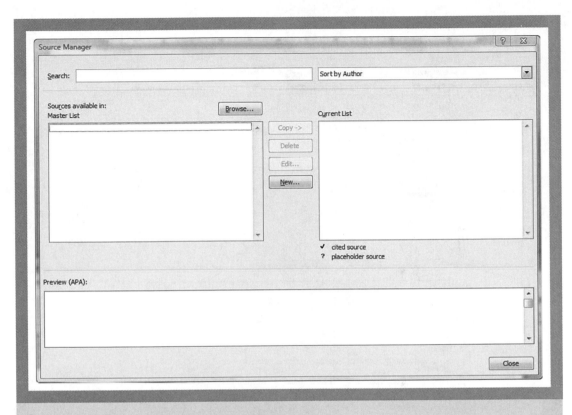

Figure 5–42 Source Manager Dialog Box for a Bibliography

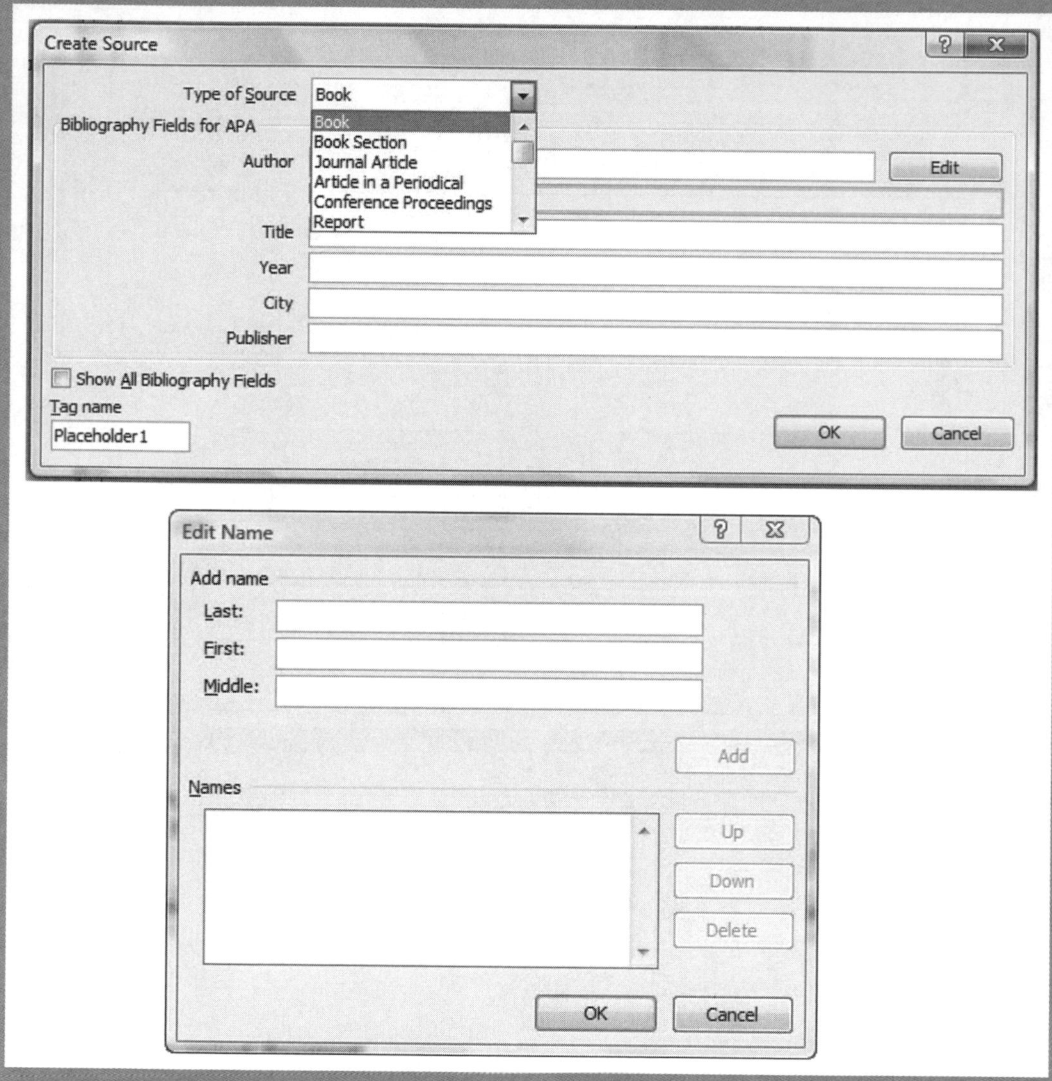

Figure 5–43 Dialog Boxes for Creating One Source and Editing One Name

Summary

Word provides unlimited possibilities for creating custom documents. This chapter has described some of the basic skills necessary for you to begin using Word features effectively and efficiently. Some of the possibilities include creating an index or bibliography, generating a table of contents, summarizing documents, working with clip art and SmartArt, making newsletters, writing blogs, addressing envelopes, and customizing and optimizing Word. To develop additional skills use one of the many Word reference books available or go to Microsoft Office Online and take advantage of the many assistance and training opportunities available. Of course, much time and diligent work will be necessary before you can take advantage of all of the program's features. However, once you have learned the basic features you will discover it is easier to learn new functions and to adapt to the newer versions of the application that arrive every few years.

EXERCISE 1 Basic Microsoft Word Functions

■ **Objectives**

1. Perform selected word processing functions.
2. Explain basic word processing terms and functions.

■ **Activity**

1. Start **Word**. (This exercise can be done using any word processing program.)
2. Create a document. Type the following text as fast as possible. Do not correct any mistakes that you make, and do not press the Enter key. Do not pay attention to spelling errors.

   Using word processing software can save many hours and much pain. It can also be very exasperating. It is important to follow a few simple rules. If the rules are ignored, disaster can strike. These are a few of the simple rules: (1) Save all work periodically. (2) Pay attention to the warnings given. (3) Always keep a second copy of the document or project on the Internet or another removable storage device or hard drive in another place.

3. Save the document.
   a. **Click** the **Office** button (image), then click **Save** (image) or press **Ctrl+S**.
   b. **Type Chap5Ex1-Lastname** in the highlighted File name text box.
   c. Go to the Location text box at the top of the Save As dialog box.

      Select the correct location (see Figure 4-11 for further help) and **click** the **Save** button. Alternatively, you can save the document by **clicking** the **Save** button (image) on the Quick Access toolbar. Once the document has a name and location, clicking the **Save** button (or **Ctrl+S**) will just update the file and not display the Save As dialog box.

4. Move around the document.
   a. Practice moving around the document.
   b. Use the arrow keys and Page Up and Page Down keys.

5. Edit text.
   a. **Highlight** the text (or **press Ctrl+A**).
   b. **Click Copy** (image) (or **press Ctrl+C**).
   c. Press **Ctrl+End** to position the insertion point below the original paragraph.
   d. **Press Enter** twice.
   e. **Click Paste** (image) (or **press Ctrl+V**). Now there are two copies of the text.
   f. **Click Undo** (image).
   g. Try doing the same thing using the **Cut** (image) and **Paste** buttons in the Clipboard group. If there is more than one copy left, delete the extra copies ending with one copy.

h. Go back to the Quick Access toolbar and **click** the **Redo Typing** button ↻.

i. Go to the clipboard. **Click** the **dialog launcher** button ⌸. A list of what was copied appears on the clipboard.

j. End this task with the document containing two of the same paragraphs.

6. Align text.

a. **Highlight** the second copy of the text. **Click** the **Align Right** button ≣ in the **Paragraph** group of the **Home** tab. Note what happens.

b. To get both right and left justification, click the **Justify** button ≣. All sentences appear flush at both margins except for the last sentence.

c. **Click** the **Align Left** button ≣.

7. Edit the document.

a. Delete any extra copies of the test, leaving only one copy.

b. Use the Tab, Indent, and Enter keys to create a document that looks like this:

> **Using word processing software can save many hours and much pain. It can also be very exasperating. It is important to follow a few simple rules. If the rules are ignored, disaster can strike.**
>
> **These are a few of the simple rules:**
>
> 1. **Periodically save all work.**
> 2. **Pay attention to the warnings given.**
> 3. **Always keep a second copy of the document or project on another disk or hard drive, and keep it in another place.**

c. **Press Ctrl+Home** to place the insertion bar at the beginning of the paragraph.

d. **Select** the **Review** tab and then **Spelling and Grammar** to correct any errors. When the dialog box appears, it will highlight misspelled words and offer corrections.

e. **Click** the **Change** button if the highlighted selection is correct and the **Ignore** button to ignore a correctly spelled word. If no suggestion is given or lists incorrect words, Word doesn't recognize the word so can't give a correct spelling. Use an appropriate dictionary for the correct spelling and type it manually if not spelled correctly.

Word will announce the completion of the spelling and grammar check and provide readability statistics if you have chosen that option under the **Proofing** section of **Word Options**.

8. Format the document.

a. Type a title above the text by **pressing Ctrl + Home**, **typing Word Processing Rules**, and **pressing** the **Enter** key twice.

b. Highlight the title.

c. **Click** the **Bold** button **B**, and **click** the **Center Text** button ≣.

d. **Click** in the text to deselect the title.

9. Print the document.
   a. **Click** the **Office** button, **select Print,** and choose an option.
   b. Alternatively, **press Ctrl+P** or **click** the **Printer** button 🖨 in the Quick Access toolbar.
10. Close and save the document.
    a. **Click** the **Save** button 💾 or **press Ctrl+S** to save the document. This will update the file saved earlier.
    b. **Click** the **Close** button **✗** on the Word application or go on to Exercise 2.

EXERCISE 2 Find, Replace, and Paragraph Borders

■ **Objectives**
1. Use a find and replace function.
2. Create a document with a paragraph border.

■ **Activity**
1. Create the document.
   a. Open a **New Blank** document and save the document as **Chap5 Ex2-Lastname.**
   b. Type the following text in the new document window:
      A descriptive survey was used to elicit information concerns of new moms as part of an evaluation of single room maternity care (SRMC) at a small Midwestern hospital. The investigators developed a list of concerns common to new moms. New moms were asked to check as many of the 16 concerns listed that they would like the nurse to help with or discuss after the birth of their baby. After a pilot study of 10 new moms, the survey was mailed to all new moms who delivered a live infant during a 12-month period.
2. Search for all occurrences of "moms" and replace them with "mothers".
   a. Press **Ctrl+Home** to go to the top of the document.
   b. Under the **Home** tab, **select Replace** ab/ac Replace.
   c. In the **Find what** text box, **type moms.**
   d. **Press** the **Tab** key, or **click** the **Replace with** text box.
   e. **Type mothers.**
   f. **Click** the **Replace All** button. What happens? (Use the Replace All option with caution, as it will change *all* words that contain the sequence of letters "moms".)
   g. **Click** the **OK** button.

   h. Use the Find and Replace dialog box again and reverse the directions.

   i. **Type mothers** in the **Find what** text box and **moms** in the **Replace with** text box.

   j. **Click** the **Replace All** button. The document will return to normal. **Click OK**.

   k. **Click** the **Close** button to close the Find and Replace dialog box.

3. Create paragraph borders.

   a. Go to the end of the document, and press **Enter** four times.

   b. Select the paragraph created in Step 1 of this exercise.

   c. Copy this paragraph and paste the copy below the first paragraph leaving two blank lines between them.

   d. Highlight the first paragraph.

   e. **Click** the **Border** button arrow ⊞▾ in the **Paragraph** group on the **Home** tab.

   f. **Choose Outside Borders** from the menu that appears.

   g. Use the same **Border** button arrow to **select Borders and Shading** ▫ Borders and Shading… . What do you think would happen if you clicked the icon and not the arrow.

   h. Under **Settings,** choose the **3-D** border box as shown in **Figure 5-44.**

   i. **Under Style, choose** the double line (heavy top, light bottom).

   j. Under **Width, choose 3 pt.**

   k. Click **OK.**

   l. Highlight the text and **choose Justify** ▤ from the **Formatting Paragraph** group. The box should look like this box, however the number of words in each line will vary:

> **A descriptive survey was used to elicit information concerns of new moms as part of an evaluation of single room maternity care (SRMC) at a small Midwestern hospital. The investigators developed a list of concerns common to new moms. New moms were asked to check as many of the 16 concerns listed that they would like the nurse to help with or discuss after the birth of their baby. After a pilot study of 10 new moms, the survey was mailed to all new moms who delivered a live infant during a 12-month period.**

4. Save and print the document.

Tip: Always leave a paragraph mark (press Enter) below the text that will be boxed or below a table to enable titles or text to be added at those location. If the last paragraph mark is within the box or table, pressing Enter will simply enlarge the box or table.

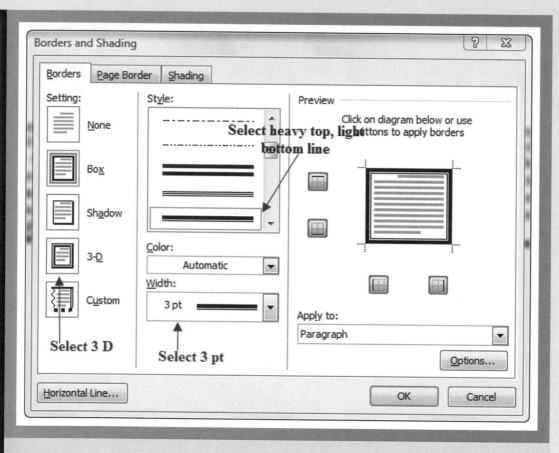

Figure 5-44 Borders and Shading Dialog Box

EXERCISE 3   Merge and Find Functions

■ **Objectives**
 1. Create main, data source, and merged documents.
 2. Use the find and replace function.
 3. Print created letters.

■ **Activity**
 1. Create the documents.
    a. Create the main and data source documents like those at the end of this exercise. Use the directions given earlier in this chapter for creating the mail merge documents.

2. Use the find and replace function and replace all occurrences of
   - "DM" with **diabetes mellitus**
   - "September 25, 2011" with **September 25, 2012**
   - "medications" with **insulin**
3. Merge the documents.
   a. Use the merge (mail merge) feature to generate and print the individual letters.
   b. Check the letters for accuracy.

The appearance of the fields depends on the word processor. The fields may be indicated with the name of the field, a number with a hyphen (-), or something else.

Main Document

Figure 5-45 shows the sample main document. Make sure you use the insert field feature; do NOT type the fields and the related chevron into the document.

<<Title>> <<FirstName>> <<LastName>>

<<Address>>

<<City> <<State>> <<PostalCode>>

(Use the automatic date function to place date with this style: Month Day, Year.)

Dear <<FirstName>>:

We invite you to attend a patient education program on adult-onset DM. The date of the program is September 25, 2011. The program time takes place from 1 to 3 p.m. in the Patient Education Conference Room, 4th floor, Computerville Hospital. We designed this program for newly diagnosed diabetics. The program will address adjusting to diabetes, diet and exercise, and medications. The guest speaker is Nellie Netscape, Nurse Practitioner. Please notify us at 624-3333 if you plan to attend. There is no charge for this program. We look forward to seeing you.

Sincerely,

Mary Data, PhD, RN

Figure 5-45 Sample Main Document

Data Source

Title	First Name	Last Name	Address	City	ST	ZIP
Ms.	Mary	Jones	325 First Street	Carnegie	PA	15102
Mr.	Robert	Tutor	45 Software Ave.	Milford	PA	15102
Dr.	Susan	Master	8997 Default Lane	Eagan	MN	55123

4. Using the information from the letter, make a flyer that you can post in the clinic where other patients might see it.

   a. Choose an **Event flyer** from MS Office Online under **Templates**, **Flyers**.

   b. Include clip art that is appropriate for the document.

ASSIGNMENT 1 Preparing a Résumé

You will need Microsoft Word and an internet connection for this assignment.

■ **Directions**

A résumé that summarizes educational and professional accomplishments is necessary when you are applying for a new job.

1. Obtain a want ad from the paper (preferably in the health field).

2. Compose a résumé using Word's Resume Template.

   a. **Choose New** under the **Office** button.

   b. Under **Templates** and **Microsoft Office Online** (you will need to have an authorized MS Word application on your computer to do this and an Internet connection):

      i. **Click Resumes and CVs** Resumes and CVs .

      ii. **Click Basic Resumes**, then **choose Professional Profile**, **Resume 1** or another of your liking.

      iii. Complete the template by replacing the text placeholders with your own information. Delete any extra placeholders. Remember that this template uses tables to hold the data, so you will need to work with tables to add or delete rows. Make sure the résumé includes the following information:

         ■ Information about the person: name, address (city, state, ZIP code)

         ■ Job/work objective (not always included)

         ■ Summary of qualifications (use the job description in the advertisement as a guide)

         ■ Education (school, degree, date, major)

         ■ Professional experience as a health professional/nurse (Begin with your most recent position and include the year, name of position, and type of unit.)

         ■ Other information: licensure, honors, student or professional organizations, volunteer activities, special skills, projects, and so on

    c. Use uppercase and lowercase.

    d. Use the spell checker as appropriate.

    e. Save the résumé as **Chap5Assign1-Lastname**.

3. Compose a cover letter applying for the position.

    a. Run the cover letter through a spell and grammar checker.

    b. Make appropriate revisions in the cover letter based on the results produced by the spell and grammar checker (if available).

4. Submit the advertisement, a letter of application (original and revised), and a résumé.

ASSIGNMENT 2 Merge Function

■ Directions

1. Write a procedure or policy for some aspect of your work or practice. This procedure or policy can be something that exists but requires revision, or it can be a new one that requires development. Use the following document format:

Margins:	Left	2 inches
	Right	1.5 inches
	Top	2 inches
	Bottom	1 inch
Header:	Flush right, procedure/policy number on each page	
Footer:	Pagination centered	
Last page:	Add your initials	

2. Use the merge function to create a form letter that will be sent with the procedure/policy to five people, along with an explanation of the attached policy/procedure, a due date for its review, and the person to contact if they have questions. Set up the letter to use the merge function. Embed the field codes in the form letter. Create a data source consisting of the following information: recipient's name (first and last), title, and hospital location.

3. Save the file as **Chap5Assign2-lastname**.

4. Turn in the procedure/policy, the letter showing its merge fields, and a copy of the merged letter in either print or electronic format.

ASSIGNMENT 3 Announcement

■ Directions

1. Prepare an announcement of a special function or party for a class.

2. Go to **Microsoft Office Online**. **Choose Clip Art**, and then **select Academic** under **Browse Clip Art**. If there is not an appropriate piece of clip

art available under the Academic heading, choose another topic, and select something that matches the announcement purpose.

3. Click the clip you have selected. Make sure that a document is open to receive the clip art.
4. Construct the announcement around the clip art. Make sure all of the relevant information is included in the announcement.
5. Turn in the announcement.

ASSIGNMENT 4 A Formal Paper

■ **Directions**

This assignment is designed to help you format a specific paper that will include a title page, outline, headers, table of contents, and bibliography.

1. Use a paper you have written for another class or download the file called **A Formal Paper** from this textbook's Web site.
2. Create a title page.
3. Outline the paper.
4. Insert a header in which your name and the page number are right justified.
5. Apply the appropriate styles to enable later generation of the table of contents.
6. Add a relevant table.
7. Add appropriate clip art, pictures, or Smart Art.
8. Generate the table of contents.
9. Create a reference list or bibliography.
10. Save the file as **Chap5Assign4-LastName** and submit it electronically to the professor.

Introduction to Presentation Graphics

Objectives

1. Define basic terminology related to presentation graphics.
2. Describe selective uses of presentation graphics software.
3. Recognize components of a quality slide and poster presentation.
4. Develop quality PowerPoint and poster presentations.

Presentation graphics programs are increasingly being used by health-care professionals and students. In many courses, students are required to use presentation graphics software for their in-class and distance education presentations; healthcare professionals use the software for presentations at conferences as well as for preparation of patient education materials; and educators use it during face-to-face training in classrooms and distance education presentations. Because these applications make it possible to view data in a variety of formats they can also be used as a tool in analyzing data. Microsoft PowerPoint is one of the most commonly used presentation graphics programs. While other applications such as word processing and spreadsheet programs typically contain some graphics capabilities, none of them has the power inherent in presentation graphics programs to prepare and deliver quality presentations.

Graphics programs include presentation software, draw programs, and computer-aided design (CAD) programs. Most presentation programs include capabilities for text handling, outlining, drawing, graphing, clip art, and special effects. They allow for the production of high-quality presentation slides, transparencies, handouts, posters, or electronic slide shows. Draw programs help users produce clip art and images that can then be incorporated into presentation programs or other applications where images might enhance the message. Computer-aided design programs assist draftsmen, engineers, and architects to produce their design plans and drawings.

This chapter focuses on presentation graphics using PowerPoint. PowerPoint and similar presentation graphics programs are typically used to present information in a pleasing visual fashion so as to facilitate decision making and to communicate a message. The inclusion of visuals that sustain the audience's interest, highlight content, and disseminate information can clearly enhance the effectiveness of presentations.

Steps in Creating a Presentation

The main purpose when using a presentation graphics program is to prepare visuals to go along with a presentation. Of course, the first step in preparing a presentation is to define its purpose or message clearly—otherwise, the presentation has no hope of conveying information effectively.

The second step is to outline or organize the content of the presentation. Many presentation programs offer an outline feature to help with this step. Be careful when using the outline feature. It is designed only to identify the essence of the presentation, the order of the slides, and some key points for each slide. All the slides should *not* just be text or bulleted lists, which is easy to do with the outline feature.

Next, decide the best medium to present the message given the time allowed. This decision requires knowledge of both the environment where the presentation will occur and the equipment that will be available.

In addition, identify the target audience. There are major differences between presentations designed for children, teenagers, or professionals; there are also differences in designing a presentation to be delivered through distance education courses. When developing a poster presentation, be sure to follow the guidelines provided by the sponsoring organization.

A variety of media is commonly used for presentations—namely, handouts, 35-mm slides, slide shows, transparencies, and posters.

Handouts

Sometimes handouts are provided to the audience to outline the presentation, define selected terms, or present complex information. Use the presentation program's handout feature when you want to provide printed copies of the slides or speaker notes for yourself or for the audience. It is easy to develop appropriate handouts and notes that go with the presentation. To prepare details not covered in the presentation or reference lists, use a word processing program. No special equipment is needed to manage handouts during the presentation, but handouts can be expensive depending on the number needed and the printing process used

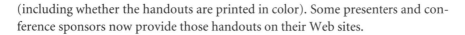

(including whether the handouts are printed in color). Some presenters and conference sponsors now provide those handouts on their Web sites.

35-mm Slides

Although not very popular now, some presenters use 35-mm slides when the appropriate graphic presentation equipment is not available, when the environment is more conducive to slides, or as a backup should something go wrong with the data projection system. Slides focus the audience on key points and present data in a pleasing and helpful manner. Depending on the slide projector, a darkened room may be required to view them. The slides need to project the text in large enough letters that the slides can be seen by all members of the audience. A remote control or another person may be needed to advance the slides. Use of 35-mm slides also increases the cost of a presentation.

Slide Shows

Using a data projector connected to a computer, PowerPoint slides may be projected on a large screen or smart board. You can create the slides in PowerPoint, and then add special effects. Adding sound makes the experience truly a multimedia event provided this is appropriate for the content and audience and provided speakers are available.

PowerPoint slide shows make it easy to adapt a presentation to different audiences and time slots without the expense of making new 35-mm slides. Data projection systems are generally available in educational and healthcare institutions as well as at convention centers. Newer models are portable, are less expensive than traditional devices, and project high-quality images that are easily seen in regular lighting.

Always have a backup plan should something happen to the data projection system, such as a burned-out light bulb or a network issue. Make sure that the appropriate software is in place or that you use the "copy your Microsoft Office PowerPoint 2007 presentation to a CD" option (**File**, **Publish**, and **Package for CD**) to avoid compatibility issues. With the latter approach, Microsoft Office PowerPoint Viewer 2007 and any linked files (such as movies or sounds) are copied as well as the presentation itself; by doing this, the presentation does not depend on the availability of the correct version of PowerPoint. (In earlier versions of PowerPoint, this capability was called the "pack and go" option.)

Save the presentation as a slide show to the secondary storage device or network drive. If using a secondary storage device, you can speed up the loading of the slides by copying the presentation to the hard drive.

Transparencies

Some presenters opt for transparencies because they are easy to prepare and use, although the equipment used for their projection is increasingly disappearing.

Document cameras, which can also show transparencies, are slowly but surely replacing overhead projectors. Transparencies can be used in rooms with normal lighting, which facilitates note taking. Because most printers can print them, transparencies are easier and less expensive to produce than slides and may work better in less technologically advanced sites. Use of laser and color printers can also enhance the effectiveness of transparencies. Transparencies, however, are not as easily revised as electronic slide shows.

Posters

Posters are used to present the results of a research study or to communicate ideas. The poster handles the presentation while the presenter stands nearby, ready to field questions. A poster is a static, visual medium that is usually prepared in color. Custom PowerPoint templates let you add content and color to the presentation and print it on larger paper for mounting on a poster board.

Once the planning process is completed, a presentation outline developed, and a medium selected, the next step is to create the graphic presentation or poster.

Key Points in Creating Graphic Presentations and Posters

Nothing is worse than using a graphics presentation that detracts from the message the speaker is trying to convey or that presents nothing but text on the screen. For poster presentations, nothing is worse than trying to cram in too much information in too small a font. A program such as PowerPoint will never be a substitute for a good speaker who is prepared and organized, speaks well, and can adjust the presentation to the needs of the audience. Likewise, a poster presenter must be knowledgeable about the topic and able to answer questions. PowerPoint will not make the speaker a great speaker, nor will it turn a poster presenter into a great presenter. Instead, the graphics program is simply a tool to aid in the development of the presentation or poster.

This section outlines some basic guidelines for preparing a graphic presentation or poster and for delivering the presentation. These guidelines should, of course, be adjusted based on the message and intent of the slide or poster.

Preparing a Presentation

- Begin the presentation with a title slide. The content of the slide should orient the audience to the topic of the presentation and identify the presenter and/or company. A subtitle, date, or clip art may also be added.
- Select a design theme and apply it to the presentation. PowerPoint comes with many preset design templates; even more options are available online

from Microsoft. Other templates are available for purchase from independent providers.

- Use an easy-to-read font. This means a simple upright font without swirls and scripts. Recommended fonts include Times New Roman, Arial, and Garamond.
- Obey the 44/32 guideline: Font sizes for titles should be between 40 and 44 points, whereas font sizes for text should be between 24 to 32 points. It is better to err by making the font too large than to run the risk of making it so small people cannot read the slides from the back of the room.
- Use a maximum of three different fonts in a presentation. Use of too many different fonts will prove distracting to the audience.
- Use both uppercase and lowercase letters for most text. Text that appears in all-capital letters is more difficult to read, although a title or word may be put in all uppercase letters for emphasis.
- Use no more than five to seven words across the slide and five to seven lines down the slide—a guideline that translates to "use phrases and not complete sentences." Use two slides if you need to include more than seven items. Be aware that speakers have a tendency to read the slides if complete sentences are used.
- Limit the use of italics. Words presented in italics are more difficult to read.
- Apply bold and shadow attributes to the text. Boldface increases the stroke weight and projects the words better than plain text. Shadowing fonts puts a crisp edge around the text. For some design templates, however, shadowing the font may produce a blurred image.
- Use bulleted lists to organize the points for the audience. Use no more than three bulleted list slides in a row. The presentation becomes very boring if all slides are bulleted list slides.
- Use clip art, shapes, and SmartArt to add interest to the slides. Make sure that these graphic elements "fit" with the message being conveyed by the slide and that they are an integral part of the slide. For example, place a definition in the "callout" shape or a list of items inside a pyramid.
- Use diagrams instead of complete sentences to describe processes. For example, you might use the shapes or SmartArt features to lay out a process that is being described. People tend to remember things when visuals are added.
- Use an interesting image to signal a break for questions and answers during the presentation.
- Keep special effects and sound to a minimum unless they enhance the presentation. If using special effects or sound, make sure the equipment that will be used for the presentation can handle these options. It can be very distracting when a speaker stops the presentation to try to deal with a special effect that is not functioning.

Preparing a Poster Presentation

There are some minor differences in the guidelines for developing posters as opposed to slide presentations, because a poster is a static visual medium that is displayed on paper and usually mounted on a board. The guidelines given in this section are intended to help you develop quality posters; sometimes, however, they may need to be altered to fit your own unique circumstances.

Planning the Poster Presentation

- How much space is permitted? Most posters are approximately 46 × 45 inches, though some may be either larger or smaller.
- What is the purpose of this poster? What is a logical layout?
- Is there a standard format? For example, a research-based poster would include a title page, introduction, objectives, literature review or theory model, methods (data sources, data collection), results, conclusions, and implications for further work. If there is a funding source, it should always be included on the poster.
- Who is the audience? How much will audience members know about the topic? Are they experts or novices, or both?

Developing the Poster Presentation

- Develop a title page that includes the title of the project, the person or persons involved in the project, and the organization represented. Many organizations also have standard formats for research poster presentations. Usually those formats include elements such as a summary of the project, introduction, research questions, methodology used, results, conclusions, and recommendations for further work. Institutions may also have standard formats for patient educational or recruitment posters.
- Select a design theme and apply it to the poster. This step helps to maintain a consistent style to the poster. Some Web sites provide free or low-cost templates for developing poster presentations. Some institutions also provide design templates for poster presentations that include the logo of the organization. Be sure to follow any applicable guidelines when using a template with an organizational logo to avoid a trademark or copyright issue.
- Use an easy-to-read font—that is, a simple upright font without swirls and scripts. Recommended fonts include Times New Roman, Arial, and Garamond.
- Use the same font throughout the poster. Using different fonts disrupts the fluency and flow of the sentences. Use bullets, bold, italic, or underline to emphasize key words or concepts.
- Make titles and headings larger than the text, but not too large—otherwise, you won't have enough space for the critical content. Text should be visible from a distance of 4–6 feet and serve to entice a person to stop by and examine the poster more closely.

- Use uppercase and lowercase letters. (The same caveats apply here as for a slide presentation.)
- Keep the material simple. Convey your message concisely and provide only pertinent information. Remember that people usually spend only 5–10 minutes at a poster station.
- Use clip art, shapes, and SmartArt to add interest to the poster, but *only* if those graphic elements add to the subject matter.
- Use diagrams to convey processes; use appropriate graphs to display data. Make sure that items are clearly labeled.
- Poster components should flow logically and be self-explanatory. Remember you are telling the what, why, how, and results of the project. Posters may consist of 8- × 11-inch printed sheets arranged on a mounting board, or they may be one sheet of a custom size, such as 48 × 36 inches (which must be printed on a special printer).
- Provide a handout that summarizes the total presentation poster for those interested in the topic. It is usually best if these are no more than one page. The handout can include the poster on the one side and the key points including contact information on the other side.

Preparing an Online Presentation

For an online presentation, follow the guidelines for a quality presentation provided earlier in this section, albeit with some alterations.

- Use a white background template with colored objects. This design results in a smaller file size than do busy, highly colored background templates; smaller files, in turn, speed up the download process.
- Keep image and picture sizes smaller for quicker download and viewing.
- Include speaker notes or narration to elaborate on the content. Remember that adding sound will increase the file size.
- Save the file as a PowerPoint slide show, PDF (Portable Document Format) file with speaker notes, package for CD, and/or Web page. The choice of how you save the file depends on the nature of the presentation and the method of delivery.

Use the spell checker for all slide, poster, and online presentations.

Delivering a Presentation

Getting ready to deliver a presentation requires the speaker to take some steps to ensure that the presentation will go smoothly and achieve its purpose:

- Know the topic and presentation well. Speak about topics on which you are knowledgeable, and practice the presentation so you are familiar with the sequence of slides. Prepare speaker notes to help keep yourself focused on what you intend to say about the slide.

- Face the audience; don't read your slides or speaker notes, but refer to them as needed to reinforce your points. Novice presenters sometimes face the whiteboard or screen and talk to it instead of addressing the audience. If you need to, look at the monitor at the speaker podium instead of turning your back to the audience. The key point here is *look*—do not *read* from the monitor.

- Be prepared to present your materials with a limited view of your slides. Sometimes the slides will appear over your shoulder (i.e., behind you) and not on the monitor in front of you. If your slides appear on the monitor, remember that the audience is looking at the projected slides. Often the projected slides are not as sharp and clear as the ones on the monitor. If the slides are behind you, look at the slides and use a laser pointer to direct the audience's attention to key points on the slides. With this approach, you and the audience are looking at the slides together.

- Use the speaker preparation rooms or student practice rooms to become comfortable with the technology that will be used. The technology—in this case, a PowerPoint presentation, computer, and data projection system— should be transparent to the audience. Remember that the technology is there to enhance the presentation, not to detract from it.

- Slow down and speak up. Nothing loses the audience more quickly than someone who talks too fast or too softly. Practicing the presentation before its actual delivery will help hone these skills.

- Have a backup plan. Technology sometimes fails, so be prepared.

- Keep to the time limit. Most presentations will have a set time for you to present your topic. Practice the timing so you aren't rushed at the end or finish too soon.

Delivering a Poster Presentation

For poster presentations, follow these guidelines:

- Arrive during the scheduled time to arrange your poster in the poster area. Make sure you have mounting supplies if they are not provided by the conference or organization.

- Be present during the scheduled time for poster presentations and be ready to answer questions asked by viewers.

- Provide handouts to further explain the project. Make sure the handouts contain your contact information. You may also have business cards available for viewers who may want additional information. These are easily produced using Word and a laser printer with business card paper or printed at a copy business.

Delivering an Online Presentation

- In an online course, post the presentation by the due date and according to the guidelines provided.
- Many online presentations can benefit from a recording of your voice explaining the slides or, if this is not an option, a script or speaker notes providing the same information.
- Respond professionally to comments made by others.
- Comment professionally about others' presentations. Be constructive and provide suggestions for improvement by giving examples.

Presentation Graphics Terminology

General Terms

Described here are general terms used when discussing presentation graphics software.

Analytic Graphics	Analytic graphics present data in graph form for analysis, understanding, and decision making. Presentation graphics, spreadsheet, or statistics programs can be used to create these graphs.
Density per Inch (DPI)	DPI indicates the pixel density—that is, the number of dots (pixels) per inch. Resolution quality increases with larger DPI.
File Format	The file format is how the program stores the graphic or image—an important consideration for importing data and developing slides. PowerPoint supports several popular graphic file formats, such as Enhanced Metafile (.emf), Graphics Interchange Format (.gif), Joint Photographic Experts Group (.jpg), Portable Network Graphics (.png), and Windows bitmap (.bmp). It also permits users to import multimedia file types such as audio video interleave (avi) and Waveform (wav) for audio and video files.
Handles	Handles are the squares that surround a selected image or block of text when it is viewed on screen. Use the handles to move, enlarge, or shrink the image or text block.
Landscape	Landscape orientation presents a slide in a wide or horizontal view. Use this orientation for on-screen presentations and to produce 35-mm slides.
Pixels	Pixels—more formally, picture elements—are the tiny dots that make up the screen image. The more pixels used, the sharper the image (resolution).

Portrait	Portrait orientation presents a slide in an upright or vertical view. Use this orientation for overhead transparencies and (sometimes) for poster presentations.
Presentation	A presentation is the group of slides that makes up the actual material to be presented. It can vary from an unlimited number of slides to only a few. Remember that more slides are not necessarily better. The general guideline is to use one slide for every 1–3 minutes of a presentation.
Resolution	Resolution is the number of pixels on the screen.
Slides	Slides are the individual screens that make up a presentation.
Slide Layout	Slide layout refers to the way in which the placeholders for the text and images are arranged on the slide. Many different slide layouts are available in PowerPoint.

Graphics Terms

The terms given in this section are used to describe and work with graphics or clip art.

Bullet	A bullet is a graphic that appears to the left of a text list. Different symbols can be used for bullets, such as a dot, arrow, block, or check mark.
Bitmapped	Bitmapped graphics images are stored and represented as pixels (tiny dots). This form is commonly used for clip art images. Examples include the GIF, PCX, and TIF formats.
Clip Art	Clip art is a library of symbols (images) prepared by others for use with specific graphics programs. Additional clip art may be obtained online at the Microsoft Web site or at other image sites. When downloading clip art from Web sites for use in your own presentations, you must obey the applicable copyright laws.
Pictures	Pictures are digital photographs that can be imported and used in a graphic presentation. They are generally in .jpg file format.
Shapes	Shapes are predesigned forms used to enhance the look of the slide. Use them in place of bulleted lists or to show processes. Shapes include rectangles, circles, arrows, callouts, and so forth.
SmartArt	SmartArt is a tool intended to make a simple list more dynamic. Use SmartArt to create graphic lists, show a process, or demonstrate hierarchies. SmartArt adds color and visual interest to slides.

Symbols	Symbols are the clip art or images that are available within, or can be imported into, a presentation program.
Themes	Themes (also called presentation styles in some programs) are professionally designed format and color schemes for a presentation.
Vector Graphics	Vector graphics are images created with lines, arcs, circles, and squares. This file format stores images as vector points. Examples include CGM and PGL.

Slide Layouts

Slide layout refers to the text or content placeholders that appear on a slide as well as the way in which these elements are arranged and formatted on the slide. PowerPoint 2007 includes nine predesigned layouts (see **Figure 6-1**). When the

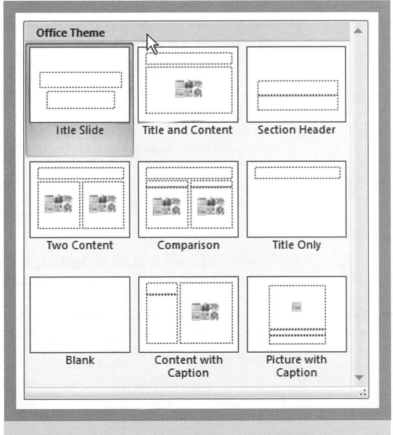

Figure 6-1 PowerPoint Slide Layouts

slide layout uses the term "content placeholder," the content to be added can include a table, SmartArt, picture, clip art, media file, or chart.

Slide Layout Schemes

Common slide layout schemes are described here.

Title Slides	Use title slides to introduce the presentation and to separate sections within the presentation. These kinds of slides are a helpful tool for orienting the audience to the topic and its parts. Title slides can have one or two placeholders.
Title and Content	This slide layout includes one text placeholder, usually for the title, and one content placeholder.
Section Header	A section header has two text placeholders. Use this layout when you have to break a presentation into separate parts.
Two Content	This slide layout includes one text placeholder for the title and two side-by-side content placeholders.
Comparison	This slide layout includes a title placeholder, two text placeholders below it, and two content placeholders below them.
Blank	There are no placeholders in this slide.
Content with Caption	This slide layout features two text placeholders, one for a title and one for explanatory text. The third placeholder is intended to hold content.
Picture with Caption	This slide layout includes two text placeholders and one content placeholder that will accept only pictures.

Charts

PowerPoint has 11 types of charts, with many variations of each being available, plus other types of graphic elements such as organizational charts. The most important point when using charts in your presentation is to pick the correct type of chart—one that visually and accurately conveys the data. The most commonly used types of charts are listed below; see **Figure 6-2** for some example charts.

Chart Types

Area	Area charts present or emphasize the total quantity (volume) of several items over time.
Bar	Bar graphs compare data against some value at a specific point in time. The categories (similar to types of antibiotics) are arranged vertically in a column on the y-axis, whereas the values (rating

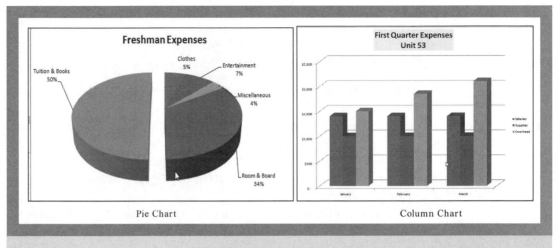

Figure 6-2 Examples of Chart Types

effectiveness) are arranged horizontally on the *x*-axis. The emphasis with this type of chart is on the comparison, not time.

Column   Column graphs show data changes over time or illustrate comparisons. The data or values are presented vertically (*y*-axis), whereas the categories appear horizontally (*x*-axis)—the reverse of bar charts. Many variations of column charts exist.

Doughnut   Doughnuts are variations of pie charts. They compare parts to the whole but can combine more than one data series.

Line   Line graphs present a large amount of data to show trends over time.

Pie   Pie graphs compare parts to a whole or several values at one point in time. They also help to emphasize a particular part or to show relationships between sets of items.

Scatter   Scatter graphs show trends or statistics, such as averages, frequency, regression, or distribution.

Chart Terms
Charts are used to visually represent data in a meaningful fashion. Chart terms describe the components used when creating charts.

Labels   Labels refer to the groups that represent the content of graph slides. They help the user to understand the graph (e.g., the names given to each pie wedge or bar).

x-**Axis**   The *x*-axis refers to the horizontal reference lines or coordinates of a graph.

y-Axis   The *y*-axis refers to the vertical reference lines or coordinates of a graph.

Introduction to PowerPoint

PowerPoint is the graphic presentation program provided as part of the Microsoft Office suite. It provides the user with the ability to design, create, and edit presentations. These presentations can be displayed to the target audience in several ways: as transparencies, using computer screens, as Web pages, as 35-mm slides, as handouts or notes, as posters, and even as workbooks. **Figure 6-3a** shows the PowerPoint screen for Microsoft Office 2007, and **Figure 6-3b** shows the PowerPoint screen for Office 2008 for the Mac.

PowerPoint screens have many similarities to Word and Excel, especially in terms of the title bar, ribbon, and groups. For a quick overview of creating presentations, click the Help icon ⓦ on the right side of the screen and type "create a presentation." Select the appropriate hypertext link for creating a presentation. Much of the help is now available only online at Microsoft's Web site, so make sure the Internet connection is active.

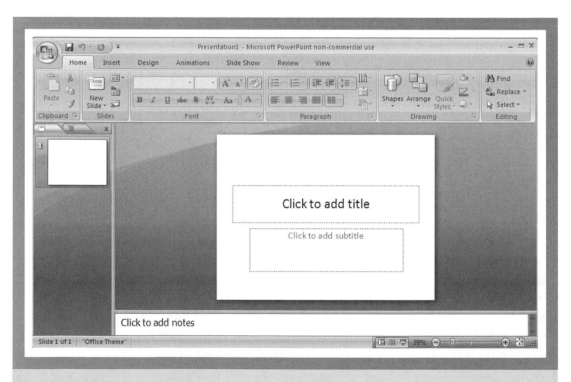

Figure 6–3a PowerPoint Screen in Office 2007

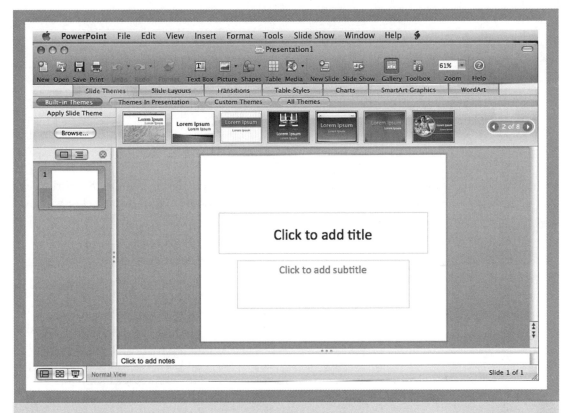

Figure 6-3b PowerPoint Screen in Office 2008 for Mac OS X

To start PowerPoint:

1. **Click** the **Start** button on the taskbar. **Select All Programs**, **Microsoft Office**, and then **click Microsoft Office PowerPoint 2007**. Some systems place PowerPoint on the Start menu in the pin area.
2. **Click** the **PowerPoint** icon in the Quick Launch area.
3. Double-click the icon of a previously prepared PowerPoint presentation.

The main PowerPoint ribbon with the Home tab selected is shown in **Figure 6-4**. Comparing Figure 6-4 with the corresponding Figure 5-4 from the Word and Figure 7-3 from the Excel chapters demonstrates how similar the ribbon is. When the pointer is positioned over one of the ribbon buttons, a box appears with the name of the command that the button represents. These floating toolbar button descriptions are called tooltips or ScreenTips.

The first two tabs (Home and Insert) and last two tabs (Review and View) are the same for PowerPoint, Word, and Excel. The middle tabs—Design, Animation

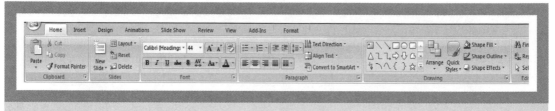

Figure 6-4 PowerPoint's Home Tab and Groups

and Slide Show—relate to PowerPoint features. The buttons to the far right end of the title bar contain window controls to restore, minimize, and close windows.

As in Word and Excel, the Quick Access toolbar can be customized in PowerPoint.

PowerPoint Ribbon Options

Home   The Home tab contains commands that are similar to those available in other Microsoft applications. They include groups such as Clipboard, Font, Paragraph, and Editing that are like those found in Word and Excel. In addition, groups specific to Slides deal with slide layouts, creation of new slides, and so forth. The Drawing group is similar to the Insert, shapes option in Word. See Figure 6-4.

Insert   The Insert tab provides options for inserting tables; illustrations such as pictures, shapes, clip art, SmartArt; links (hyperlinks); text such as text boxes, headers and footers, and WordArt; and media clips. See **Figure 6-5**.

Design   The Design tab contains options for changing the page setup, themes, and background.

Animations The Animations tab contains commands for previewing a slide show, adding animations, and adding the transitions between slides. See **Figure 6-6**.

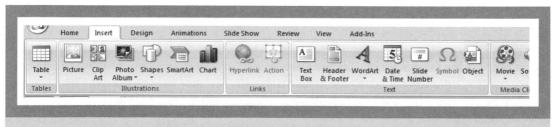

Figure 6-5 PowerPoint's Insert Tab and Groups

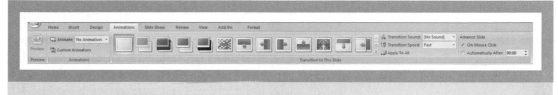

Figure 6-6 PowerPoint's Animations Tab with Groups

Slide Show   The Slide Show tab has options for starting the presentation, setting it up, and determining how it will be displayed. These commands provide for inserting sounds, animation, special effects during transitions between slides, and automation. See **Figure 6-7**.

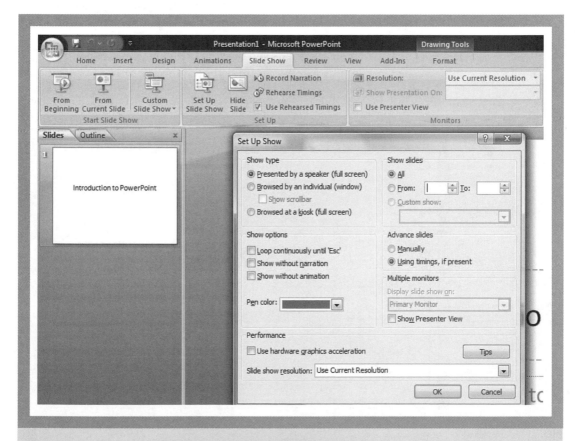

Figure 6-7 Slide Show Tab with Set Up Slide Show Selected

Review   The Review tab is similar to the tab in Word but includes only proofing, comments, and protect commands.

View   The View tab is also similar to Word's View tab but includes a presentation view instead of a document view, as well as show/hide, zoom, window, and macros options. It also contains a group of commands for changing the color to a gray scale and black and white.

Like Word and Excel, PowerPoint includes additional tabs that appear during certain functions, such as when you use the table and drawing tools.

Creating a New Presentation

Before creating a new presentation, consider your audience, think about what information you want to share with them, and decide the best way to present that information. Create an outline of the major points to be covered.

1. Start PowerPoint. The PowerPoint main screen opens. By default (clicking on the New Slide icon), the user is presented with a title slide layout screen using a blank presentation template (**Figure 6-8**).
2. **Click** the **Title** placeholder, and **type** the **title** of the presentation.
3. **Click** the **Subtitle** placeholder, and **type** the **subtitle** for the presentation.
4. **Click** the **New slide** button down arrow on the Home tab, Slides group.

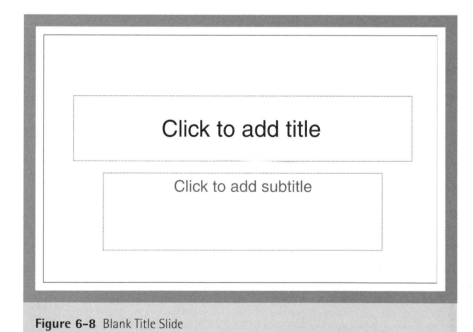

Figure 6-8 Blank Title Slide

5. **Select** a **layout** from the Office Theme dialog box. (See Figure 6-1.) By default, the next slide will be a title and content slide unless you change it.

6. **Type** the **text** and continue adding new slides until the presentation is complete.

PowerPoint has many templates and themes. To access them, **click** the **Office** button, and then **click New** on the menu that appears. Some of the options available are blank and recent templates, installed templates and themes, and Office Online. See **Figure 6-9** for examples of the options that appear when the installed templates option is selected. You might want to access the Introducing Power-Point 2007 template, which provides an overview of some of the new capabilities available in the 2007 version of PowerPoint.

Blank Presentation   This is the default template used when PowerPoint opens. Slides that use this template have minimal design and no color applied to them. Replace the text in the title and subtitle placeholders with appropriate content,

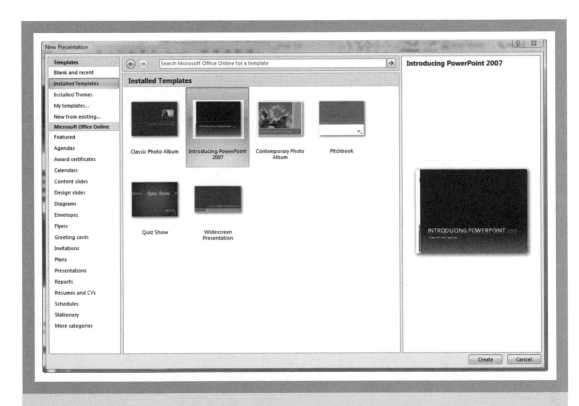

Figure 6-9 Options for Themes and Templates

and then **click** the **New Slide** button to continue adding slides. The ribbon provides options to change the design, layout, and background of the presentation and/or slides as well as options to add and format graphics and apply transitions and animation.

Template

This option presents a variety of templates to apply to the presentation. Think of it as being a sort of "starter document." A template is a pattern or blueprint of a slide or group of slides that is saved as a .potx file. **Figure 6-10** shows examples of the templates available from Microsoft's Web site. Many helpful templates reside on the

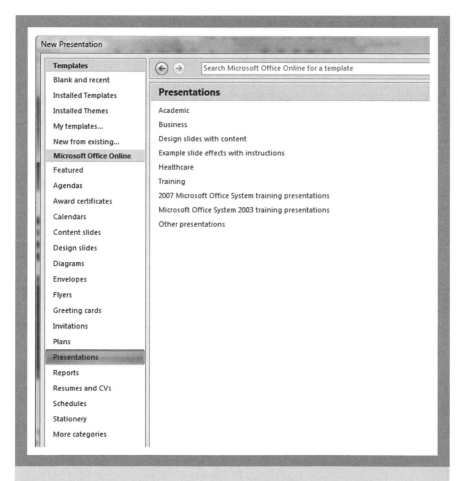

Figure 6-10 Example Templates from Microsoft's Web Site

Web site, so make sure you have an active Internet connection and a legal copy of the software to access them.

Templates generally include layouts, a theme color and fonts, background styles, and, in some cases, suggested content. Users can also design their own template or use one created by their institution. Under Office Online's "More categories" are a few poster presentation templates.

No matter which template is selected, it should not be too busy or distracting. The template should match the topic of the presentation and help to reinforce what is being discussed in the presentation.

Themes   Themes are displayed in the Themes gallery in the Design tab. Every document created in Office 2007 has a theme attached to it. Themes do not contain text or data, but rather certain colors, fonts, or effects that are applied to each slide. Themes replace the slide designs found in earlier versions of PowerPoint. They contain multiple master slides for title slides, speaker notes, and audience handouts.

Existing Presentation   This option creates a copy of an existing presentation so that it can be changed without altering the original file. The user is free to change the design, delete or add new slides, or change the content of existing slides.

New slides can also be inserted into a current presentation from another presentation. With the current presentation open, **click Insert** on the menu bar, and then **click Slides from Files**. Browse to the presentation from which the slides will come, and select the slides to insert.

Developing a Presentation

Most users will start with either a blank presentation or select a template from the gallery of templates installed on the computer or available online. After clicking the template desired, the user can also choose to change the color scheme of that template (**click** the **Design** tab, and then **click** a **Theme**) or add an animation scheme (**click** the **Animation** tab, **click** a **transition** type, and **click Apply to all**). Most users select the template and then move to the slide layout.

To develop a presentation, first complete the title slide information, and then click **New Slide**. To apply the default layout (title and content), **click** the **New Slide** button. To select a different slide layout, click the down arrow button. Pick one of the layouts from the menu of options.

Now begin typing the presentation. Typing can be done directly on the actual slide or in outline view, which works well for organizing the presentation and ensuring a logical flow of ideas. If you choose the second approach, it is easy to add or delete parts of the outline. The decrease and increase indent buttons in the Paragraph group promote and demote content or slides. The Tab key and Shift + Tab key combination also do the same thing. If you right-click on a slide in outline view, a menu of options appears for working with slides and slide content; see **Figure 6-11** for a list of the commands. Slides may also be reordered or deleted.

Objects on the slide do not appear in outline view, nor does text created as an object or with TextArt. The only text that shows in this view is that found in text placeholders. Beware that outline view may lead you to use all text slides, which violates good design guidelines.

As you continue to develop the presentation, you may find that you need to use the table, chart, or graphic slide layouts.

To change or select a new slide layout:

1. **Click** the **New Slide** button, and then select the correct slide layout from the Office Theme dialog box.

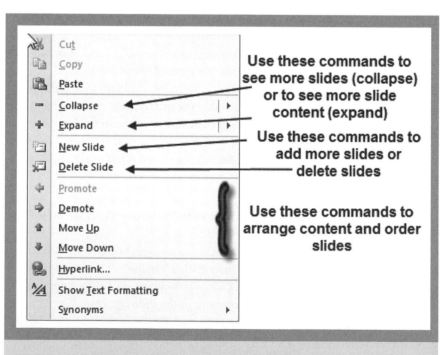

Figure 6-11 Shortcut Menu When Working in Outline View

2. Alternatively, select the correct slide layout from the **Layout** button [Layout ▾] in the Slides group of the Home tab. The screen shown in Figure 6-1 appears, and the correct slide layout is chosen.

You can also move back and forth between the Outline and Slides tabs. In fact, after typing an outline segment, you can go to the tab and review the entire slide presentation. View buttons make this easy to do.

View Buttons

The view buttons [⊞ ⊞ ☐] located at the lower-right side of the screen are used to scroll through the different views of the slide presentation. These choices (and a few others) can also be found under the View tab in the Presentation group. Use these buttons to move between different views of the presentation.

The **normal** view [⊞] is used by default. It contains three parts: the slide, the notes pane at the bottom, and the left pane for seeing all of the slides or outline view. The user works on one slide at a time in this view. The chevron keys at the bottom of the right scroll bar allow you to go back and forth between slides.

The **slide sorter** view [⊞] displays the entire presentation so that slides may be easily rearranged. This view gives you an opportunity to view the presentation in its entirety. To move a slide, simply click it and drag it to a new location. Slides may also be selected and easily duplicated in this view. Transition effects can also be added in the slide sorter.

The **slide show** view [☐] is the best way to view the slide show. Transitions from one slide to another or any special effects or sounds can easily be seen in this view. Press the **Esc** key or right-click the mouse to end the slide show.

To access the **outline** view, click the **Outline** tab in the left pane of the window; the notes page view can be accessed at the bottom part of the screen. The notes section of the normal view is used to create and edit the presentation speaker's notes.

To see and edit the total **notes page** view, **select** the **View** tab, **Notes page** option. At this point, the slide may be made smaller, making more room available for notes. The text placeholder can also be enlarged, making it easier to see. Similarly, the font may be enlarged.

The **View** tab also contains the **master view** options. Use this tab to alter the master slide; it includes both a title slide and subsequent slides. Altering the master view affects all of the slides in the presentation. If you want to alter all of the notes pages or handout pages, click those options in the Presentation Views group of the View tab.

Adding Clip Art, Pictures, and Sound

Several hundred clip art pictures are included with PowerPoint as well as some sounds and movies; thousands more are available online. A Search feature is available that can help you locate a particular piece of clip art. Pictures may also be added to the Art Gallery from CD collections, from the Web, or even from a scanned photo.

To add clip art:

1. **Click** the **New slide** button . The title and content slide should appear by default. If not, **click** the **New Slide down arrow** and **select** a **Title and Content** option.
2. **Click** the **Insert clip art image** in the add text placeholder (**Figure 6-12**); the Clip Art task pane opens on the right side of the screen.
3. **Type** the **word** that represents the clip art in the search box, and **click Go**. Either a gallery of clip art or a message saying "No results found" appears.

Clip art and pictures may also be inserted in the normal view from the Insert tab when they are not to be placed in an object placeholder. In the normal view, **select** the **Insert** tab, and then **choose Picture or clip art** from the Illustrations group. When using the Clip Art Gallery for the first time, PowerPoint must create a clip art database; to do so, click **Yes** in the dialog box if it comes up.

Several choices are available to you when searching for clip art. First, you can search for a specific type of clip art by typing a name of something such as "cat" or "dog" (see **Figure 6-13**); all clip art of a cat or dog will then appear. Second, you can locate clip art by using the Organize Clip Art option on the

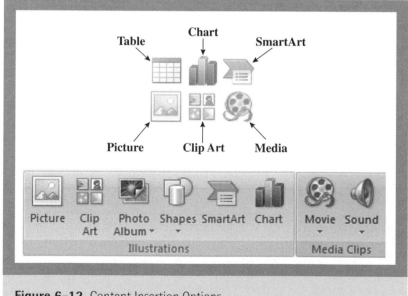

Figure 6-12 Content Insertion Options

task pane; it provides the ability to look for clip art by categories such as "business," "technology," and "health." Finally, you can find clip art on the Internet either at Microsoft's Web site (by selecting Clips Online) or by going to other Internet sites and saving the images found there. Always pay attention to copyright issues when selecting clip art online. Clip art found from other Web sites may be inserted by using the Insert tab and selecting the appropriate pictures: Locate the picture, click it, and then click **Insert**. Clip art from any file can be inserted into PowerPoint as long as the graphic is saved in a compatible graphic file format.

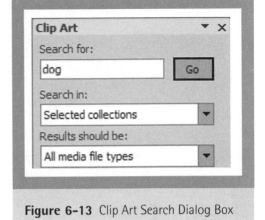

Figure 6-13 Clip Art Search Dialog Box

Digital pictures may also be inserted into Power-Point presentations. To do so, follow the same procedure used to insert clip art from a Web site. These files should be saved before you try inserting them into the presentation. Be aware that digital pictures can dramatically increase the size of the presentation. Pictures may also be inserted in current slides by **clicking** the **Insert** tab, and **selecting pictures** in the Illustrations group.

To add pictures:

1. **Click** the **New slide** button ![New Slide]. The title and content slide should appear by default. If not, **click** the **New Slide down arrow** and **select** a **Title and Content** option.
2. **Click** the **Insert picture** image ![icon] on the Insert object placeholder (Figure 6-12). The Insert Picture dialog box appears.
3. **Select** the **Location and File name** for the picture.
4. **Select** the picture file and **click Insert**. The picture is now inserted into the slide.

Pictures and clip art may be moved and resized.

Movies and **sounds** may also be inserted into and played as part of a PowerPoint presentation. Movies are video files that have extensions such as .avi, .mov, and .mpeg. Animated files include motion; they carry a .gif file extension. These files contain multiple images that are streamed together to produce the effect of animation. Although not technically a movie, animations can demonstrate a process or motion.

To add a movie or sound:

1. Display the slide to which the sound or movie is to be added.
2. **Select** the **Insert** tab and then either **Movie** or **Sounds** from the Media Clips group.

3. **Select** the location and file that contains the movie or sound.
4. At the prompt, choose whether the sound or movie is to play automatically or with a mouse click.

A few sounds and animated .gif files come with the installed version of Power-Point. Others can be found at Microsoft's Web site or on the Internet. Movie and sound files are linked files; in other words, they are linked to the presentation, but are not embedded in it like clip art or pictures. When the presentation has linked files, those files must be copied along with the presentation if another computer will be used for the presentation.

Adding a Table

Use tables to summarize data, place information in categories, show research results, or help the viewer make comparisons between items.

To add a table:

1. **Click** the **New Slide** button in the Slides group of the Home tab. A new title and content slide appears.
2. **Click** the **Insert** table option in the new slide. **Figure 6-14** shows the Insert Table dialog box.
3. **Type** in the number of columns or use the arrows to select a number.
4. **Press** the **Tab** key, and **type** the number of rows or use the arrows to select a number.
5. **Click OK** when you are finished.
6. When the table contents are completed, **click** outside the table on the slide.
7. **Select** the **Title** placeholder and **type** the title of the slide.

A table created in PowerPoint functions just like a table created in a Word document. That means you can use the Tab key (or Shift+Tab) to move around the table. When working in the table, a Table Tools tab appears with two additional tabs: Design and Layout. You add rows and columns to the PowerPoint table in the same way you would do so in Word.

Remember, however, that a slide contains a limited amount of space. Having too many rows or columns in a table will render its contents unreadable.

Adding a Chart (Graph)

As mentioned earlier in this chapter, charts are pictorial representations of data. In PowerPoint (unlike in Excel), you choose the type of chart you want first and then either add data or import data from Excel.

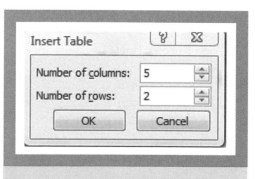

Figure 6-14 Insert Table Dialog Box

To add a chart or graph:

1. **Select** the **New Slide** button. The new title and content slide appears.
2. **Click** the **Insert Chart** option 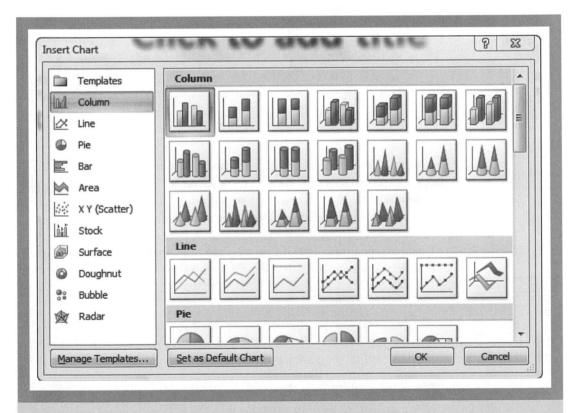 in the new slide. The window in **Figure 6-15** appears, allowing you to select the type of chart to insert.
3. **Select** a type of chart and **click OK.** The window splits in two, with Power-Point appearing on the left and a spreadsheet on the right. See **Figure 6-16**.
4. **Type** the correct data in the spreadsheet screen, replacing what is there by default. As the correct data and labels are entered, the chart changes on the left side of the screen. Filling in the data sheet is much like completing an Excel spreadsheet.
5. Once data are entered, if the data sheet has too many columns, clear the ones not needed. You may also add rows and columns if necessary.

Pie charts are good choices for comparing parts to the whole. Bar and column charts compare different items over time. Line charts show progress over time or multiple data sets.

Figure 6-15 Types of Charts Available in the Insert Chart Dialog Box

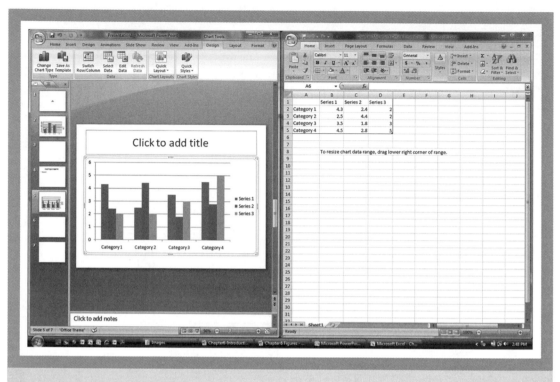

Figure 6-16 Adding Data to a Graph

When you single-click the graph, you can then move or change it as desired. **Right-click** the graph and **select Edit data** option or **select** the **Design** tab, **Edit Data** option to make the data sheet return. Note that three additional tabs are available under the Chart tools tab—Design, Layout, and Format—that enable you to adjust the graph.

There is much more to learn about graphs and charts, of course. Be sure to look at the documentation that comes with PowerPoint and keep experimenting!

Adding a Hyperlink

Hyperlinks are used to take the user someplace else or to provide additional information about a topic. PowerPoint permits the use of hyperlinks to go directly to a specific slide within the presentation or to go to a place on the Internet.

To add a hyperlink:

1. **Select** the text or object that will be used to access the linked site or slide.
2. **Select** the **Insert** tab, **Hyperlink** option in the Links group. **Figure 6-17** shows the Insert Hyperlink dialog box.
3. Make the appropriate selections and **click OK**.

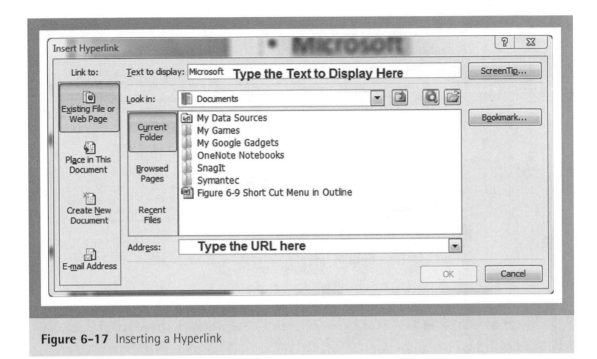

Figure 6-17 Inserting a Hyperlink

The hyperlink will not work unless you are in slide show view; if the hyperlink goes to an Internet site, you must also have an active Internet connection. A link to other slides in the presentation can also be made from the Insert Hyperlink dialog box.

Adding SmartArt

SmartArt graphics provide the ability to add visual representations of information and ideas. Their many different layouts provide a quick way to communicate a message without a lot of text. Such illustrations and graphics help the audience understand and remember the information better than text-only presentations can. They are also more visually interesting. Some of the SmartArt options are shown in **Figure 6-18**. You do not need to spend time creating these illustrations; simply select the appropriate one and type in the content.

To create a SmartArt graphic:

1. **Click** the **New Slide** button. A new title and content slide appears. Alternatively, click the **Insert** tab, **SmartArt** button in the Illustrations group.
2. **Click** the **Insert SmartArt** option ⬛. Figure 6-18 shows the Choose a SmartArt Graphic dialog box.
3. **Select** the type and layout of the SmartArt to be inserted.
4. Enter the text by clicking in a shape and typing the text or by clicking the [**text**] placeholder in the text pane and typing or pasting the text. Text may also be copied from another program and pasted into the text pane.

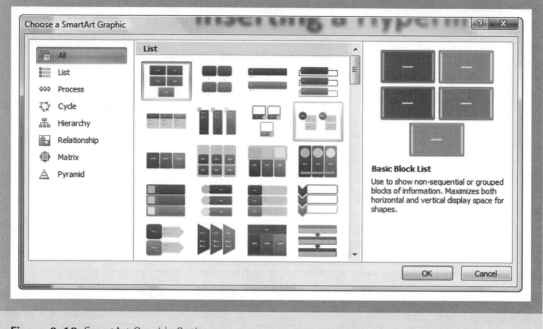

Figure 6-18 SmartArt Graphic Options

Adding Transitions to a Slide Show

When graphic presentations are prepared as an electronic slide show, transitions (animations) can be added to parts or all of the slide show to make it flow more smoothly. Slide transitions are animation-like effects that appear when moving from one slide to the next during an on-screen presentation. A custom animation lets each object on the slide appear separately. The speed of each slide transition and any associated sound can be controlled as well.

As a general rule, transitions should move the presentation along without distracting from the key points of the presentation. For this reason, it is usually more effective to use the same transition or complementary transitions throughout the presentation unless a specific transition is being used to reinforce a specific point.

Figure 6-19 shows the choices for slide transitions. They include no transition, fade, cut, dissolve, and wipe, with variations on these options also being available. To see additional transitions, **click** the **More** arrow ▼.

To add the same slide transition to all slides in the presentation:

1. With the presentation open, select the **Animations** tab.
2. **Click** the transition effect to apply.
3. **Click** the **Apply to All** button 🔲 Apply To All in the **Transition to slide** group.

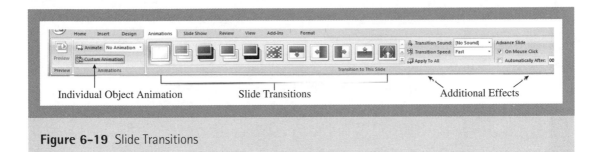

Figure 6-19 Slide Transitions

4. **Click** the **Transition speed down arrow** ⬛ Transition Speed: Fast ▾ to set the transition speed to fast, medium, or slow.

To add different transitions to a specific slide or group of slides:

1. In the slide sorter view, **click** the **slide** to which the transition will be applied.
2. **Click** the **transition** effect to apply.
3. **Click** the **next slide** to which to apply a transition.
4. **Click** the **transition** effect to apply.
5. Repeat this process until all slides that need a transition have one.

Adding Custom Animations

Custom animations apply a special visual effect or sound to text or other objects on the slide such as diagrams, clip art, and charts. For example, each bulleted item may appear in an animation by "flying in" or "dissolving in," giving you an opportunity to discuss the point before the next bulleted item appears.

Custom animations can be applied using a preset animation scheme or can be applied to each item individually on the slide. Be careful to ensure that any animation used adds clarity to the message, rather than detracts from it. Most users carefully select items for custom animations and do not apply them to the total presentation. This provides some variety and interest to the presentation without boring the audience.

To activate the custom animation option:

1. **Select** the part of the slide to animate by clicking the object, such as a bulleted list or clip art.
2. **Click** the **Animations** tab and then the **Custom Animation** button ⬛ Custom Animation. The Add Custom Animation task pane appears on the right side of the screen.
3. **Click** the **Add Effect** button, and then click **Effect**. See **Figure 6-20** for the available options.
4. **Click** a specific effect.

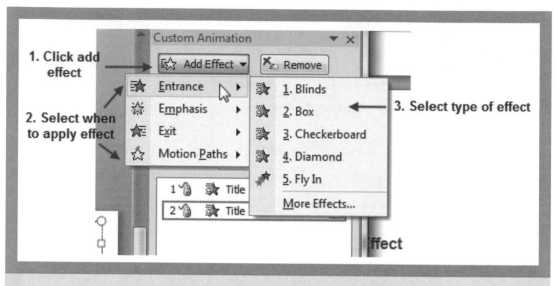

Figure 6-20 Custom Animation Options

Some of the many animation choices include options for playing a sound, adding one letter at a time, and adjusting the speed of the animation. In addition, previous bulleted items may be dimmed as each new one appears.

Changing a Presentation Design

The theme of a presentation can always be changed.

With the presentation open, to change the theme:

1. **Click** the **Design** tab.
2. **Choose another theme** from the options in the **Themes** group.

When you place the mouse pointer over a different theme and hold it there without clicking, the slide displays the new look. You can check out all the possibilities before choosing the one you like.

To change text or objects for all slides in the presentation, use the master slide. This template is used for all slides in the presentation and is the place where items such as corporate or university logos are added to all slides. You can also change the text properties of all slides by modifying the master slide.

To change text or objects for all slides:

1. **Select** the **View** tab, then **Slide Master** from the **Presentation Views** group.
2. **Click** the specific **master slide** from the left pane.
3. **Select** the **text** or **text placeholder** on the master slide that is to be changed.

4. Change the text properties (e.g., bold, shadow, font size, color).
5. **Click** the **Close Master View** button 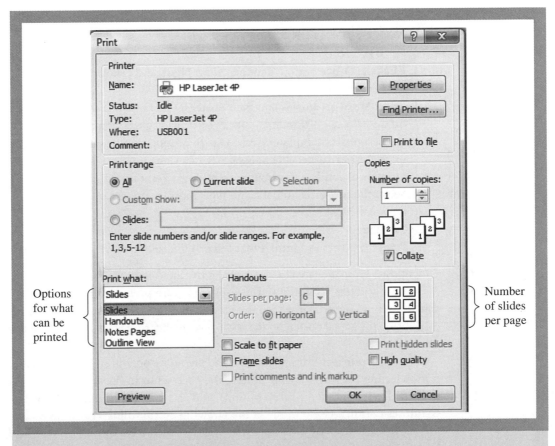 to exit the slide master view.

Printing with PowerPoint

PowerPoint has many options for printing various parts of the presentation.
To print overheads, audience handouts, notes, or a presentation outline:

1. **Click** the **Office** button and then **Print. Figure 6-21** shows the Print dialog box.
2. **Select Slides, Handouts, Notes page**, or **Outline**.
3. Check the other settings to make sure that they are correct, and then **click OK**.

The Slides option prints the entire presentation using one slide per page. The default option uses 8½- × 11-inch paper. The **Handouts** option prints a smaller

Figure 6-21 Print Dialog Box

version of the slides, with the number of slides selected per page (i.e., 1, 2, 3, 4, 6, or 9 slides per page). The **Notes page** option prints a slide at the top of the page, with the notes appearing on the bottom half of the page; this option prints one slide per page. The **Outline** option prints all of the text shown in the outline view. Make sure the outline is expanded to see all the text in the outline.

Be sure to choose the correct option before printing so that only what is needed is printed. If you are printing handouts, print one page of three or six slides to a page to decide which format will work the best for your audience. Avoid printing handouts before the presentation is complete and all revisions have been made. Always run the spell checker, and consider using AutoCorrect to handle misspellings as you work.

Developing a Poster Presentation Using PowerPoint

Use PowerPoint to develop professional-level poster presentations. Make sure you follow the guidelines given earlier in the chapter when doing so.

To create a poster from a template:

1. Open PowerPoint.
2. **Click** the **Office** button, and then **New. Figure 6-22** shows a list of the categories available.
3. **Select More categories** and then **Posters**. (You must have Internet access for this choice.) A thumbnail sketch of available posters appears.
4. **Select** a poster template. A message may appear stating that only legitimate users can access the templates. **Click Continue** and follow any screen prompts to confirm that your copy of PowerPoint is legal.
5. **Select** the text placeholders, and type appropriate text or add graphics to replace them.
6. **Save** the file.
7. **Print** the poster to a printer that will print in color and handle larger paper.

Other poster templates are also available on the Internet.

Some templates, as noted in the zoom area, are presented at 18% of their actual size so that you can see the total layout and design of the template. When working on the actual poster, set the zoom level higher so that you can see the text placeholders.

You can create a custom poster size and layout by opening a blank presentation, selecting the blank layout, setting the page setup to the width and height desired (**Design** tab, **Page setup** option), and showing the gridlines (**View** tab, **Gridlines** option). Use options in the Drawing group to insert text boxes and format them as desired. Be aware that creating such a customized poster will be much more time-consuming than simply finding and adjusting an already designed poster template.

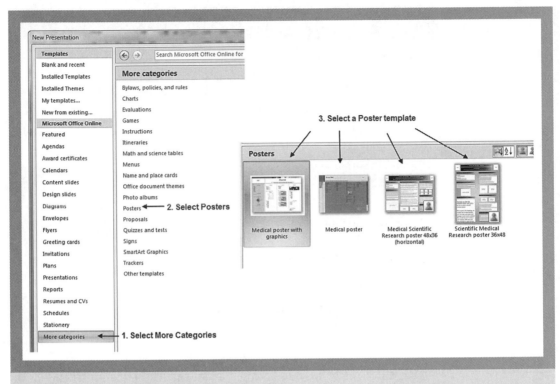

Figure 6-22 Poster Templates

Summary

PowerPoint is a powerful program that can help you produce presentations and posters that are professional and make the appropriate points with the audience. This chapter has outlined the beginning steps you need to follow to produce a PowerPoint slide presentation or poster.

EXERCISE 1 Creating a PowerPoint Presentation*

■ **Objectives**

1. Create slides using correct information.
2. Create a bulleted list slide.
3. Edit slides by altering the formatting and placement of objects.
4. Insert and adjust clip art from the clip organizer and from Microsoft's Web site.
5. Save the presentation.

■ **Activity**

1. Create a title slide.
   a. **Start** PowerPoint. A blank title slide appears.
   b. **Click** the **Design** tab and then **select** the **Flow** theme in the **Themes** group.
   c. **Click** the mouse over each one to see the name.
   d. **Type Using Technology in Health Care**.
   e. **Click** the **subtitle placeholder**.
   f. **Type By** and press the **Enter** key.
   g. **Type your name**.

2. Add a bulleted list slide.
   a. **Click** the **New slide** button [New Slide] on the **Home** tab under the **Slides** group. A new title and content slide appears.
   b. **Click** the title placeholder.
   c. **Type Information System: What Is It?**
   d. **Click** the text placeholder.
   e. **Type Hardware**.
   f. Press the **Enter** key, and **type Software**.
   g. Press the **Enter** key, and **type Data**.
   h. Press the **Enter** key, and **type Communications**.
   i. Press the **Enter** key, and **type People**.
   j. Press the **Enter** key, and **type Policies and Procedures**.
   k. **Click** outside the bulleted list placeholder.

3. Edit the title slide.
   a. **Click** the **title** slide in the left pane.
   b. **Click** the **subtitle** placeholder.
   c. **Click** the **border** of the subtitle placeholder.
   d. **Select Garamond** and **20** points from the **Font** group on the **Home** tab. The name and font change.

---

*This exercise was modified from one used at La Roche College, IST105 Online. It is used with the permission of Irene Joos.

e. With the subtitle placeholder still selected, place the cursor along a border unit until it turns to a four-headed arrow. Drag the placeholder down farther on the slide.

4. Edit the bulleted list slide.
   a. **Click** the **bulleted list** slide in the left pane.
   b. **Click** the **text** (content) placeholder **border**.
   c. With the double-headed arrow on the right border, **drag** the **right text placeholder border** to the left about 2 inches. The text placeholder is now smaller.
   d. With the double-headed arrow on the right border, **drag** the text place-holder to the right until the "H" in "Hardware" is under the "f" in "Information."

5. Insert clip art and pictures.
   a. **Click** the **title slide** in the slide pane on the left.
   b. **Click** the **Insert** tab, and select **Clip Art** in the **Illustrations** group.
   c. **Click** the **Organize clips** option ⬜ Organize clips... at the bottom of the task pane.
   d. If necessary, **click** the + signs next to the words "Office Collection" and "Technology." **Click** the word technology.
   e. **Select** one of the clip art images by clicking the down arrow on the right side of the image. Select **Copy**.
   f. **Click** the title slide and then click the **Paste** button in the **Clipboard** group in the **Home** tab.
   g. Adjust the placement of the object so that it is arranged on the slide attractively. **Close** the **clip art task pane** on the right.

6. Change the slide layout and insert clip art into a placeholder.
   a. **Click** the **bulleted** slide in the left pane.
   b. **Click** the **Home** tab, **Layout** option in the **Slides** group.
   c. **Click** to select the **Two Content** layout. The slide changes, moving the bulleted list to the left and inserting a content holder on the right.
   d. **Click** the **Clip Art** option ⬜ in the content placeholder.
   e. **Type data** in the search text box, and then **click Go**. If this produces no results, use the word information.
   f. **Click** a clip art down arrow key and **select Copy**.
   g. Enlarge the clip art to be about the same size as the bulleted list content area (click the image and drag the handles).

7. Insert clip art from the Microsoft Web site.
   a. **Click** the **New Slide down arrow** button. The Slide Layout dialog window appears.
   b. **Select Title only slide** from the layout options.
   c. **Click the title placeholder**, and **type Hardware**.
   d. **Click** the **Insert** tab and then the **Clip Art** option.

e. In the clip art task pane, click the **Clip art on Office Online** text 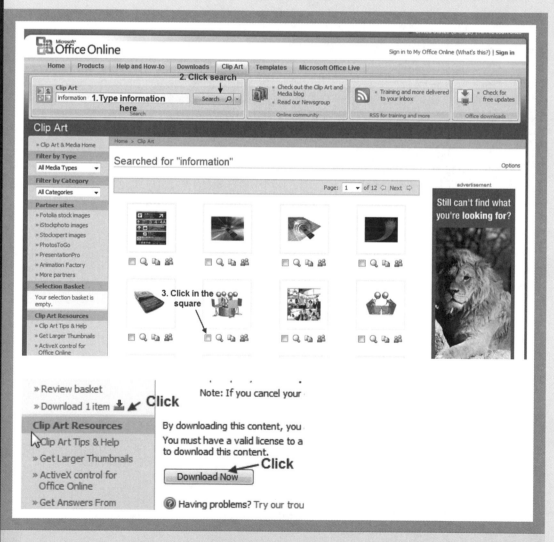 at the bottom of the task pane. Make sure that there is an active Internet connection.

f. Once you are connected to the Internet, type **information** in the search text box and then **click** the **Search** button.

g. **Click** the **square** next to the gold figures with the computers (j0439359.jpg) image. See **Figure 6-23**. You can hover over the images to see their file name. You may also click the image to obtain a pop up window with details about the file. Here you may also click to add the image to the

Figure 6-23 Microsoft's Online Site for Finding Clip Art

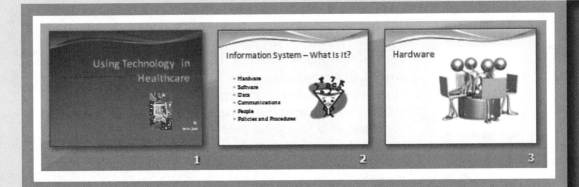

Figure 6-24 Exercise 1: Finished Slides

      download basket and then close the window. Alternatively, you may select any other image desired.

    h. **Click** the **Download 1** item button in the left pane. If necessary, respond to any prompts from Microsoft.

    i. **Click** the **Download Now** button. A message may appear about opening the file. **Click Open**. If any other messages appear, click **Allow** or **Yes**. A window appears with the new clip art in it.

    j. **Click** the **down arrow** next to the new clip art and **select Copy**.

    k. **Click** the slide and **select Paste**. The image now appears in the slide.

    l. Size and move the clip art to fit as shown in Figure 6-24.

8. Save the presentation.

    a. **Click** the **Save** button on the Quick Access toolbar or click the **Office** button, **Save** option. The Save As dialog box appears.

    b. **Click** the **Computer** option on the left and **select** your **USB storage device** on the right.

    c. If you are saving the presentation to a specific folder, select that folder.

    d. **Type** the name of the file (**Chap6-Ex1-Lastname**).

    e. **Click** the **Save** button.

The slides just created should look like those in **Figure 6-24**.

EXERCISE 2   Inserting a Picture and Printing Handouts*

■ **Objectives**

    1. Add a picture to a slide.

    2. Print handouts.

---

*This exercise was modified from one used at La Roche College, IST105 Online. It is used with the permission of Irene Joos.

■ **Activity**

1. Insert a picture from Microsoft's Web site.
   a. **Open** the presentation you created in Exercise 1, and go to the end of it.
   b. **Click** the **New Slide down arrow** button. The Layout dialog box appears.
   c. **Select** the **Title only** layout.
   d. **Click** the **title placeholder** and **type A Picture with Clip Art**.
   e. Find a piece of clip art that is a map of your state. Go to **Clip Art** on Microsoft's Web site and **search** for this map.
   f. **Download** and **copy** the map of your state to the slide.

2. Adjust the location and size of a picture.
   a. **Move** the **map** to the lower-left side of the slide.
   b. **Size** the **map** to be approximately 4 inches.

3. Add another picture to the slide and adjust it.
   a. Find a digital picture of something related to your state or to health care. For example, you might use a picture of some part of your state or city, some part of your campus, or a piece of equipment at a technology center.
   b. **Click** the **Insert** tab, **Picture** option from the **Illustrations** group.
   c. **Select** the drive and folder where the .jpg picture was placed.
   d. **Select** the file, and **click Insert**.
   e. **Enlarge** the picture, if necessary, and **move** it to the upper-right side of the slide, below the title.

4. Insert a text box and use a line tool.
   a. **Click** the **Insert** tab and then the **Insert Textbox** option.
   b. **Drag** the mouse to form a box on the state image, indicating the location where the picture was taken. Type a capital letter **X** in the text box.
   c. **Click** the **Home** tab and the **Line tool** ╲ in the **Draw** group.
   d. **Draw** a line between the X and the Picture.
   e. **Save** the file as **Chap6-Ex2-Yourname**. If your instructor requests it, also print the slide. The slide should resemble that shown in **Figure 6-25** but with your state and picture.

5. Print handouts.
   a. **Click** the **Office** button and then the **Print** option or **click** the **Printer** icon on the Quick Access toolbar. The Print dialog box appears.
   b. **Select Handouts** under the **Print What** options.
   c. **Select** the option to print six slides per page.
   d. **Click OK**. One page containing six slides is printed.

6. Print a set of speaker's notes.
   a. **Click** the **Office** button and then the **Print** option or **click** the **Printer** icon on the Quick Access toolbar. The Print dialog box appears.
   b. **Select Notes page** under the **Print What** options.
   c. **Click OK**. Four pages of notes are printed.

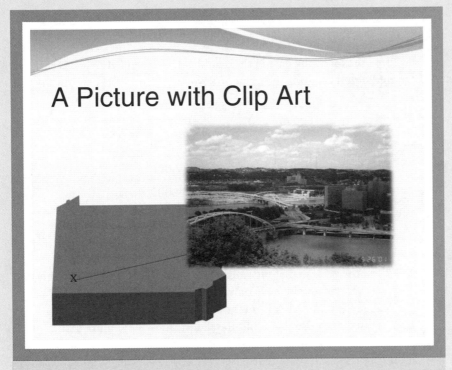

Figure 6-25 Slide with an Imported Picture and Clip Art

EXERCISE 3 Table, Line, Pie, and Bar Graphs

This exercise can be done with PowerPoint or Excel, although our preference is to have you practice with PowerPoint. The table can also be created in Word.

- **Objectives**
  1. Create a computer-generated table, bar, pie, and line graph for use in PowerPoint presentations.
  2. Save and print the presentation.

- **Activity**
  1. Create a table and then convert it to a line chart.
     a. **Start** PowerPoint and **select Title and Content** from the **Layout** button. Remember that all presentations start with a title slide; this one is just for demonstration purposes.
     b. **Select** the **title text placeholder**, "Click to add title" and **type Projected FTE Requirements and Supply of RNs in the U.S.**

c. **Click** the **Insert Table** icon in the middle of the slide. The Insert Table dialog box appears.
d. **Set** the size of the table to **3 columns** and **6 rows. Click OK.**
e. **Type** the following data in the data sheet. (Remember that it is easier to enter numbers using the numeric keypad.)

Year	Requirements	Supply
2010	2,232,000	2,214,000
2015	2,391,000	2,277,000
2020	2,575,000	2,284,000
2025	3,450,000	2,110,000
2030	4,001,000	2,001,000

f. **Adjust** the table so that the words **Year, Requirements,** and **Supply,** the years, and the numbers are right justified.
g. **Change** the font to **Arial** and the size to **18 points.**
h. **Enlarge** the table so that it fills the slide as shown in **Figure 6-26.**

2. Convert a table to a line chart.
   a. If necessary, **click** the slide, and look at it. You will change it to a line chart and compare the two slides for easiest interpretation of the data.
   b. **Click** the **Insert New Slide** button. A new slide appears.
   c. **Click** the **Insert Chart** icon in the middle of the slide.

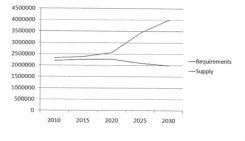

Figure 6–26 Comparison of a Table and a Line Chart

d. **Double Click Line** on the left-hand side and **Line** on the right-hand side. See **Figure 6-27**.

e. **Size** the **right pane window** in the data sheet to cover cells A1 through C6. Use the double-headed arrow at the lower-right corner of the blue line and drag it until the blue lines border all dummy data.

f. **Delete** the dummy data.

g. **Click** the table chart, and then **select** all the data in the table. **Click** the **Copy** button or **press Ctrl+C**.

h. **Click** the chart slide data sheet, and then **click** the **Paste** button or **press Ctrl+V**. The data from the table now appear in the data sheet. Resize the data sheet so that all of the data are visible.

i. **Copy** the title of the slide from the table slide to the chart slide. See Figure 6-26 for the end results.

j. **Save** the file as **Chap6-Ex3-LastName**. If requested to do so by your instructor, print the two slides.

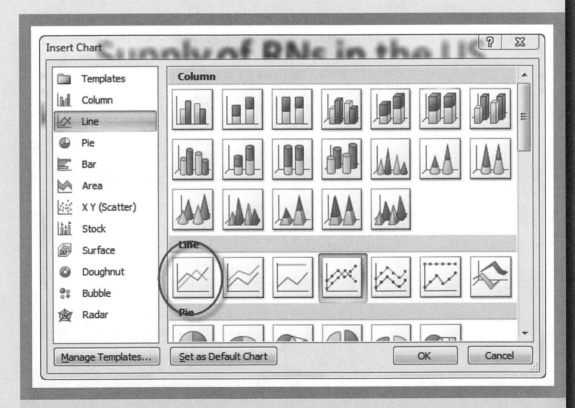

Figure 6-27 Insert Line Chart Options

  k. Which slide presents the data in the clearest manner or a more visually
     pleasing manner that makes it easier to see the trend?
3. Create a pie chart.
  a. Follow directions given previously but create a **3-D Pie chart**. The title
     of the slide should be **How the Money Is Spent**.

Chart title:	**Medicaid/Medicare Expenditures Fiscal Year 2010**	
Items:	**Home Care**	**34%**
	Physician	**18%**
	Hospital	**23%**
	Skilled Care	**24%**
	Others	**1%**

  b. Save the file as **Chap6-Ex3A-Lastname** and print it.
  c. How might you modify this pie chart to enhance it?
4. Reformat a pie chart.
  a. **Click** the **Layout** tab under Chart tools. If you don't have this contextual
     tab, click the chart object and it will appear.
  b. **Click** the **Data Labels** button in the **Labels** group.
  c. **Select More data labels** at the bottom of the menu.
  d. **Place** check marks in **Category name**, **Percent**, and **Show leader lines**,
     and then **click** the **Close** button.
  e. **Click** the **Legends** button and select **None**. The legend disappears from
     the chart.
  f. **Click** the labels once, and pause and **click** again. The labels should sepa-
     rate, and one should be selected.
  g. **Drag** each label a little distance from the pie wedge. Each label will need
     to be moved separately.
  h. **Click** the pie wedge called **Hospital** once; then pause and **click** it again.
     Drag the wedge away from the other wedges. (This format is called
     exploding the wedge.)
  i. **Right-click** the **Hospital** wedge, and select **Format Data Point**.
  j. **Select Fill**, **Gradient fill**. **Click** the **down arrow** for present colors. Select
     the **Gold** option and **click** the **Close** button.
  k. **Change** the colors of the other wedges. See **Figure 6-28** for an example.
  l. **Save** the changes, calling the file **Chap6-Ex3B-Lastname**.
5. Create a bar chart.
  a. **Click** the **New Slide** button. A new slide appears. It should use the title and
     content layout. If it isn't, **click** the **Layout** and **Title and Content** options.
  b. **Click** the **Chart** option in the middle of the slide.
  c. **Select Bar** and then **Clustered bar in 3D**.
  d. **Click OK**.

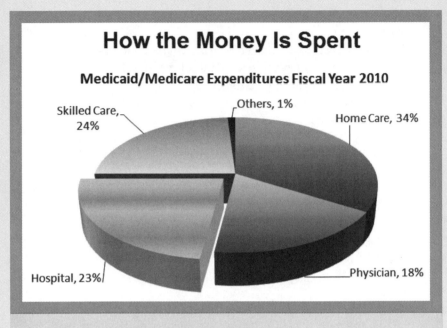

Figure 6-28 Exercise 3: Pie Chart

e. Enter the data into the cells in the same way as done previously. A bar graph appears in PowerPoint.

Dell	8.9
IBM	8
Gateway	7
HP	6.5
Compaq	3

6. Modify a bar chart. The revised chart will have no legend and no title above the chart.
   a. **Click** the **Layout** tab and **Chart Title** in the **Labels** group. Make sure the chart is selected for the Chart tools contextual tab to appear.
   b. **Select** the **Above chart** option and type **Rating***. A chart title appears.
   c. **Click** the data series chart wall. Handles appear around it.
   d. **Click** the **Layout** tab and **select** the **Chart wall down arrow** from the **Background** group.

e. **Select More wall options**; select **Gradient** fill, and type **radial. Click Close** button.

f. **Select** the chart bars (which have handles around them).

g. **Click** the **Format** tab and **select** a fill color of **red**. The bars turn red.

h. **Click** the **Insert** tab and **Textbox** in the **Text** group.

i. **Draw** a rectangle at the bottom of the chart to hold the following text: ***Rating based on price, reliability, performance, warranty, and service**. Adjust the size of the rectangle as needed (see **Figure 6-29**).

j. Save the file as **Chap6-Ex3B-LastName**.

7. Convert a bar chart to a column chart.

a. **Right-click** the bar chart. A shortcut menu appears.

b. **Click Change Chart Type.**

c. **Select** the **Column, 3-D Clustered** chart type.

d. Adjust the chart, applying what you learned from the lesson, practice, and textbook.

e. **Save** the file as **Chap6-Ex3C-LastName**.

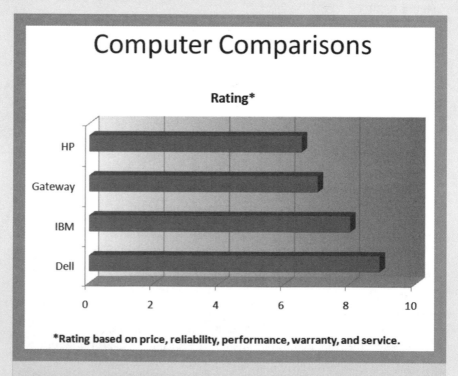

Figure 6–29 Exercise 3: Bar Chart

EXERCISE 4 Shapes, WordArt, and SmartArt

■ **Objectives**

1. Use shapes, WordArt, and SmartArt to enhance the message on a slide.

■ **Directions**

1. Create a new presentation using a design template.
   a. **Open** PowerPoint. A blank presentation appears.
   b. **Click** the **Office** button, and **select New**. A list of options appears.
   c. Under the **MS Office Online** section, click **Design Slides**. A list of design slide categories appears. Make sure you have an active Internet connection.
   d. **Click** the **Healthcare design styles** and other design styles. You can use the back arrow above Healthcare to return to the main list.
   e. **Type Blue Fade Elegance** in the search box and **press Enter**. Accept any Microsoft message that might appear.
   f. **Click** the **Download** button on the lower-right side of the window. The new design slide appears.

   HINT: If you see Microsoft's "Genuine Advantage" message, click **Continue.** The software will check whether you have a legal copy of the software on your computer before it will download the template.

   g. With PowerPoint opened and the new design on the screen, click the **Layout** button in the **Slides** group. **Select** the **Title Only** option (third column, second row) in the Slide Layout window. The title-only slide appears.
2. Add information to a slide.
   a. **Click** the title placeholder "Click to add title" and **type What Does a Computer Do?** The text appears in the title placeholder. (You could also use "What Does a Nurse Do?", "What Does a Radiology Technician Do?", and so forth, substituting appropriate text as necessary.)
   b. If needed, adjust the title size to fit on one line.
   c. **Select** the **Textbox** button in the text group from the **Insert** tab.
   d. **Drag** the mouse to create a text box under the title placeholder.
   e. **Type Convert data to information through processing**. Make sure the text appears on one line and is centered under the title.
3. Make and format a box shape.
   a. **Click** the **Shapes** button in the Illustrator group on the **Insert** tab ribbon. A menu of options appears.
   b. **Select** the **Rectangle** icon (left) under Rectangles category.
   c. With the + cursor, drag on the slide to create a 1½- × 1½-inch box.

    d. With the box selected (handles around it), **click** the **Format** tab under the **Draw Tools** tab. The ribbon changes to reflect the formatting options available.

    e. **Click** the **More** arrow in the **Shape Styles** group. This means to **click** the **More** arrow at the bottom right of the **3 Visual Shapes** not the down arrow to the right of the **Shape Fill** words. Hover over the colors to see their name. A menu of color options appears.

    f. **Click** the **Light Blue** option (Subtle Effect 1—Accent 4). The rectangle changes color.

    g. **Click** the **Shape Outline** button in the **Shape Styles** group. A list of options appears.

    h. **Select No Outline** from the options menu. The outline disappears.

    i. **Click** the **Shapes effects** button. A list of options appears.

    j. **Select** the **Bevel**, **Circle** option. The shape changes.

4. Create additional shapes.

    a. With the shape selected, click the **Copy** button on the **Home** tab, **Clipboard** group.

    b. **Click** the **Paste** button three times. Objects appear stacked on top on each other.

    c. **Drag** one shape to the right side of the slide and the other shape to the left side of the slide. **Drag** the next shape to the top, center of the slide and last one to the bottom, center of the slide. **See Figure 6-30.**

5. Create text for each shape.

    a. **Click** the **Textbox** button on the **Insert** tab, **Text** group. The text box button is selected.

    b. **Drag** inside the left shape to create a text box.

    c. **Type Sends data to processing unit**. Adjust the text to fit the shape and center it in the text box. (Note: You can add text appropriate to what a nurse does or what a radiology technician does if you changed the label earlier.)

    d. Repeat the process for the other three shapes:
- Center, top: **Type Stores data and programs**
- Center, bottom: **Type Executes instructions**, **press** the **Enter** key, **type Memory holds programs and data**
- Right: **Type Makes processed data available**

6. Format the text for each shape.

    a. **Select** the left shape. Click the **Bold** button on the **Home** tab. The text appears in bold.

    b. **Click** the **Center** button on the **Home** tab. The text is centered within the text box.

    c. Repeat this process for each shape.

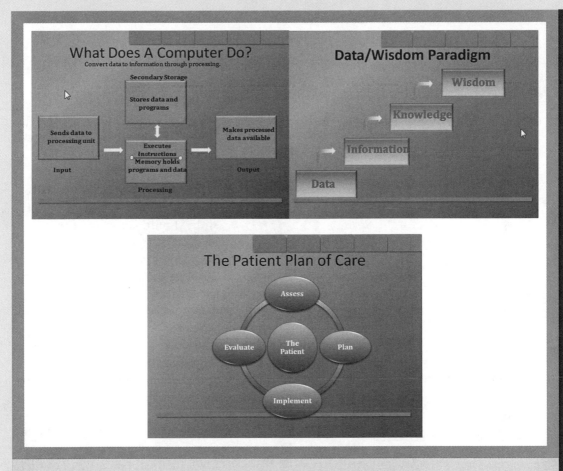

Figure 6–30 Shapes, WordArt, and SmartArt Slides

7. Create a title for each shape.
    a. **Click** the **Textbox** button on the **Insert** tab, **Text** group.
    b. **Drag** the text box under the left shape. Type **Input**.
    c. Repeat the process for each shape:
        ■ Top, center: **Secondary Storage** (Place the text box above the rectangle.)
        ■ Right: **Output**
        ■ Bottom, center: **Processing**
    d. Make each of the shape titles bold.
8. Insert flow arrows.
    a. **Click** the **Shapes** button on the **Insert** tab, **Illustrations** group. A menu appears.
    b. **Select Block arrows**.

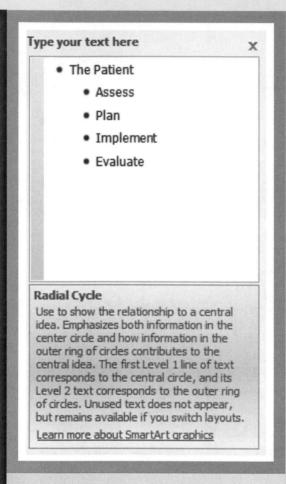

Figure 6-31 Inserting Text in SmartArt Slide

c. Using what you learned earlier while creating the rectangles, **create three arrows** as shown in Figure 6-30. **Recolor** the arrows and adjust them as shown in the slide.

9. Draw a line.

   a. **Click** the **Line draw** tool located under the shapes icon on the **Insert** tab, **Illustrations** group.

   b. **Draw** a line between "Executes" and "Memory" in the "Processing" shape.

   c. **Recolor** the line and enlarge it. The slide should look like the one in Figure 6-30.

   d. Using what you learned here, create the slide shown in Figure 6-30. This slide uses WordArt in the rectangles; you should be able to figure out how to insert WordArt. Use the same design theme as with the previous slide, except make the rectangles gold and the WordArt red. The arrow shapes can also be gold.

10. Create a slide with SmartArt.

    a. **Create** a **new slide** with the Title and Content layout.

    b. **Click** the **Insert SmartArt** button in the middle of the slide.

    c. **Click Cycle** in the left pane and then **Radial cycle** (first column, third row); click **OK**. The SmartArt diagram appears with a screen to the left in which you can type the content.

    d. **Type** the text as shown in **Figure 6-31**.

    e. **Type** a title for the slide: **The Patient Plan of Care**.

    f. **Adjust the size** of the font and make it bold. If the circle needs to be enlarged to fit the text, do so. The end result should match the slide shown in Figure 6-30.

    g. What is the major part missing from this slide? HINT: A connection between the outer circles and Patient circle. Add that connection.

    h. Save the file as **Chap6-Ex4-LastName**.

ASSIGNMENT 1 Create Pie, Line, and Bar Charts

■ **Directions**

1. Create a pie chart.
   a. Find research data that provide information about something related to health care or the nursing shortage. Make sure the information compares parts to a whole (e.g., a comparison of the budget items for a clinical unit).
   b. Create a pie chart using PowerPoint.
   c. Move the legend to the bottom of the slide.
   d. Enhance the title of the slide.
   e. Experiment with different styles of pie charts for presenting the data. Pick the one that most clearly shows the data in the best light.
   f. Save the file as **Chap6-Assign1-1-LastName** and print the slide.
   g. Under which conditions would a pie chart be an appropriate choice?
2. Create a bar chart.
   a. Find research data about the educational levels of practicing nurses from three different years (e.g., 2007, 2008, and 2009) and create a bar chart.
   b. Give the bar chart a title: "Educational preparation of registered nurses: diploma, associate degree, and baccalaureate."
   c. Create a slide with only a title on it so that there is more room for the bar graph and its legend.
   d. Save the file as **Chap6-Assign1-2-LastName** and print the slide.
3. Create a line chart.
   a. Find research data for a clinical trial or clinical problem in your area that would be appropriately depicted as a line chart.
   b. Create a line chart.
   c. Save the file as **Chap6p-Assign1-3-LastName** and print it.
   d. Under which conditions would a line graph be an appropriate choice?
4. Submit the research articles containing the data, the printouts, and the files to your instructor.

ASSIGNMENT 2 Preparing a PowerPoint Presentation

■ **Directions**

Prepare a PowerPoint presentation on a topic related to technology in health care that you will present to the class using a computer and data projector. Use your creativity and the knowledge gained from this chapter to produce quality slides; follow the good design tips given in the chapter.

1. Include a minimum of 10 slides, with at least one of each of the following:
   - Title slide
   - Bulleted list slide
   - Mixed-format slide with a bulleted list and clip art that is integral to the slide
   - Altered clip art on a slide
   - Table slide
   - Graph slide
   - SmartArt slide
   - Recolored shape slide
   - Imported clip art slide
   - Imported picture slide (generally .jpg files)
2. Introduce some variety into the layout of the slides. For example, avoid more than three bulleted list slides in a row. Use some of the shapes to enhance the slides.
3. Create a transition between slides. **Save** the presentation as **Chap6-Assign2-LastName**.
4. **Print** an outline of the presentation and a handout displaying three slides to a page. Prepare at least one notes page. Turn in the printouts or an electronic version of the presentation if instructed to do so.
5. Make sure you add a footer to the slides alerting the audience to the altered clip art, sources of the imported clip art and picture, and altered shape.

Introduction to Spreadsheet

Objectives

1. Identify uses of the spreadsheet in general as well as for healthcare applications.
2. Define basic terminology related to spreadsheets.
3. Review selected functions for using Excel 2007.

Common Spreadsheet Terms

Spreadsheets do for numbers and charts what word processors do for writing. Although their strength is their function as numeric calculators, most spreadsheets also have a database management component for organizing, sorting, and retrieving data and a chart component for creating and printing graphs. This chapter explains how a spreadsheet can be used to process and display numerical information.

The advantages of computerized spreadsheets include their accuracy and speed. Spreadsheets also have the capacity to recalculate formulas automatically when any numbers used in the calculation are changed. Spreadsheets have many uses; for example, they can manage inventories, tax returns, statistical procedures, grade records, personnel files, budgets, and quality assurance information.

Figure 7-1a shows Excel 2007 for Windows with the Home tab selected; **Figure 7-1b** shows Excel 2008 for the Mac computer. Note the differences in the two interfaces. No matter which version you use, however, the basic concepts are the same.

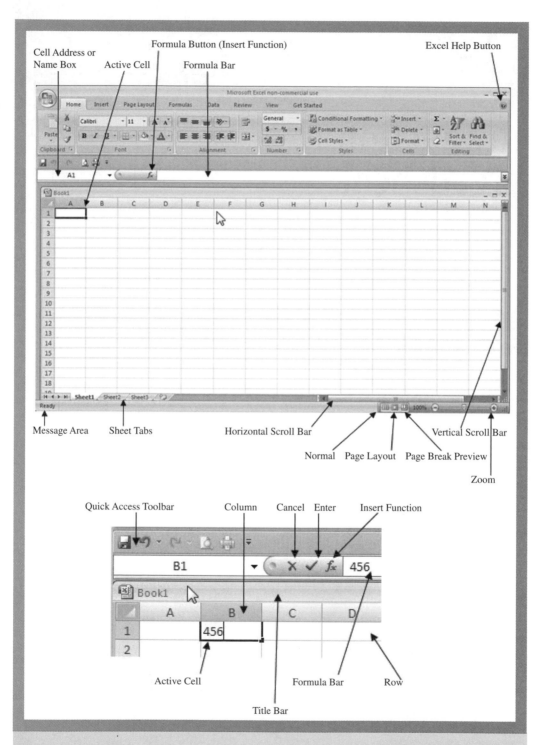

Figure 7-1a Excel Window in Office 2007 for Windows with Home Tab and Groups Selected

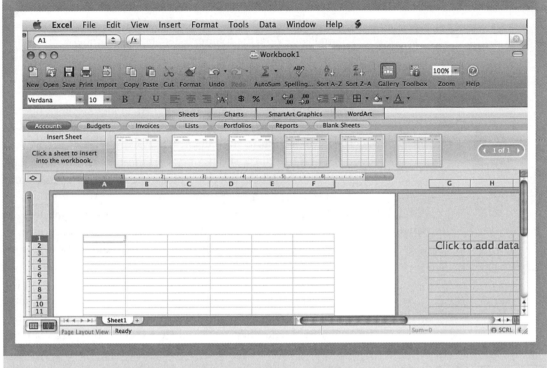

Figure 7-1b Excel Window in Office 2008 for Mac OS X

The various parts of a spreadsheet window are described next.

Rows	Rows run horizontally across the spreadsheet. Beginning with 1, they are numbered down the left side of the worksheet. Although the maximum number of rows varies with different spreadsheets, more than 1 million rows are available in Excel 2007.
Columns	Columns go vertically down the worksheet. They are labeled from A to Z, going from left to right. After Z, labeling continues with AA to AZ, BA to BZ, and so on. More than 16,000 columns are available in Excel 2007.
Cell	A cell is a placeholder for data. Each cell occurs at a specific intersection of a row and a column. Cells are labeled by the column letter followed by the row number (e.g., A1 or T112).
Cell Address (Cell Reference)	The cell address is the label for each cell. It is used to reference the cell when creating formulas or using functions.

Active Cell	The active cell is the cell currently being used; it is outlined or highlighted so that it can be located quickly on the worksheet. In Figure 7-1a, the column letter and row number for the active cell are marked by a different color. The address of the active cell appears in a designated location on the spreadsheet screen.
Range (Block)	A group of cells in a rectangular pattern defined by the upper-left and lower-right corners is called a range or block of cells. For example, the range of cells from A1 to E6 would include all of the cells in columns A, B, C, D, and E in rows 1, 2, 3, 4, 5, and 6. A block of cells on a worksheet is identified as a dark rectangle. Blocks of cells may also be noncontiguous or may include all rows or columns.
Workbook (Notebook)	A workbook or notebook is a collection of spreadsheet pages. Workbook pages are called worksheets in most programs. In Excel they are called Sheet1, Sheet2 until otherwise renamed. In some spreadsheet programs, pages in a workbook are numbered; in others, they are labeled by a letter. All of the worksheets are saved together in one file. In some programs, when the workbook is blank, it is called a sheet. When they contain data, they are called worksheets. In Figure 7-1a, the worksheets are labeled Sheet1, Sheet2, and Sheet3. Worksheet names can be changed to more effectively reflect the worksheet content and type of data contained on the worksheet. For example, if the worksheet contains charts, the worksheet could be labeled Chart-Freshmen Expenses, Chart-Nursing Shortage, and so forth. Spreadsheet programs have a default number of worksheets in each workbook (Excel has 3); the user can add more worksheets to a workbook or delete the unused ones if desired.
Worksheet	A worksheet is made up of labels (letters), values (numbers), lines or borders, and formulas. It can also contain charts, illustrations, tables, links, and special text like WordArt and text boxes.
Template	A template is a spreadsheet that has been formatted with labels and formulas but no specific data; it is helpful when multiple uses of the same spreadsheet are needed. You might use a template for a yearly personal budget or for the budget of a health-care unit, for example. In this kind of application, the labels and the calculations used remain stable from one year to the next; only the values change. A variety of interesting templates are available from the Microsoft Web site related to health care. See **Figure 7-2** for two examples of health-related templates.

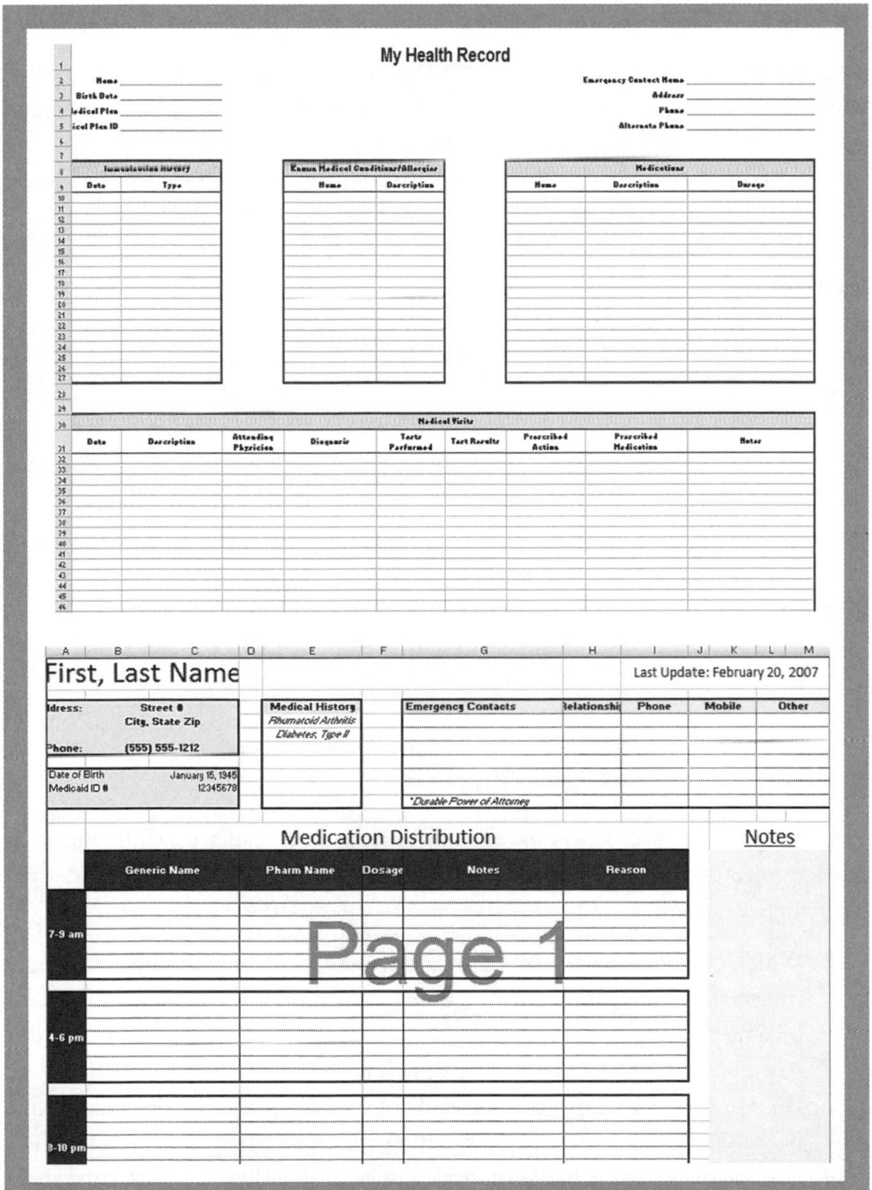

My Health Record

Name _____	Emergency Contact Name _____
Birth Date _____	Address _____
Medical Plan _____	Phone _____
Medical Plan ID _____	Alternate Phone _____

Immunization History

Date	Type

Known Medical Conditions/Allergies

Name	Description

Medications

Name	Description	Dosage

Medical Visits

Date	Description	Attending Physician	Diagnosis	Tests Performed	Test Results	Prescribed Action	Prescribed Medication	Notes

---

First, Last Name

Last Update: February 20, 2007

Address:	Street #		Medical History		Emergency Contacts	Relationship	Phone	Mobile	Other
	City, State Zip		Rhumatoid Arthritis						
Phone:	(555) 555-1212		Diabetes, Type II						
Date of Birth	January 15, 1945								
Medicaid ID #	12345678				*Durable Power of Attorney				

Medication Distribution

Notes

	Generic Name	Pharm Name	Dosage	Notes	Reason
7-9 am					
4-6 pm					
8-10 pm					

Page 1

Figure 7-2 Two Sample Health-Related Templates

Spreadsheet Screen Display

The screen displays for most spreadsheets are similar. Spreadsheets look like pages from an accountant's ledger (or columnar pad), containing many rows and columns. A series of letters, denoting columns, go horizontally across the screen; a series of numbers, denoting rows, run vertically along the left side of the screen. Like other Office 2007 applications (previously discussed in Chapters 4, 5 and 6), Excel has a ribbon, tabs, and buttons (see Figure 7-1a). Scroll bars appear along the right and bottom sides of the screen, along with the View buttons and the Zoom slider. Features specific to the spreadsheet screen display include the current cell address, the active cell (indicated by a black border), the formula bar or input line, sheet tabs, and the message area.

Current Cell Address	The current cell address indicates the *active cell* and is displayed on the left side of the formula toolbar.
Formula Toolbar	The data or formula entered appears in this location on the screen.
Message Area	The message area shows which actions will occur when a function or button is activated. It may also show error messages. It is usually located in the bottom left corner of the status bar.

Getting Ready to Use a Spreadsheet

Before beginning spreadsheet use, it is important to consider carefully the goals of the project so that an optimally useful spreadsheet is developed. Consider the following questions:

1. Which type of data is needed in the spreadsheet (e.g., inventory supply information, infection control, home medication tracking, or numbers for income or expenses)?
2. Are monthly, quarterly, or yearly time intervals needed?
3. Is there a need to make comparisons of data between units or across time periods?
4. How many data elements or time intervals are there? Is one worksheet adequate or would it be better to divide the data elements or time intervals among several sheets? For example, if you were doing an inventory of computer equipment in an organization you might put all of the computers by type or location on one page and all of the printers by type or location on another page. However, if the same inventory was being done for your personal computer-related equipment, one worksheet might be fine. If this were a budget, you might divide the budget into monthly or quarterly worksheets.

It is often most logical to place categories of data in columns because the width of columns can be customized to fit the data. The specific data for each record, situation, or individual can then be entered in each column under the category headings.

Once the goals of the project have been determined, the general process for creating the worksheet includes the following steps:

1. Create a file name that reflects the type of data maintained in the file. For example, UNIT 93 Budget 2009–2010.
2. Enter spreadsheet-identifying information on the first few rows. This information includes data such as name of the organization, department or division, the project (quarterly budget, inventory), and spreadsheet originator.
3. Enter labels that identify the columns and rows.
4. Enter the data.
5. Enter formulas and functions.
6. Format the data and labels (e.g., fonts, size, justification, number format).
7. Format the worksheet (e.g., borders, shading, color).
8. Create charts or graphs.
9. Print worksheets and/or charts.

Accomplishing Tasks in the Worksheet

Moving about the worksheet is accomplished by using the mouse or arrow keys alone or in combination with other keys on a keyboard (more details are provided later in this chapter). As the mouse is moved, the active cell is highlighted and noted as the cell address. To accomplish a task, select commands from the ribbon tabs or groups or click command icons. Using the scroll bar to move around the spreadsheet does not change the active cell; it simply changes the view of the spreadsheet until a cell is clicked in the worksheet area.

Entering Data

Spreadsheets allow the user to enter two types of data: constants and formulas. Constants include dates, numbers, text, logical values, and error values. Formulas perform mathematic operations such as calculating the mathematical relationships between the constants on the worksheet. When constants are changed, the formulas are still there, and the results on the worksheet are recalculated to keep the spreadsheet up-to-date.

To enter data:

1. **Click** the cell in which the data will be entered. The cell address will be displayed, and the cell will be highlighted or outlined.
2. **Type** the data into the cell.

3. **Press** an arrow key to go to another cell, press the tab key, **click** in another cell, or **press Enter**. Which key you use depends on the location of the next cell for which data will be entered.

When data are typed, they appear in the formula bar. For example, in Figure 7-1a 456 has been typed into cell B1, the active cell. Additional data values can be entered by pressing the Enter key (goes to the cell below the current cell), using the Tab key (goes to the cell to the right of the current cell), or clicking in another cell to move from one cell to the next cell. If new data are entered into a cell that already holds data, the new data will overwrite the original data. In Excel, continuous data such as a column of dates are entered using the AutoFill feature.

Typically, in spreadsheets, text is aligned to the left, and numeric values are aligned to the right. However, this alignment can be changed.

Unless otherwise indicated for data such as a social security number, phone number, or street number, the digits 0 to 9 and certain characters are treated as numbers in Excel. Other characters that are commonly treated as numbers include the following symbols: $- + . ( ) \$ \% / *$. Any number is treated as positive (+) unless a negative sign (−) is placed in front of it. Unless the user changes the format, the spreadsheet will use a standard default approach to displaying numerical data. For example, when a percent sign (%) is placed after a number, the number may appear converted to a decimal. For example, 45% may appear as .45. Some spreadsheet programs automatically convert any numbers beginning with a dollar sign ($) to include two decimal spaces. For example, $12 would be displayed as $12.00. While all spreadsheet programs will use default approaches to displaying data, the user can alter the way percentages, currencies, and other data types are displayed.

The following numeric operators are commonly used in formulas:

Symbol	Meaning	Symbol	Meaning
^	exponentiation	=	equals
*	multiplication	+	addition
/	division	−	subtraction
<	less than	>	greater than

When multiple numeric operators appear in a formula, the formula is calculated using certain ordering rules. Most often the standard rules of precedence are used: The first operator evaluated is exponentiation, followed by multiplication and division, and finally addition and subtraction; if there is a tie, calculation proceeds from left to right. Calculations enclosed in parentheses will always be calculated before other operations. For example:

5 * 4 + 3 would be calculated as 20 + 3, or 23
5 * (4 + 3) would be calculated as 5 * 7, or 35

Saving Worksheets

Each spreadsheet program has specific conventions for saving workbooks. Similar to word processing programs, spreadsheets replace newer versions of a workbook by overwriting older versions. The cautionary warnings given in regard to saving word processing documents are equally important with workbooks.

To save a workbook, first open it, **choose Save** (or **Ctrl+S**), name it, and decide where to save it. Save your work often and before you try something new! Excel 2007 saves files in the **.xlsx** format, which is XML based. This format ensures that Excel data may be integrated with outside data sources and keeps the sizes of the files relatively small. Files containing macros are saved in the **.xlsm** format. Data can also be saved in a variety of formats including HTML or older versions of Excel (**.xls**). A file name can contain letters, numbers, and spaces but not any of the following characters: / \ : * ? " < >. Excel automatically adds a file extension (usually.xlsx) to the file name when you save it. As in Word 2007, Excel work-books can be saved as Excel 97–2003 workbooks.

Using Charts

Charts are often effective ways to display spreadsheet data and illustrate trends. Because the data in a spreadsheet can often be more easily understood in graphic form, spreadsheets come with the ability to create charts. A good chart lets the reader instantly see the point being made by the data; it graphically compares and contrasts data.

Some terms related to charts are defined here:

Axis	The horizontal (x) and vertical (y) plane or line on which the data are plotted is the axis. It provides a comparison or measure-ment point.
Categories	Categories are labels given to the x-axis and y-axis.
Chart Type	The chart type refers to the way the chart will display the data. Examples include pie and bar charts.
Data Series	A data series is a group of related data points on a chart that orig-inated from rows and columns in the worksheet. These values are used to plot the chart.
Legend	The legend is the information that identifies the pattern or color of a specific data series or category.

The best choice for the type of chart depends on the data to be displayed. For example, when comparing parts to a whole, such as a department's budget to the total budget for the organization, a pie chart might be useful. The following questions will help you make design decisions when creating a chart:

1. Is this the right chart to convey the data in the worksheet?
2. How would a viewer expect to see these data displayed?
3. Does the chart add to the understanding of the data and help the audience to make decisions?
4. Which questions or solutions does the chart suggest?

The process of creating a chart is discussed later in this chapter.

Introduction to Excel 2007

This chapter focuses on Excel 2007. Excel is available for both the Windows Vista and Macintosh and earlier operating systems. This chapter provides specific information about the Office 2007 version of Excel for Windows Vista, which looks significantly different from previous Office versions and versions for the Macintosh operating system. Specifically, the menus, toolbars, and task pane have been removed from Excel 2007, just as they have been from other Office 2007 applications and replaced with the ribbon. The basic functions remain the same, however. Chapter 4 described the basics of applications running in a Windows Vista environment; those basics apply to Excel as well. Thus many of the skills learned in Chapters 4 and 5 will carry over into Excel.

Starting Excel proceeds just like starting other Windows programs. **Click** the **Start** button at the lower-left corner of the screen, **select All Programs**, and **highlight** and **click** first **Microsoft Office** and then **Microsoft Excel**. Figure 7-1a shows the Excel window. Alternatively, if an Excel icon appears in the Quick Launch area to the right of the Start button, click it to open Excel immediately (see Figure 4-8).

The Ribbon in Excel: Microsoft's "Fluent User Interface"

The menu bar in Excel has been replaced by a ribbon, as described in Chapters 4 and 5. The ribbon is made of task-oriented tabs and groups that are organized to keep like tasks together (see Figure 4-3). Each tab contains a different group of commands or tasks that help you use Excel. No matter which tab is chosen, the Office button and Quick Access toolbar are always available. The Office button in Excel contains the same commands as it does in Word (see Figure 4-2). It is helpful to compare the ribbons in Word and Excel on your computer screen to see the similarities and differences between them.

A brief description of each tab and its groups in Excel 2007 appears next.

Home   The most commonly used commands and features in Excel are found on the Home tab (**Figure 7-3**). The cut, copy, and paste commands appear in the Clipboard group. The Font group

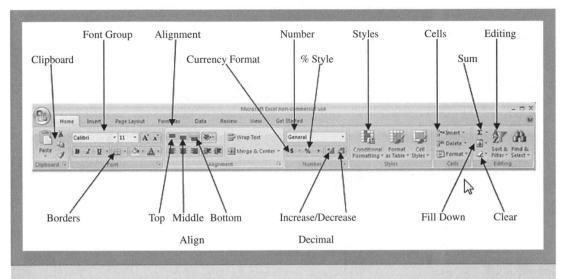

Figure 7-3 Home Tab and Its Groups in Excel

looks very similar to that in Word; it also has a Borders icon. The Alignment and Number groups appear next, followed by the Styles, Cells, and Editing groups. Clicking the dialog launcher arrow box ▣ opens a dialog box. The Quick Access toolbar appears above the ribbon in the Title bar; it can be moved below the tabs and customized to suit the user's preferences.

Insert   The Insert tab (**Figure 7-4**) provides quick access to groups related to tables, illustrations, charts, hyperlinks, and text objects. Seven large icons represent the various chart types. The Chart Tools ribbon (**Figure 7-5**) appears when a chart shape is selected for the data and provides access to Design, Layout, and Format ribbons for customizing charts. As long as a chart is selected in a worksheet, the Chart Tools tab appears on top of the screen.

Page Layout   Groups in the Page Layout tab (**Figure 7-6**) include Themes, Page Setup, Scale to Fit, Sheet Options, and Arrange. Here you can quickly change a document's theme to match a similar theme available in Word and PowerPoint. The Page Layout commands help you arrange items on the worksheet and prepare it for printing.

Formulas   The Formulas tab (**Figure 7-7**) is used to build formulas, check formulas, and create names for cells and tables. Groups include Function Library, Defined Names, Formula Auditing, and Calculation.

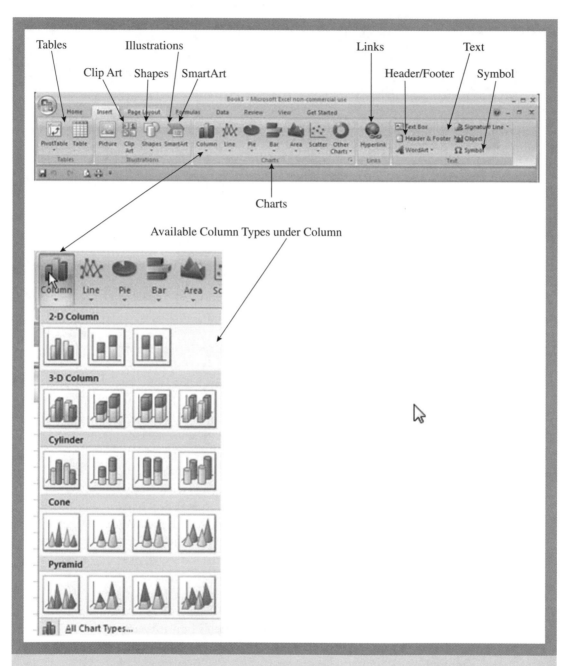

Figure 7-4 Insert Tab and Its Groups

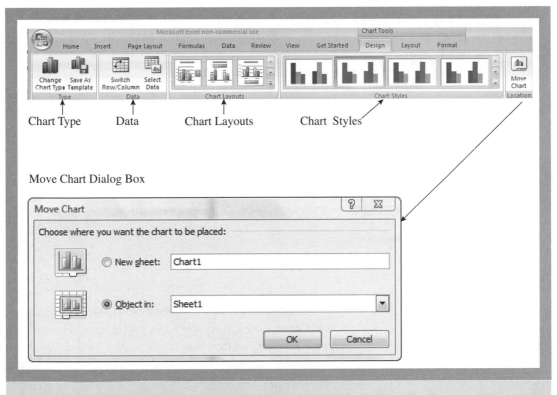

Move Chart Dialog Box

Figure 7–5 Chart Tools Ribbon

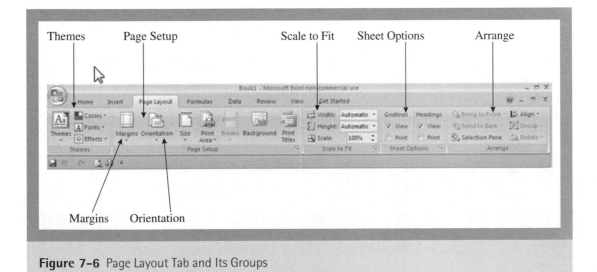

Figure 7–6 Page Layout Tab and Its Groups

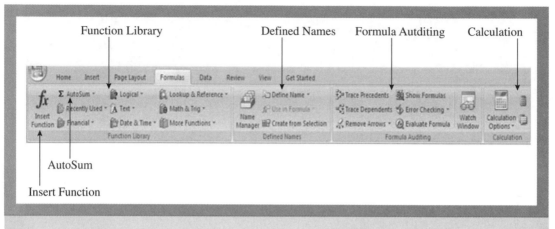

Figure 7-7 Formulas Tab and Its Groups

Data   The Data tab and groups (**Figure 7-8**) allow you to import external data, view linked spreadsheets (Connections group), sort and filter data, outline data, and use data tools. Some of the same icons for sorting and filtering appear in drop-down menus on the Home ribbon.

Review   Functions related to proofing, commenting on, and protecting or sharing the contents of the active Excel sheet appear in the Review tab and its groups (**Figure 7-9**). Spelling, Research, the Thesaurus, and the new Translate feature are part of the Proofing group.

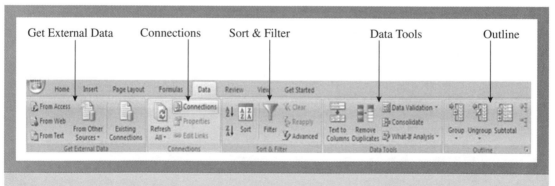

Figure 7-8 Data Tab and Its Groups

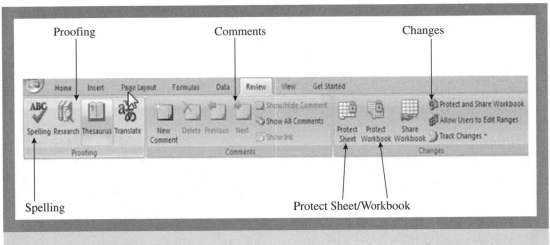

Figure 7-9 Review Tab and Its Groups

View   Most of the options that appeared in the Window menu in Excel 2003 are now found on the View tab (**Figure 7-10**). The groups in the View tab are similar to those in Word, with some exceptions. Many refer to how spreadsheets are viewed in preparation for printing, as drafts, or arranged in the window.

Get Started   The Get Started tab (**Figure 7-11**) provides pathways to commands, online training, and demos and videos for Excel 2007. It may or may not appear on laboratory computers.

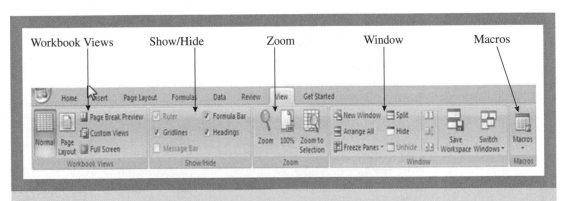

Figure 7-10 View Tab and Its Groups

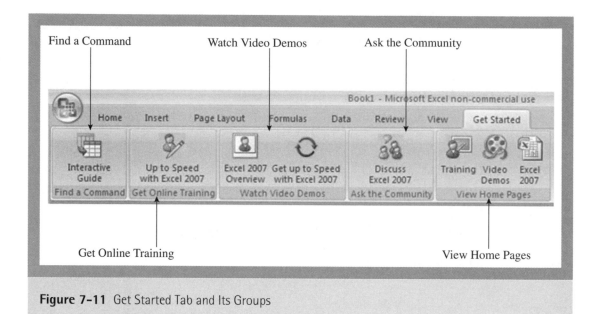

Figure 7-11 Get Started Tab and Its Groups

Excel also has contextual tabs that appear when necessary. Editing a header or footer will bring up the Header & Footer Tools tab, for example. Other context-sensitive tabs include Chart Tools, Drawing Tools, Picture Tools, Pivot Chart Tools, SmartArt Tools, and Print Preview Tools.

Entering Data and Correcting Errors

In Figure 7-1a, the message area appears at the lower-left corner of the screen. It says "Ready" when data can be entered. After typing the data and before doing anything else, the message area says "Enter." Entering data is accomplished several ways, including the following:

1. **Press Enter**.
2. Use the mouse, Tab key, or an arrow key **to move to another cell**.
3. **Click** the **Enter** button ✓ on the formula bar when entering formulas.

When an error is noticed after entering data, it may be changed in one of three ways:

1. **Retype** the data, and **press Enter**. This will automatically overwrite the error.
2. Place the cursor in the cell where the error occurs and right-click. **Figure 7-12** shows the dialog box that appears. **Choose Delete** to simply remove the data; **choose Cut** if you want to place the contents somewhere else in the spreadsheet.

3. Place the cursor in the cell to be changed. **Double-click** and then make appropriate changes to the cell contents.

The Mouse Pointer

Inside the spreadsheet the mouse pointer takes on different appearances that could be described as crosses.

- The "wide plus sign white cross" ✛ is used to select cells that you want to work within the spreadsheet.
- The "four-headed arrow" ⊕ is used to move cells or groups of cells from one place to another.
- The "two-headed cross" ↔ is used to widen rows or columns.
- The "little black plus sign" ⌐ is used with AutoFill and is found only on the lower-right corner of a cell.

Using AutoFill

AutoFill is a built-in, time-saving feature in which Excel automatically inserts data by following a pattern you have begun in a worksheet. For example, when months are needed as headings, follow these steps:

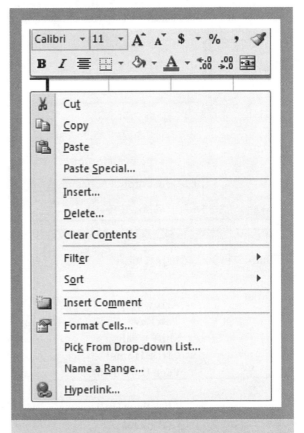

Figure 7-12 Menu That Appears When a Selected Cell or Section in the Worksheet Is Right-Clicked

1. **Type January** or the first month needed.
2. **Press Enter**.
3. Place the cursor at the lower-right corner of the cell with the month just typed; a black plus sign ("little black cross") will appear. See **Figure 7-13a**.
4. **Hold down** the mouse button and **drag** the cursor along the row until you have all 12 months listed. **Release** the button.
5. You can also **click** the right mouse button over the symbol ▦▾ below the last cell selected; a menu box will appear, as shown in **Figure 7-13b**. More choices then become available.

As you drag the black plus sign across the cells, the month will appear below the cell so you can see what will be inserted there when you release

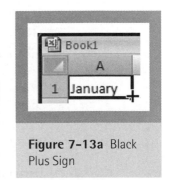

Figure 7-13a Black Plus Sign

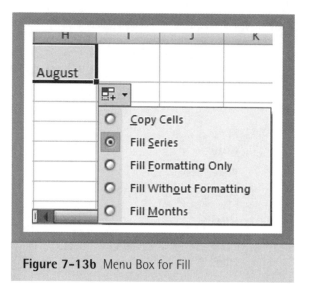

Figure 7-13b Menu Box for Fill

the mouse button. To AutoFill a series of numbers, type the first two values in adjacent cells such as 1 and 2 in cells A10 and A11 or 5 and 10 in cells A10 and A11. Select both cells, and then use the AutoFill box to highlight the cells. The AutoFill function will count by 1 or 5 as you AutoFill to cells A12, A13, and so forth.

Moving Around in the Worksheet

Navigating in the worksheet may be done with the mouse, arrow keys, or key combinations. The simplest way to move is to place the mouse in the desired cell and click. Other ways to move include the following:

Arrow Keys	Move one cell in the direction of the arrow key used.
Tab Key	Move one cell to the right.
Shift + Tab	Move one cell to the left.
Ctrl + Home	Move to the beginning of the worksheet (cell A1).
Page Up/Down	Move to the cell one screen up/down in the same column.
Alt + Page Up/Down	Move left/right one screen in the same row.
Ctrl + End	Move to the intersection of last row and column containing data.
Home	Move to the beginning of the row.

To go to a specific cell:

1. **Type** the **address** in the cell address area, and **press Enter**.
2. Alternatively, **press F5** or **Ctrl+G** for the **Go To** dialog box. **Type** the desired **cell address** in the reference box, and **press Enter** or **Click OK**.

Viewing the Worksheet

The View tab (Figure 7-10) provides options for changing how the workbook is viewed on screen such as in normal page layout or in full screen. Gridlines, the formula bar, and headings can be turned off and on. Other choices relate to the Zoom feature, adjusting windows, and macros.

When working in the worksheet, clicking the arrow keys on the scroll bars will move the worksheet one row or column at a time in the direction of the arrow. For example, clicking the down arrow on the vertical scroll bar moves one row down in the worksheet; clicking the right arrow moves one column to the right. Clicking in the blue area between the scroll bar and the arrow moves the display by an entire screen either vertically or horizontally, depending on the scroll bar selected. The Pg Up and Pg Dn keys move the screen view up or down to the next section that fits onto the screen. Note that this does not change the active cell; it just changes the view of the worksheet.

Common Commands

To create a new worksheet:

1. **Click** the **Office** button.
2. **Click New** and choose **Blank Workbook. Click Create** or **double-click Blank Workbook.**

Existing templates or ones from Microsoft Office Online appear to the left of Blank Workbook icon. If the **New** button appears in the Quick Access toolbar, simply click it. Selecting the New button opens a new blank worksheet. Pressing **Ctrl+N** also opens a new workbook.

To access an existing worksheet:

1. **Click** the **Office** button. Note that a list of Recent Documents appears in the right window pane. Choose the desired workbook
2. .If the workbook is not there, **click Open** and then choose the workbook from the file/folder in Documents in Vista (My Documents in XP) or wherever the file is stored.
3. **Click** the desired **file.**

To select cells:

To Select	Do This
A single cell	**Click** the **cell.**
A range of cells	**Click** a **cell** at one end of the series and **drag** the mouse to highlight the desired range of cells. Make sure the pointer is the white plus sign when you are holding down the mouse button to drag. If it is a four-headed arrow or a black plus sign, the data will be moving or autofilling, respectively.
Entire rows/columns	**Click** the row or column **heading** (the shaded horizontal or vertical area containing row numbers or column letters); the black arrow appears (see **Figure 7–14**). **Drag** to include more than one row or column and to delimit the area selected.
Multiple cells, columns, or rows that are not contiguous	**Hold down** the **Ctrl** key while **clicking** all desired cells, columns or rows; then release the Ctrl key.
Entire worksheet	**Click** the rectangle at the left of the columns just under the formula bar.

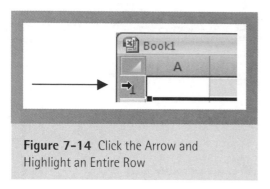

Figure 7-14 Click the Arrow and Highlight an Entire Row

If you need to clear cells, cut, copy, and change cell formats or to apply formulas to a series of cells, first select the cells.

The clear command acts as an eraser and eliminates information or formats from a worksheet. One or more cells may be cleared at one time. The cells are left on the worksheet and retain a value of zero.

To clear cell contents:

1. **Select** the **cell** or range of cells to be cleared.
2. Under the **Home** tab, in the **Editing** group, select the **Clear icon** .
3. Choose the appropriate command – clear all, formats, content, or comment.

Here is another way to delete the contents of a cell:

1. **Select** the **cell** or range of cells.
2. **Right-click** the selection.
3. Choose **Clear Contents**.

To delete the contents of a cell:

1. **Select** the **cell**.
2. **Press** the **Del** key to erase the cell contents.

To change the size of a column:

1. At the top of the worksheet along the column letters, place the cursor on the vertical line (called a separator) to the right of the column to be widened or made smaller. The cursor will appear as a vertical line ↔ with arrows pointing left and right.
2. **Drag** the column lines to the size desired *or* double-click to use the "size to fit" option.

If more numbers are entered than can be shown in the cell after you **press Enter**, the cell will look similar to this: 2.34568E+11. If a calculation results in a number bigger than the cell can hold, the cell will appear like this: ####### .

To insert a cell, row, or column:

Cell: Place the cursor where the new cell is desired; right-click. Figure 7-12 shows the menu that appears. **Choose Insert**; then select the appropriate option in the dialog box (**Figure 7-15**).

Column: Right-click the **column heading** (such as "C" or "E"), and choose **Insert** from the pop-up menu.

Row: Right-click the **row number** (such as "5" or "8") and choose **Insert**.

Rows are inserted *above* the current row and columns to the *left* of the current column. More than one row or column may be inserted by highlighting the row or column headers equal to the number to be inserted and following the steps described above.

The Insert, Delete, and Format commands appear under the Home tab in the Cells group. To use them, place the cursor in a cell or a column or row heading. If you click once on Insert, for example, a cell, column, or row is added depending on what you have selected.

If you click on the drop-down arrow ▾ next to Insert, a menu appears. See **Figure 7-16**. A similar menu appears if you click on the drop-down arrow beside Delete.

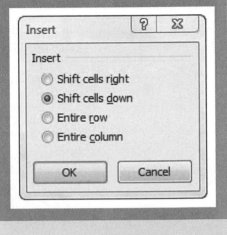

Figure 7-15 Insert Dialog Box

To delete a row/column:

1. **Place** the cursor on the row or column heading to be deleted, and **click** to **highlight** it. **Press Delete**.
2. **Right-click** the row or column header, and **select Delete** from the menu that appears.
3. **Select** the row or column header, and **click Delete** in the **Cells** group under the **Home** tab.

The save, save as, print, cut, copy, and paste functions work the same in all Office 2007 applications and have been reviewed in earlier chapters. It is always a good idea to use the Print Preview feature before printing a worksheet. There are many options for presenting data in an interesting print format by adjusting headings, color, alignment, type size, SmartArt, and so forth.

Working with Multiple Worksheets

Excel, by default, includes three worksheets in a workbook file. (See the sheet tabs in Figure 7-1a.) To move between worksheets, click the labeled sheet tab at the lower-left corner of the worksheet. Worksheets may also be added or deleted, and the default number of worksheets added can be changed.

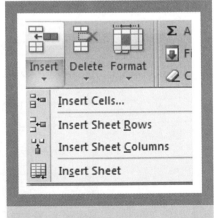

Figure 7-16 Home Tab, Insert Drop-Down Menu

To change the default number of worksheets:

1. **Click** the **Office** button.
2. **Click Excel Options** at the bottom of the Office button menu, and **choose** the desired number of worksheets under the "When creating new workbooks" section of the menu. See **Figure 7-17**.

To add a worksheet to the workbook only:

1. **Click** the arrow next to **Insert** in the **Cells** group under the **Home** tab and **choose Insert Sheet**. A new worksheet is added to the left of the selected worksheet.
2. **Click** the rectangle next to Sheet 3 at the bottom of the worksheet to add another sheet. (Pressing **Shift+F11** will have the same effect.)
3. **Right-click** the **sheet tab** and **choose Insert** from the pop-up menu. Make sure **Worksheet** is selected in the Insert dialog box, and then **click OK**.

To reorder worksheets:

1. **Right-click** the **worksheet tab**.
2. **Select Move or Copy**; then select the order desired from the dialog box and click **OK**.

Worksheets may also be reordered by dragging the sheet tab to the correct location.

To delete a worksheet:

1. **Click** the arrow next to **Delete** in the **Cells** group under the **Home** tab and choose **Delete Sheet** Delete Sheet .
2. **Right-click** the sheet label and **choose Delete** from the pop-up menu that appears.

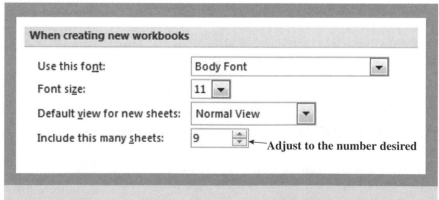

Figure 7-17 Increasing the Number of Worksheets for the Default Workbook

Data may be copied and pasted between the sheets in a workbook. Any formulas based on data in one worksheet that are not copied to another will result in the error message #REF, however, because the formula will be looking for the reference data in the cells of the new worksheet.

Working with Multiple Workbooks

Just as in Word, where it is possible to have multiple documents open, so multiple workbooks may also be open in Excel at the same time; data may be copied and pasted between them as well. Open workbooks are shown in the taskbar at the bottom of the screen and can be selected from there.

To view two worksheets from the same workbook:

1. Under the **View** tab in the **Window** group, **click** the **New Window** button ⬚ New Window .
2. On the **View** tab in the **Window** group, **click View Side by Side** ⬚ .
3. In the Workbook window, click the worksheets that you want to compare.
4. To scroll both worksheets at the same time, **click Synchronous Scrolling** ⬚ in the **Window** group on the **View** tab. This option acts like a toggle switch and can be turned off and on as needed.

To view two worksheets from different workbooks:

1. **Close** other documents.
2. **Open** the first workbook, and then **open** the second workbook.
3. **Click View** in the **Window** group; **choose Arrange All**.
4. **Select tile**, **horizontal**, **vertical**, or **cascade** from the dialog box.
5. **Click OK.** The tile option will arrange the windows side by side in small, even rectangles to fill the screen; the horizontal option arranges windows one above the other; the vertical option arranges windows side by side; and the cascade option creates a stack of windows with only the title bar of the inactive windows showing.

The save, save as, print, cut, copy, and paste functions work the same way in Excel as they do in all Office 2007 programs (see Chapters 4 and 5 for a review of these functions).

Numbers and Formulas

Cell entries are considered to be either labels or values. Values can be numbers or formulas. The first character typed determines the type of cell entry. In addition to the numbers 0–9, Excel treats the following characters as values: $- + / *$. E e ( ) $ and %. An equal sign signals a formula or function.

The default format for numbers is general. Any numbers entered into Excel appear exactly as typed. Number formatting can be changed to signal that the values are decimals, percentages, currency, time, or other types of numbers. As different selections are made, examples are presented in the dialog window to allow a view of the effects of the format.

To format cells:

1. **Select** the cells to format.
2. Under the **Home** tab, go to the **Number** group.
3. **Select** the desired format from the shortcut icons in the Number group. (See Figure 7-1a for examples of formatting types.)

If you click the down arrow beside **General**, a Number Format menu appears that provides more choices. (See **Figure 7-18**.) To see even more options, **click** the **dialog launcher arrow** in the **Number** group or **More Number Formats** in the Number Format menu. **Figure 7-19** shows the Format Cells dialog box that appears.

The changes that can be made to a worksheet, particularly after it is complete, are nearly endless. For example, you can modify the font type and size, color, spacing, alignment, and styles. **Figure 7-20** shows the Cell Styles menu that appears after you select the drop-down arrow Cell Styles in the **Styles** group of the **Home** tab.

Formulas and Functions

Formulas help you analyze the data on a worksheet. With formulas, it is possible to perform operations such as addition, multiplication, and comparison and to enter the calculated value on the worksheet. A function is a more complex preprogrammed formula.

An Excel formula or function always begins with an equal sign (=). Entering a formula is just like typing an equation on a calculator.

To build a formula:

1. **Type** an = sign in the cell where the formula will be placed.

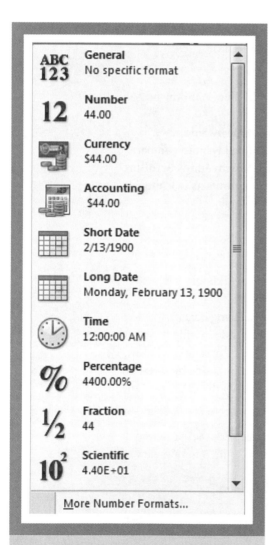

Figure 7-18 Number Format Menu Available in the Number Group, General

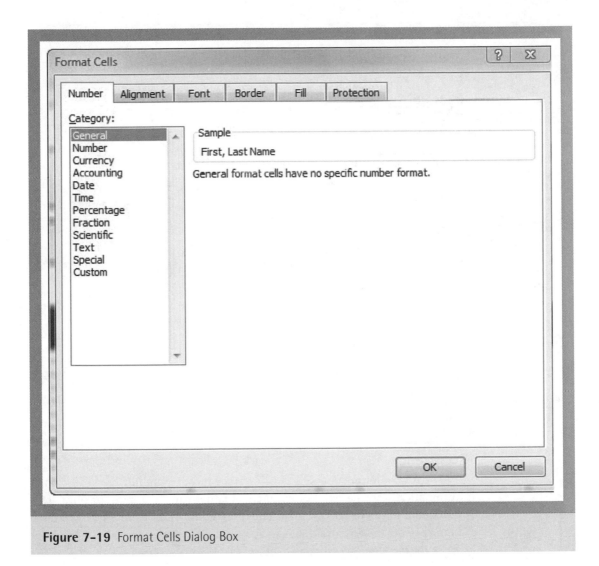

Figure 7-19 Format Cells Dialog Box

2. **Enter** the formula by typing cell addresses or selecting cells by clicking on them with the mouse and including the desired math calculation symbol where appropriate (e.g., + - * /).

3. **Press Enter** or **click** the **Enter** icon ☑ in the formula bar.

In **Figure 7-21**, two cells were added by typing = and then clicking on cells D2 and D3. Note that the formula appears in the cell and formula bar in the top example. After the formula is entered, the total appears and the formula shows only in the formula bar.

When using formulas in Excel, the standard rules of precedence listed earlier in this chapter dictate how the mathematic calculation proceeds.

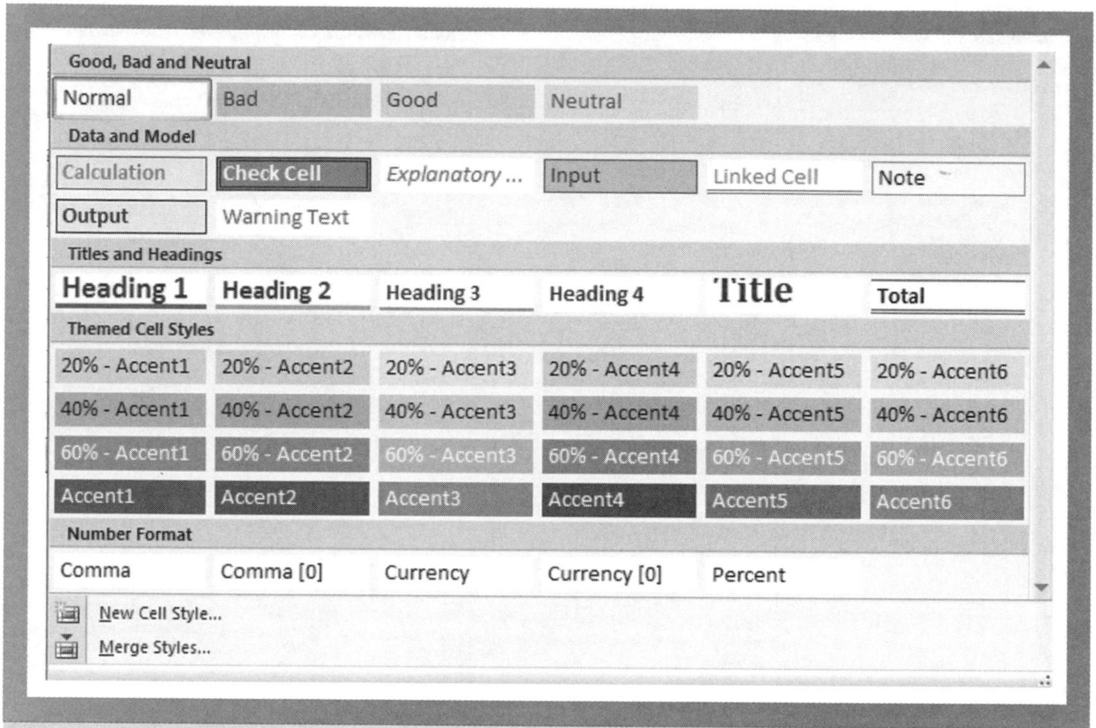

Figure 7–20 Cell Styles Menu

The AutoSum function ∑ AutoSum ▾ is the most commonly used function; it automatically adds a series of numbers in either rows, columns, or both. This function is found in the Home tab under the Editing group and in the Function Library under the Formulas tab.

To use the AutoSum function:

1. **Highlight** the cells to be summed and include a blank space at one end of the series.
2. **Click** the **AutoSum** icon ∑ ▾; the sum will be displayed.

Another way to use this function is by following these steps:

1. **Click** an **empty cell** where the sum will be displayed.
2. **Click** the **AutoSum** icon.
3. Confirm that the range of cells to be added is correct, as shown in **Figure 7-22**.
4. **Press Enter** or **click** the **Enter** icon ✓.

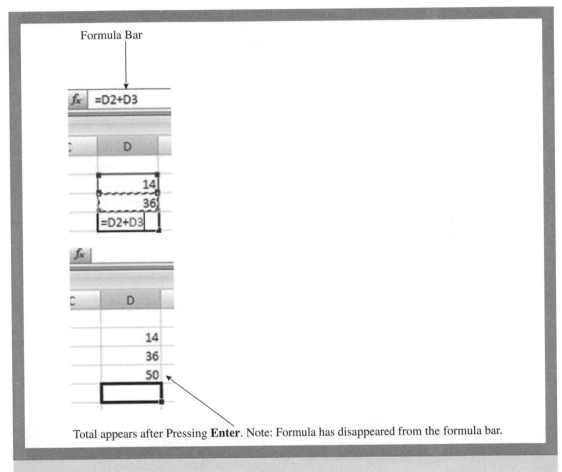

Total appears after Pressing **Enter**. Note: Formula has disappeared from the formula bar.

Figure 7-21 A Simple Formula for Adding Values in Cells D2 and D3

Some commonly used formulas have been included in numeric functions; this eliminates some of the steps required for writing a formula. Excel 2007 includes 356 built-in functions that are useful in finance, mathematics and statistics, and engineering.

To access these functions:

1. **Click** the **Formulas** tab.
2. **Choose** the appropriate function from **Function Library** group.

Figure 7-23 shows the Statistical Functions menu found in the Function Library when you **click More Functions** and then **Statistical**.

Commonly used functions include the following:

Function Name (Attribute)	Purpose
=SUM(range)	Sums the values indicated
=AVERAGE (range)	Averages the values indicated
=COUNT(range)	Counts the number of cells within a range that contains numbers
=MAX(range)	Returns the largest value within a range
=MIN(range)	Returns the smallest value within a range
=STDEV(range)	Computes the standard deviation for the range
=VAR(range)	Determines the variance for the range
=IF(condition, true, false)	Returns a true value if condition is met; returns a false value if the condition is not met

The most commonly used function in Excel is the Sum function. It adds two or more values together and displays the result in the selected cell. If any values change, so does the sum.

The parts of a function include the following components:

= sign + function name + parentheses ( ) + arguments within the parentheses

Examples
=SUM(B3:B5)
=AVERAGE(F1,F4,G1,G3,G5)

If the cell addresses to be included in the function or formula are adjacent to each other, a colon is used to separate them (B3:B5). The colon (:) can be thought of as a vertical ellipsis; in other words, you have left something out—in this case, cell B4. If the cell addresses are not adjacent, then a comma is used between them. Both adjacent and non-adjacent cells can be combined in the same function. The result of the calculation appears in the selected cell, but the function appears in the formula line, as shown in **Figure 7-24**.

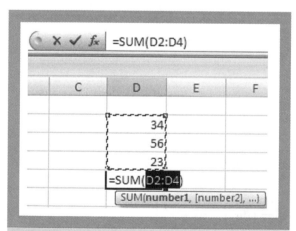

Figure 7-22 Confirm Range of Cells with the AutoSum Feature

To sum cells:

1. **Click** the cell below or to the right of the values you want to total.
2. **Choose Home, Editing,** and then **AutoSum Σ ▾**. Alternatively, **choose Formulas, Function,** and **AutoSum**.
3. **Press Enter** or **click Enter icon** on the formula toolbar.

If you want to select cells different from the ones that Excel chooses for a formula or function, select them with the mouse or type them in. You will need to add the colon or commas as necessary.

Absolute Cell Addresses

Relative addresses are cell addresses in formulas that are designed to change when the formula is copied to other cells. **Absolute addresses** are cell addresses in formulas that remain the same despite other changes in the worksheet; they are indicated by a dollar sign ($) preceding the part of the address that is to remain absolute. For example, if the number in C5 is to be the divisor in a formula no matter where the formula is moved, that address should appear in the formula as C5.

The following combinations are used to keep certain parts of an address constant:

CR   Both the row and column addresses always remain the same.

$CR   The row changes, and the column address always remains the same.

C$R   The column changes, and the row address always remains the same.

Sorting Data

Excel allows data to be sorted after those data have been entered, thereby enabling you to specify the order of the data records. It is possible to sort data alphabetically or by numerical order. All data relevant to the sort must be included in the sort area.

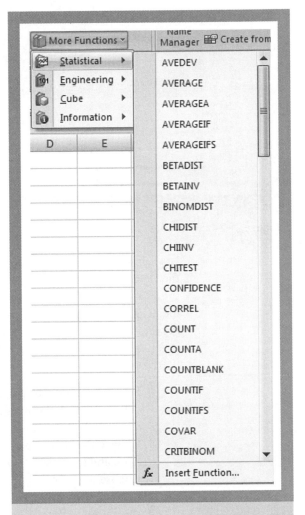

Figure 7-23 Statistical Functions Menu Found in the Function Library under More Functions

To sort data:

1. Using the mouse, **highlight** all **data** involved.
2. **Click Sort & Filter** in the **Editing** group under the **Home** tab (**Figure 7-25**), and designate whether data should be sorted in ascending (1, 2, 3 or A, B, C) or descending order (10, 9, 8 or Z, Y, X). Choose **Custom Sort** to see other sorting options.

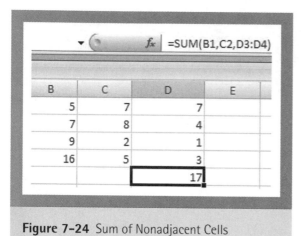

Figure 7–24 Sum of Nonadjacent Cells

If the data have a "header," exclude the header from the data range so it is not sorted, or include the header and use custom sort and then **select My data has headers**. When you use the Sort By option, you will see the headers and will not have to remember what they were.

Figure 7-26 shows the Sort & Filter Group under the Data tab and the Advanced Filter dialog box.

Filtering allows you to select specific records for review. It does not rearrange data, but rather hides rows you do not want displayed. This feature makes it easier to manage large lists. When **Filter** is selected under the Data tab, a drop-down arrow appears in the selected column(s). **Figure 7-27** shows a list of hours with the drop-down arrow; clicking the arrow brings up the menu shown in this figure. You could first filter the data desired, and then sort the filtered data by smallest or largest order. In the example, Number Filters was selected to show the filter choices that are available.

To create a chart:

1. **Select** the **data** to be graphed on the worksheet. Include the appropriate column and row headings.
2. **Click** the **Insert** tab.
3. **Choose** the chart type from the **Chart** group—Column, Line, Pie, Bar, Area, and so forth.
4. **Choose** one of the options available in that group. (Figure 7-4 shows the options when Column is selected.) The graph then appears in the worksheet along with the **Chart Tools Design** tab (see Figure 7-5).
5. **Choose** a Quick style in the Chart Tools, Design tab if the graph style needs adjusting. If the chart type is not what you want, **click Change Chart Type** and **choose** another chart type. When you have a chart type you like, **click** one of the options in the **Chart Layout** group. See which one works best with the graph.
6. **Click** the **Chart Title** icon in the **Chart tools, Layout tab**.
7. **Type** the title. It will appear in the Formula bar as you type.
8. **Press Enter**.
9. **Choose** a location for the chart—the open worksheet or a new one. Clicking inside the **Graph** box (4-headed arrow) allows you to move the box within the worksheet. If you want to move the chart to another worksheet, **click** the **Move Chart** box at the right end of the Chart Tools ribbon.

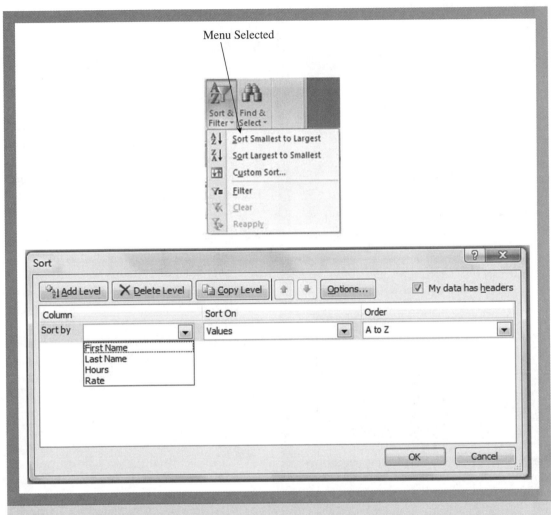

Figure 7-25 Sort & Filter Option in the Home Tab, Editing Group

10. The Move Chart dialog box appears (see Figure 7-5). Choose another location.

Scenarios

Scenarios are a type of what-if analysis tool. A scenario is a set of values that Excel saves and can substitute automatically in the worksheet. Scenarios are used to forecast the outcome of a worksheet model. Different groups of values can be created and saved in a worksheet; users can then switch to any of these new scenarios

Lowest Values at Top

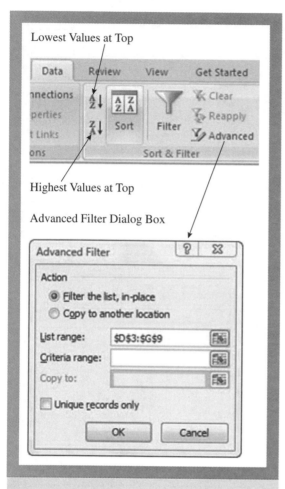

Highest Values at Top

Advanced Filter Dialog Box

Figure 7-26 Sort & Filter Group in the Data Tab

to view their results. For example, when creating a budget with uncertain revenues, scenarios can be defined with different values for the revenue. It is then possible to switch between the scenarios to perform what-if analyses.

The What-If Analysis button appears in the Data Tools group under the Data tab. When using the Scenario Manager, it is possible to have as many as 32 variables that change from scenario to scenario.

Summary

Spreadsheets can make tasks such as budgeting, inventory tracking, quality assurance documentation, and many others involving numeric calculations much easier and more accurate. This chapter has provided basic information about using spreadsheets—specifically, building simple formulas, using common functions, and developing charts to represent data visually in Excel 2007.

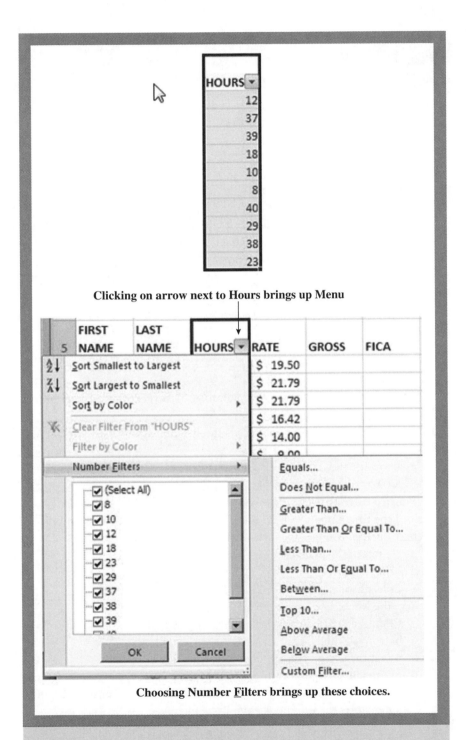

Figure 7-27 Filter Example Using the Data Tab

EXERCISE 1 Create a Simple Salary Worksheet

■ **Objectives**

1. Create a simple spreadsheet.
2. Use simple formulas and functions.
3. Format a worksheet.
4. Print, save, and retrieve a spreadsheet.

■ **Activity**

1. Access Excel.
   a. Click **Start**, **Programs**, **Microsoft Office**, and **Microsoft Excel**. An **Excel** button ⊠ may also appear in the Quick Launch area of your taskbar or in another area of the Start menu.
   b. Once you see the spreadsheet on the screen with "Ready" `Ready` in the message area, you can begin. Be certain that you are in the correct cell for performing the remaining actions in this exercise.
2. Practice moving the cursor.
   a. Practice moving from one cell to another using the mouse and the arrow keys.
   b. Move from cell **A1** to cell **C5**.
   c. What happens to cell C5 when you moved the cursor there?
   _____
   d. What shape does the pointer assume when it is inside the worksheet?
   _____
   e. Look for the current cell address in the Name box on the Formula toolbar. What do you see? _____
3. Practice entering data.
   a. **Type first name** in cell **C5** using lowercase letters and **press Enter**.
   b. **Type Last Name** using lower case letters, and **press Enter**.
   c. Go to cell **C6**, **press** the space bar, and then **press Enter**.
   d. What happens? _____
   e. **Erase** the name from cell **C5**.
4. Save the worksheet.
   a. **Click** the **Office** button, then **Save** or press **Ctrl+S** or **click** the **Save** button 🖫 on the Quick Access toolbar.
   b. **Select** the correct storage location for the file.
   c. In the File name box at the bottom of the screen, **type Chap7Ex1-Last Name; click** the **Save** button or **press Enter**. Remember that the computer stores the workbook as an Excel file.
5. Enter spreadsheet ID information.
   a. **Click** cell **A1**.
   b. **Type UNIT BUDGET**, and press **Enter**.

6. Use the process in this step to enter the labels on your spreadsheet. Do not waste your time about making the data look nice at this point. Formatting comes after the labels and data are entered.

   a. **Highlight** the range of cells **A3:G3**.

   b. **Press** the **Caps Lock** key.

   c. **Type LAST** in cell **A3. Press Alt+Enter. Type NAME** and **press Enter**. Since you highlighted the range of cells, the Enter key will move you to the next cell.

   d. **Type First. Press Alt+Enter.** Type **NAME** and **press Enter.**

   e. **Type Social. Press Alt+Enter. Type Security. Press Alt+Enter. Type Number** and **press Enter.**

   f. **Type CARE. Press Alt+Enter. Type LEVEL** and **press Enter.**

   g. Continue typing the labels as shown in **Figure 7-28**. Be sure to **press Alt+Enter** after entering each word and press **Enter** for the last word to move to the next cell.

7. Enter the data.

   a. **Press** the **Caps Lock** key to turn off the caps lock function. **Click** cell **A5**.

   b. **Type** the following data in the cell as indicated and press **Enter** after each name:

Row	Column A
5	Henderson
6	Nightingale
7	Barton
8	Wald
9	Dock
10	TOTALS

   c. Complete the rest of the data as shown here. Remember if you highlight the range of cells you can use the enter key to enter all these data items from the numeric keypad.

Row	B	C	D	E
5	Veronica	123-45-6789	1	32290
6	Felicity	345-80-6543	4	47664
7	Connie	234-68-6789	1	8432
8	Larry	456-98-5678	2	32450
9	Laverne	342-87-9807	1	43250

8. Create formulas. Project a salary increase of 5% for each healthcare worker.

   a. **Click** cell **F5. Type =(E5*1.05)** and **press Enter**.

   b. **Click** cell **F5**.

   c. **Place** the pointer at lower-right corner of the cell until it turns to a black plus sign $\boxed{\$\quad 33,905}$.

   d. **Drag** through cell **F9** and **release** the mouse button.

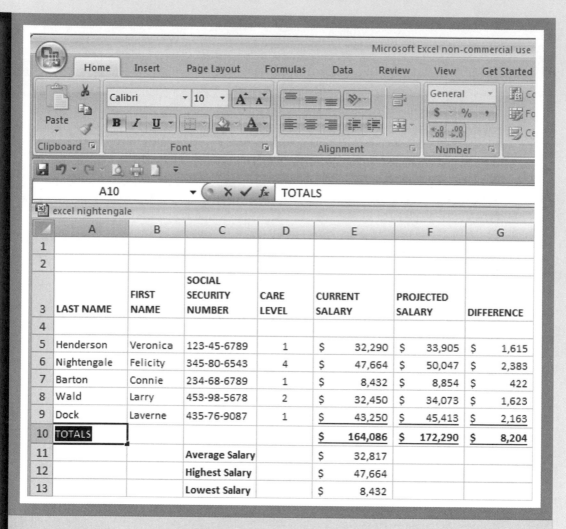

Figure 7-28 Exercise 1: Labels and Data Unit Budget

e. Which formula appears in cell F7? _____
f. **Click** cell **G5**. **Type** =. **Click** cell **F5**. **Type** −. **Click** cell **E5**.
g. **Click** the **check mark** ✓ on the formula toolbar or **press** the **Enter** key.
h. **Place** the pointer at lower-right corner of the cell until it turns to a black plus sign.
i. **Drag** through cell **G9** and **release** the mouse button.
9. Use functions. Use the Sum function to total the salaries and differences in the budget.

a. **Click** cell **E10**.

b. **Click** the **AutoSum** button twice. What total do you get?
_____

c. Do the same thing in cells **F10** and **G10** to total the projected salaries and differences.

d. Add the following labels in the designated cells:

Cell C11: **Average Salary**

Cell C12: **Highest Salary**

Cell C13: **Lowest Salary**

e. In cell **E11**, type =**average(E5:E9)**. **Press Enter**.

f. In cell **E12**, type =**max(E5:E9)**. **Press Enter**.

g. In cell **E13**, type =**min(E5:E9)**, **Press Enter**.

h. Change Henderson's salary to 33,000 by typing **33000** in cell **E5**.

i. What total do you see now in cell E12? _____

j. Change Henderson's salary back to the original value.

10. Format labels, numbers, and the worksheet as a whole.

a. **Click** cell **A1**. If necessary, **click** the **Home** tab.

b. **Click** the **Font down arrow** and select **Times New Roman**.

c. **Click** the **Size down arrow**, and select **10**. **Click** the **Bold** button **B**.

d. **Select** cells **A1:G1**.

e. **Click** the **Merge and Center** button.

f. **Select** cells **A3:G13**.

g. **Select** the **Format** button in the cells group and then **choose AutoFit Column Width** from the drop-down menu. See **Figure 7-29**.

h. **Select** the range **E5:G5**. Hold down the **Ctrl** key and **select** the range **E10:G10** and **E11:E13**.

i. **Click** the **Currency** button **$** on the formatting toolbar.

j. **Click** the **Decrease decimal** button twice.

k. **Select** the range **E6:G9** and **click** the **Comma** button.

l. **Click** the **Decrease decimal** button twice.

m. **Select** cell **A10**. **Click** the **Bold** button **B**.

n. **Select** the range **E9:G9**. **Click** the **Underline** button **U**.

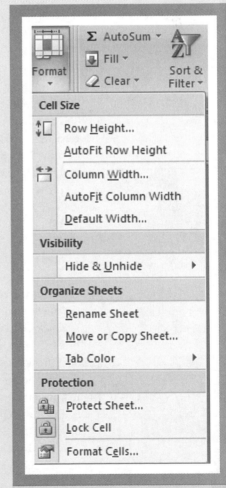

Figure 7-29 Format Dialog Box

o. **Select** the range **E10:G10. Click** the **Underline** button **U**.

p. **Click** the **Bold** button **B**.

q. **Highlight Average**, **Highest**, and **Lowest Salary. Click** the **Bold** button **B**.

r. If you still need to make adjustments in how the data fit into cells, place the pointer on the vertical line between the columns and adjust their width.

s. The last formatting that you need to do is to center the labels. Think about how you would accomplish this task using Word. What will you do in Excel? Do it now.

If all of these steps have been completed correctly, the spreadsheet should look like the one in Figure 7-28.

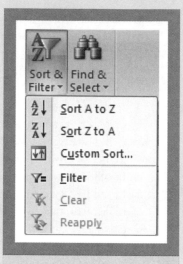

Figure 7-30 Sort & Filter Menu

11. **Save** the worksheet.

12. Sort the information by last name.

a. **Highlight** cells **A3 to G9. Click** the **down arrow** in the **Sort & Filter** menu in the **Editing** group on the **Home** tab. (See **Figure 7-30.**) **Click Sort A to Z.**

b. What do you notice about the column letters and the row numbers? **Click** the **Undo** button.

c. Sort the information by first name.

d. Make sure cells **A3 to G9** are still highlighted.

e. **Select Custom Sort** from the **Sort & Filter** menu.

f. The Sort dialog box appears. Choose **Column B** under **Column**.

g. **Click OK.** Now the worksheet is sorted by first name.

h. **Click** the **Undo** button.

13. **Sort** the worksheet by last name and then save the worksheet, as in Step 11 but change the name to Chap7Ex1Sort-Lastname.

14. Exit Excel.

a. **Click** the **Office** button, and then **Close.**

b. **Click** the **Close** button **x** in the upper-right corner of the screen to close Excel.

15. Reopen Excel and find the sorted file.

a. Which steps will you use to see where you stored the budget file?

b. What is the full file name of the sorted budget file? _____

c. **Click** the **Office** button.

d. **Click** the sorted file from the Recent Documents list.

e. **Click** the **Printer** button 🖶 or **click** the **Office** button, and then choose the appropriate Print options.

f. Exit the program. Be sure to exit Windows fully, and turn off the equipment as instructed.

EXERCISE 2 Create a Six-Month Budget

■ **Objectives**

1. Create a six-month budget using selected spreadsheet commands.
2. Use selected functions and simple formulas.
3. Add color to highlight selected information.

■ **Activity**

1. Create the identifying information.
   a. **Open Excel** and **save** the worksheet as **Chap7Ex2-Lastname**.
   b. In row 1, **type** the heading for the spreadsheet: **6-MONTH BUDGET**.
   c. In cell B2, type **BUDGET**. In cell C2, type **ACTUAL**. In cell D2, type **DIFFERENCE**.

2. Add the labels.
   a. Type **JAN** in cell **A3**.
   b. Use the AutoFill function to fill the labels through cell A8. Place the cursor in the lower-right corner of cell **A3**. Using the black plus sign [JAN ⌐], drag through cell **A8**.

A3	A4	A5	A6	A7	A8
JAN	FEB	MAR	APR	MAY	JUN

3. Enter the data. For each month, under the headings, enter the data as indicated here:

Month	Budget	Actual
JAN	950	843
FEB	950	795
MAR	925	889
APR	985	949
MAY	950	878
JUN	975	934

4. Add functions. Use the Sum function for finding sums in row 9, columns B and C.

5. Which formulas would you use to compute the differences between the budgeted amounts and the actual amounts for JAN?
   Enter this formula in column D3.

6. Which feature would you use to copy the formula to compute differences for each month? _____ Copy the formulas to the appropriate cells.

7. How would you write the function to determine the average for the six-month BUDGET and ACTUAL amounts? In cell A11, **type Averages**, and then enter that function to determine those averages in cells **B11** and **C11**. (Click cell **B11** and click the **Sum** function Σ . **Click** on the **down arrow** and **choose Average**. Make sure the correct range is selected. If not, select the correct range. HINT: The range should not include the total for either column. **Press Enter** or click the Enter button on the formula toolbar once the correct range is selected. Drag to cell **C11**.)

8. Format the numbers.
   a. **Highlight** the numbers in the worksheet.
   b. Go to the **General** option in the **Number** group under the **Home** tab.
   c. **Click** the **down arrow** and **choose Number**.
   d. Now look at the numbers. Format the first and last row as currency, no decimal points. Format the remaining numbers as comma, no decimal points.

9. Highlight cell **B9, click** the **down arrow** beside the **Fill Color** button, and **choose yellow. Highlight** cell **C9**, and add a color fill of your choice.

10. **Save** and **print** (if requested to do so) the spreadsheet.

EXERCISE 3 Create a Chart

■ Objectives
   1. Use the Chart Wizard to create several chart types.
   2. Print several chart types.

■ Activity
   1. Create a spreadsheet.
      a. Create a spreadsheet representing the expenses for three months.
      b. Save the file as **Chap7Ex3-Lastname**.
      c. Include the following categories in the spreadsheet: utilities, rent, food, car expenses, and personal expenses. Either use the figures below or fill in your own.

Expenses	JAN	FEB	MAR
Utilities	225	195	175
Rent	550	550	550
Food	294	305	325
Car Expenses	95	85	105
Personal Expenses	185	166	153

2. On the spreadsheet, **highlight the labels and data** for expenses for the month of January.

   a. **Click** the **Insert** tab.
   b. **Select Pie** in the **Chart** group.
   c. **Choose** the **3-D pie** 🥧.
   d. Go to **Chart Layout** and **click** 🥧.
   e. **Click** the **chart title**. **Right-click** and **choose Edit Text** from the menu that appears.
   f. **Type Expenses** after "January." Your pie chart should look like **Figure 7-31**.
   g. With chart selected, **click Layout** tab under **Chart** tools.
   h. In the labels group, **click Legend** icon and **click Show legend** at the top.
   i. **Click Data labels** icon in the Labels group and **click More Data Labels** option.
   j. Remove the check mark from the category name and **click close**.

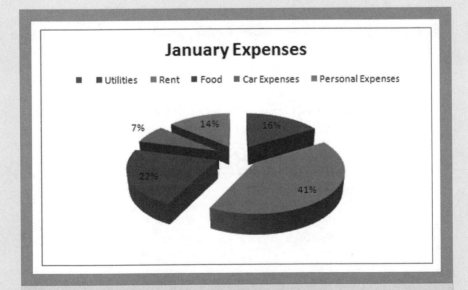

Figure 7-31 Exercise 3: Pie Chart for January Expenses

   k. Experiment with different chart types. Is there one that presents all of the data in a better way?

3. Using the steps learned here, create and print a column chart (any subtype) that compares all of the expenses for the three-month period.

ASSIGNMENT 1   Create a Simple Spreadsheet

■ Directions

1. Create a spreadsheet for any of the following:
   a. A unit budget that includes last year's costs, this year's costs to date, and cost projections for next year if costs increase 5%.
   b. A drug worksheet that lists the dose by weight for a class of drugs (e.g., emergency drugs for premature babies or for cardiac arrest, a comparison sheet giving safe doses of narcotics) and formulas for calculating the drugs for persons weighing different amounts.
   c. A personal budget of your living costs for the past year, the current year, and projected for next year if all costs increase by 3%.
   d. A special topic approved by your instructor.
2. Submit both the printed spreadsheet and the electronic file naming it **Chap7Assign1-Lastname** showing what happens with formulas and "what if" questions.

ASSIGNMENT 2   Create a Grade Sheet

■ Directions

1. Use a spreadsheet to create a grade sheet that includes headings for students' first and last names, ID numbers (Social Security numbers), and the test scores for a midterm exam, a project, a final exam, and the final grade.
2. Enter the data under the headings as they appear here:

ID	Last Name	First Name	MIDT	PROJ	EXAM	FINAL
123-45-6789	Titmouse	Martha	95	98	87	
125-12-4534	Finch	Jerry	87	75	90	
124-65-9087	Cardinal	Sam	65	70	67	
124-65-9087	Robins	Sally	85	80	90	
125-65-1234	Nuthatch	Jamie	85	90	95	
127-12-1234	Wren	Timothy	90	95	90	

3. The midterm exam and project are each weighted to be 30% of the final grade, and the final exam is weighted to be 40% of the final grade. Enter formulas to calculate the final grade for each student.

4. Using the appropriate functions, enter formulas to calculate the highest and lowest grades and the average for the midterm, project, and final exam grades.

5. Give each grade a percentage weighting so that all three grades total 100%. Place those percentages in a row you add between the headings and the first row of data.

6. Using the percentages and grades, determine the final numerical grade for each student.

7. Adjust the columns so that the spreadsheet is visually pleasing.

8. Practice creating a scenario showing how Martha's grade would change if she earned a 95 on the final exam.

9. Sort the spreadsheet in alphabetical order by the last names of the students.

10. Save the spreadsheet as **Chap7Assign2-Lastname**. Print the spreadsheet. Turn in the spreadsheet and the electronic file to your instructor.

ASSIGNMENT 3 Create a Chart

■ **Directions**

1. Use the data from Assignment 2 to create a chart that compares all five students' grades on each of the three different parts that determine the grade for the course.

2. Print the graph. On the back of the paper, indicate why you selected the chart that you did.

3. Save the chart as **Chap7Assign3-Lastname**.

Introduction to Databases

Objectives

1. Identify the data types that are best managed through databases.
2. Identify the advantages and uses of databases.
3. Describe the characteristics of databases and their associated features.
4. Define terms related to database applications.
5. Describe the database design process.
6. Interpret basic directions for operating a database program.
7. Perform selected queries.

Electronic databases are widely used in all aspects of modern society. For example, libraries catalog their collections in databases. Businesses track inventory, manage customer information, and maintain accounting data in databases. Healthcare institutions use a variety of database programs to manage and track patient information, employee data, research data, and trends. Educational institutions track applications and enrollments, drop and add students to courses, and produce class lists using databases. These databases reside on all levels of computers, from large mainframes to small home personal computers. This chapter introduces basic database concepts and terms with an appreciation of how they are used in health care. The chapter then introduces basic database skills, with a small sample database exercises to reinforce these skills.

Database management systems are used to organize, store, and retrieve data. These programs permit the user to create table structures, modify these structures, store data, and retrieve data in a variety of ways. They act as efficient file systems; they are, however, only as effective and efficient as the accuracy of the data and the structure of the tables within them. Most end users do not create the data structures, but rather use the database input and query forms and reports that have been previously designed. A basic understanding of these data structures is critical to assisting in the development of the database that meets the end user's needs.

Electronic databases offer the following advantages for managing data:

- A reduction in data redundancy (duplicate data in a variety of places)
- A reduction in data inconsistency (data stored differently in the same file, such as the format use to store a person's name—full name, including first and middle names, or first name, middle initial, and last name)
- Increased data access

Some professionals believe that automated databases offer a data security advantage. They believe that with centralized data, control over access is much easier. Others believe that automated databases create a data security disadvantage because the increased access to data results in increased security concerns. To counter this disadvantage, decisions about who has access to which data and at which level must be made. Should everyone have the ability to correct and add data or do some users only need access for viewing data but not changing those data? In the healthcare arena, should receptionists at the information desk have access to a patient's diagnosis and physician's name, or do they need access to only the patient's name and room number? Should executive administrators have the ability to chart medications on all patients, or should only the nurses on the unit have that ability? These are the types of questions that must be answered by healthcare providers working with the IT department in the clinical setting.

Effective information systems produce accurate (free of errors), timely (available when needed), and relevant (useful and appropriate for the decisions to be made or the task at hand) information that can be used for effective decision making.

Database and Database Management Characteristics

A database is a collection of stable stored data that can be accessed and interrelated to provide a total picture of the entity, as well as to answer questions and make decisions. In this definition, "entity" means the focal point of the database. It can be a person (a patient or a healthcare worker), a thing (e.g., medications, vital signs), a place (hospital), or an event (admission). "Stable" means the data elements do not change. The stored data are used to calculate values that do change such as a patient bill. Each time a bill is produced, it relies on the stable data elements to make its calculations of the total cost of care.

As mentioned earlier, a key characteristic of the data found in a database is that the data are shared with those users who need to have the information produced by the database. This requirement means that many healthcare providers must be able to access this database at the same time. However, only one user at a time will be able to edit data elements.

Finally, the data in the database are interrelated by connections to the various entities in the database and the relationship of those entities. For example, patients are prescribed treatments ordered by providers based on their diagnoses, which in turn is based on symptoms monitored by staff.

Database Models

A database model or schema refers to the structure of a database, which includes how that database is organized and used. These structures are generally stored in a data dictionary and many times are depicted in a graphical way. The database model defines a set of operations that one can perform on the data stored in the database; as a consequence, each model structures, organizes, and uses data differently. For example, hierarchical and network models are commonly used on mainframes and minicomputers, whereas personal computer database programs use a relational model. **Table 8-1** describes these models in more detail. No matter which structure is selected, the model underlying the design of the database program influences or limits the searching options permitted. It also influences the maintenance of the database.

The first generation of database models (1960s) was a single flat table. **Table 8-2** presents a security example flat model. Note that there is one user for one login, password, security question, and security answer for each record. The second generation of these models developed in the 1970s; two examples are the hierarchical and network models described in Table 8-1. The third generation of database models is the relational database, which is based on tables that link the various entities around which the tables are designed. The fourth generation of database models, as seen in the examples in Table 8-1, was developed to deal with task-specific data. These structures include the object-oriented and Internet models.

Data Relationships

Another important concept in understanding databases is relationships—that is, how the data in the database are related.

The simplest of these forms is the one-to-one relationship. For example, in **Figure 8-1** there is one healthcare provider in Table B with one security entry in Table A. No two healthcare providers have the same ID, password, security answer, and so forth. However, most data relationships are not this simple.

The next relationship type is one-to-many. In Figure 8-1, at 8 A.M. one patient in Table A receives multiple medications from Table B (the medication table). Thus an entity from one table (Patient A) has multiple entries in a second table (Medications).

TABLE 8-1   DATABASE MODELS

Model	Description
Flat table	A flat model consists of a single table with columns and rows of data elements. Columns identify the data that will be entered into the cell in each row. Most of the time the type of data (e.g., numbers, text, date) expected in the column is also identified.
Hierarchical	A hierarchical model is like a tree or organizational chart. During searching, the program searches each root and branch in sequence, checking for a match. This process is commonly called traversing the tree. Some terms commonly associated with this model include "root," "parent," "child," and "siblings." When designing the database, each child in the hierarchical model can have only one parent.
Network	The network model was developed to solve problems caused by the hierarchical model's inability to store certain types of data easily. The network model permits more than one parent per child. However, it requires multiple links to the various fields, making it much more difficult to revise or edit. Two constructs are important here: records and sets. A record contains fields and sets that define the one-to-many relationships between records. As a consequence, lower levels of a branch can be connected to multiple upper branches or nodes.
Relational	A relational model relies on flat tables for its structure. Designers use only one data element per field, which means tables must be reduced to their simplest form. The term used for this process of reduction is "normalizing the table." For example, a parent with two children would become two tables that are linked based on a common field. Each table has rows (records) and columns (fields). Each entity is its own table, and columns describe this entity. For example, a patient table might include the patient's name, address, phone number, age, sex, insurance number, and so forth. All columns describe the entity—the patient—in some way. Each database consists of multiple linked tables.
Object-oriented	The object-oriented model deals with defining and manipulating objects. Traditional databases are not structured to handle drawings, images, photographs, and recordings well. In contrast, the object-oriented structure stores data and procedures that act on those data as objects. This approach has been especially useful in health care where images such as X rays or pictures of wounds can be key to tracking a patient's progress.
Dimensional	The dimensional model represents data in a data warehouse so that data can be easily summarized. It is a task-specific database model.
Hypertext	One task-specific model is the hypertext model encountered on the Internet. This design relies on objects linked to other related objects. The object may be text, pictures, data files, or sound files. This structure is particularly useful for organizing large amounts of diversified data as seen in an electronic health record (EHR). The disadvantage to this setup is that it is not possible to perform numerical analysis on the data, nor can it be certain how people will access each part of the database.

TABLE 8-2	FLAT MODEL EXAMPLE: SECURITY TABLE			
User	Network Login	Network Password	Security Question	Security Answer
Nurse A	Nightif1	Jt34kd10	1	Center
Nurse B	Henderv1	Hgt567k	3	healy
Doctor C	Watsonj1	Tor438d	2	Smithton
Pharmacist A	Winterp1	Zwqf95t	1	Modern
Lab Technician	Dragulc1	Lhk5d18	3	camry

There are also times when the relationship between entities is a many-to-many relationship. This means that many entities (patients) from one table may have many relationships with entities from the second table (Medications). For example an individual patient may be receiving several different medications. At the same time several patients may also be treated with many of these same medications.

When healthcare professionals work with database designers, it is the healthcare professional's responsibility to help the designer identify how the entity in one table relates to the entities in other tables.

Database Terms

The following terms describe the structure of a database from smallest unit to largest. Recall from Chapter 2 that data are stored in the computer as bits. Bits are organized into bytes, which represent a character or symbol. When discussing databases, the bytes are further organized into fields, records, files, and databases. (See **Figure 8-2**.)

Bit	A bit is a zero (0) or one (1).
Byte	A byte is a combination of 0s and 1s that represents a character or symbol. For example, H may be given by the byte sequence 0100 1000 and I by the byte sequence 0100 1001, making the word "HI."
Data	Raw facts consisting of numbers, letters, characters, and dates are data. They are the contents of fields. Other names used for data include "data items" and "elements." Examples of data include Jones, 200-23-1234, and Chicago.
Data Types	Data types refer to the description of which data should be expected to appear in a field. These types are software dependent;

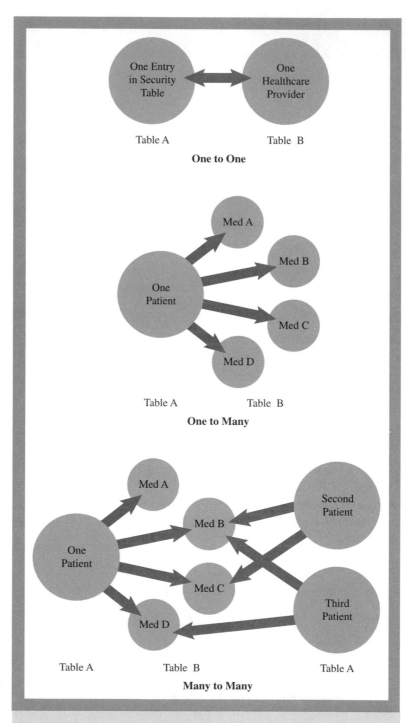

Figure 8-1 Database Relationships

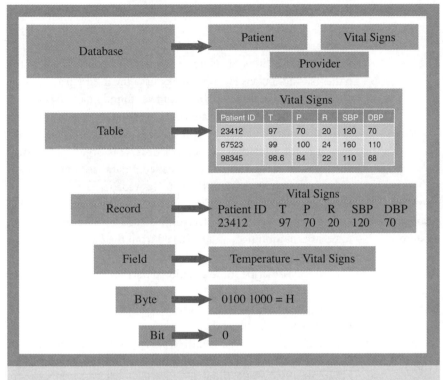

Figure 8-2 The Data Hierarchy in a Database

each program defines them. Most programs support alphanumeric (characters and numbers), numeric (numbers), short numeric (short, whole numbers), currency (money), character (letters), date and time, logical (equal to, greater than, or less than), memo (comment), and object (pictures or objects) data types.

Field   A field (also called an attribute) is a space within a file that has a predefined location and length. Only one data item is placed in each field, a concept referred to as the use of atomic data. For example, a patient's temperature, pulse, and respiration data should be stored in separate fields; do not place them together in one field such as a "vital signs" field. Examples of field names include last name, first name, city, state, diagnosis, systolic blood pressure, diastolic blood pressure, pulse, and height. Use a field name that reflects the data to be stored in that location.

Record   A collection of fields related or associated with a focal point makes up a record. For example, a patient is a focal point around

	whom certain data are collected and stored. A patient chart is a record. A college transcript is a record. Each row of a table, in most programs, is a record.
File	Files are collections of related records. For example, all of the patients in St. Luke's Hospital make up a file. Many people compare a file in a database with a file drawer found in a filing cabinet. Continuing this analogy, related data are kept in the same drawer.
Database	A database is a collection of files that is analogous to a file cabinet; it holds related drawers of records. It is organized in such a way that a computer program called a database management system can quickly retrieve the data desired.
Database Management System	Database management systems (DBMSs) are the programs that enable users to work with electronic databases. They permit data to be stored, modified, and retrieved from the database.

The following definitions describe some additional database concepts:

Key Field	One or more fields with a unique identifier constitute key fields. Using key fields ensures that no duplicate records will appear in this database, because a key field accepts only one record with that combination of text and/or numbers. One of the most commonly used key fields in healthcare systems is a Social Security number or some other unique patient number.
Link	A link is a logical association between tables based on the values in corresponding fields; it is a connection between two tables in a relational database program. The existence of a link permits you to query or ask questions of multiple tables and extract only the data desired from these tables. The linked field must be of the same data type and the linked field must appear in both tables.
Table	The table is the structure that is used to store the data. It consists of fields and records. The vertical columns are fields, and the horizontal rows are records.

Database Functions

Commonly available database functions allow users to create table structures, edit data or records, search tables, sort records, and generate reports. In the healthcare arena, healthcare professionals, in consultation with the information system department, design, create, and maintain a variety of databases. Once these databases are designed and populated, healthcare providers may or may not be able to edit clinical patient data or records that have been entered and verified in the system; if they can see records but not change them, the type of permission is called read-only access. If they are able to edit and view these data, an audit trail is maintained. While healthcare providers may not be able to edit or change patient data, they may be able to search, sort, and generate reports from the databases.

The rest of this chapter focuses on a small desktop database program, called Access, to demonstrate the functions commonly found across database programs.

Creating the Database

There are two steps to creating the database: designing the structure (sometimes called the schema) and entering the data. Entering the data will populate the data fields in the database.

Designing the Structure

Designing the structure of the table requires identifying the field names, field types, and field widths. This structure design is generally stored in a data dictionary, which is a file that defines the basic organization of a database. The data dictionary lists all of the tables associated with the database as well as the names and data types for each field. In addition, it often includes comments about the range of acceptable data. For example, it may require that state names be entered as a two-letter abbreviation such as "PA" or "OH."

Entering the Data

Data are entered using the designed structure. Sometimes this task requires redesigning the structure to facilitate entry of all data. Most databases provide options for verifying the accuracy of the data entered. These utilities (i.e., tools) permit users to set data ranges and data images to help ensure the accuracy of the data entered.

Editing Data or Adding Records

Editing data or records involves adding records, deleting old records, or changing data in active records. In health care, policies and procedures are usually established that govern what you can change in a patient record. These guidelines may not apply to nonclinical databases, however. For example, an employee record may need to have the phone number and address changed to reflect the employee's current information; a patient registration form must reflect any changes since the last admission; and so forth.

Add	The add function permits placement of additional records into the database.
Delete	The delete function permits the user to remove records from the database.
Change	The change function permits the user to alter the contents of a record.

While most databases will let you replace or override the previous data with new data, this practice is much less common in health care. Frequently all data are retained with a time stamp, thereby preserving an audit trail of what has been modified, when it was modified, and who modified the data.

Searching the Database

Searching is the process of creating data subsets or locating specific records in the database. Terms used to describe this process include "search," "query," "find," and "ask." The power of a database derives from this search function and the ability to extract data. Additional terms related to searching are described next.

Answer Table

In some databases, the answer table is a temporary table in which the program stores search results. It is overwritten when you conduct a new search or deleted when you exit the program. In other databases, the answer tables or results are automatically saved in the Queries object.

Boolean Searching

Boolean searching is one of the most commonly used features for searching any database; it provides the ability to narrow or expand a search as well as to eliminate some records. Three of the most often used Boolean operators are AND, OR, and NOT, whose basic uses are described here. Additional discussion is presented in Chapter 12.

AND   This strategy provides records that include both terms on either side of the AND. For example, a search for "computer AND health" elicits only records that include both terms. If one term is missing, that record does not show in the search results. The match must be exact. If a record includes the terms "computers" and "health," it will not be included in the search results. The singular term "computer" is not considered the same as the plural term "computers."

OR   This strategy provides records that have either term. For example, a search for "hepatic OR liver" finds records that include either the term "hepatic" or the term "liver."

NOT   This strategy provides records that exclude the term following NOT. For example, a search for "computer NOT bedside" elicits records containing the word "computer" and eliminates records that include the word "bedside."

Other operations, such as NEAR and ADJACENT, are also available, although they are used less commonly than AND, OR, and NOT. What is important is that the search strategy is refined to make it as efficient as possible for eliciting the information desired.

Exact Match	This search finds only entries that are an exact match for a specified word. Any minor difference results in exclusion of that entry from the results. For example, when searching for "child," the query finds only "child" and not "children," "infants," or "teenagers."
Pattern	This type of search permits the use of wild cards in place of a character. For example, "nur*" would match the string "nur" and any word with "nur" as the beginning string. Thus, this query would find "nurse," "nurses," "nursing," "nursery," "nurture," and "nurturing."
Range	Operators such as greater than, less than, equal to, or some combination of them are called logical operators. Searches with these operators return records that fit the operator, such as "all patients with a pulse greater than 110."
Select Fields	This type of search uses some mark to select the fields to be displayed in the search results. All of the fields or only selected ones may be chosen. For example, a healthcare worker may choose to display only the patient name and room number in the results or may choose to display additional fields such as diagnosis, doctor, primary nurse, and laboratory test results.
Calculated Fields	Calculated fields are generated by performing mathematical operations on other fields. For example, a calculated field may be used to sum the total cost of five different medications based on their associated prices.

Sorting the Database

The sorting function permits you to arrange records in a variety of ways and to work with some subset of those records. For example, a list of patients on a clinical unit may be sorted in alphabetic order and then sorted by the names of the primary nurse assigned, thereby creating subsets of these patients. This feature allows you to arrange the data in the order that makes sense for the result desired. Two terms used when sorting are "ascending" and "descending." An ascending sort puts the items in alphabetic or numeric order from A or 1 to Z or NN (the highest number). A descending sort puts the items in the reverse order, going from the highest value to the lowest.

Generating Reports

Another powerful feature of databases is the ability to generate multiple reports from the same database or data subset. Most programs permit multiple report formats to be used to display the same data. This is a significant advantage in health care, where a datum such as the patient's weight may be included in several different reports; with a database, staff do not need to record the same measurement on each of these reports.

Other Terms Related to Databases

As automation has continued to increase the ease of data generation, additional strategies to deal with the wealth of generated data have developed. Some are discussed here.

Data Mining	This concept refers to database applications that look for patterns in already-created databases. Do not confuse data mining with the use of software that presents data in new ways. Data mining software actually discovers new relationships between the data items that were not previously known. This class of database software has great potential for discovering new patterns of patient responses, including which patients respond to which type of treatment, and which patients are at greater risk for developing certain conditions or side effects.
Data Warehouse	A data warehouse is a collection of data designed to support decision making. Its purpose is to present a picture of the general conditions of the entity both at a particular time and historically. With this type of structure, software extracts data from other systems and places them in the warehouse database system. Along the way, many different databases from the institution are collectively scanned for the data relevant to or supportive of decision making. Generally, a warehouse supports summary data, not detailed data; it does not deal with the day-to-day operations of an institution. Use of the data warehouse's contents supports analysis of trends over time.
Data Mart	A subset or smaller-focus database designed to help managers make strategic decisions is termed a data mart. Sometimes it comprises a subset of a data warehouse. Like a data warehouse, a data mart combines aspects of many databases within the institution, but with a focus on a particular subject, department, or unit. In health care, many individual clinical departments will maintain a data mart specific to that department while sending the same data forward to the institution's data warehouse.
Distributed Database	A distributed database is stored in more than one physical place instead of in a single, central location. This is done

in one of two ways: Either parts of the database are stored in different locations, or the data are replicated in multiple locations. This practice of deploying the database speeds up service to local users while simultaneously reducing the vulnerability of the database. The downside is related to increased security issues and the potential for noncompliance with standards. Distributed databases are one of the approaches used to build an electronic health record (EHR), where the latest reports (such as lab or radiology results) are pulled to the patient's record from the departmental system (lab or radiology) as needed.

A Few Database Design Tips

The most difficult task in developing any database is to create the database structure. This time-consuming task requires the designer to pay attention to detail. As a healthcare professional, it will be your responsibility to effectively convey your database needs to the professionals designing the database. What information do you need? In what form? These are two key questions that need to be answered. Remember the purpose of the database is to help you provide efficient, quality care.

Here are some questions to answer before creating table structures:

1. What kind of output is desired? Which reports or screen outputs are needed? For example, which information needs to be on the daily plan of care?
2. Which search questions will be asked? What questions do you have when caring for patients?
3. Which fields are needed to produce the desired output and to answer the search questions? When asking these questions, what are the details you need to know?
4. What is needed to define the record accurately?
5. Which field names are desired? What are the common terms used to identify these data? For example, what is the difference between "list of diagnoses" and "problem list"?
6. Which data type will be placed in each field? For example, blood pressure (BP) is a number or numeric data, so you would never record text data or a letter in the BP field.
7. What serves as the unique identifier for each record? How do you ensure that patient records are never mixed, even if patients have the same name? Another important example is provided by the administrative simplification provisions of the Health Insurance Portability and Accountability Act of 1996 (HIPAA), which mandates the adoption of standard unique identifiers for all healthcare providers and health plans that accept Medicare.

8. How will this table or file relate to other tables or files? What are the relationships?
9. Are there any redundant (duplicate) data in this table? Are healthcare providers charting the same data twice because of problems in how the database was designed?

Common Uses of Databases in Health Care

Databases have many uses in health care. For example, they are frequently used by healthcare administrators who deal with staffing, scheduling, personnel records, and inventory control issues. Clinical databases are used to hold patient records such as lab, radiology, and pharmacy data. Educators use databases for test banks, student experiences, and student records. Research-related databases are utilized for literature access, data collection, data storage, and data retrieval. Additional databases specific to information literacy are discussed in Chapter 12.

Introduction to Access

The remainder of this chapter describes a relational database program called Access. While many larger databases use Oracle, learning about Access will provide you with a basic understanding of the process of working with databases. If you need to learn additional functions, remember to use the help system or refer to the many Access books available at bookstores.

An Access database can contain tables, forms, reports, queries, macros, and modules. This section focuses on tables and queries, as well as providing information about forms and reports.

If you have the Home or Student edition of Microsoft Office 2007, you will not have Access as part of the package; you will need to use Access in the computer lab or purchase the software separately. Alternatively, your faculty may provide you with a different database experience.

Starting Access

There are many ways to start this program:

- **Double-click** the **Microsoft Access icon** on the desktop if present.
- **Click** the **Start** button, **All Programs**, **Microsoft Office**, **Microsoft Access**.
- **Double-click** an **MS Access file**.
- **Click** the **MS Access icon** on the Quick Launch area of the taskbar.

In the Getting Started window, you will choose either to open an existing database or to create a new blank database. Just as in Word, Excel, and PowerPoint,

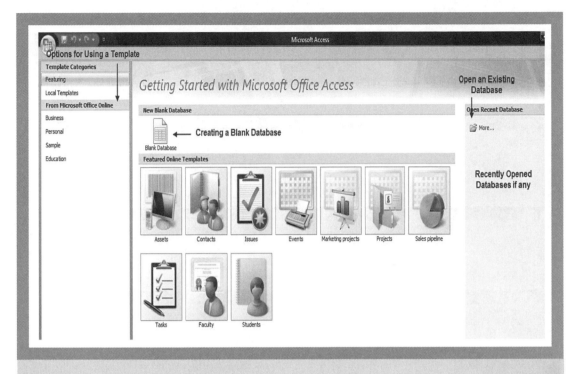

Figure 8-3 Access: Opening Screen

you have the option to select a template. You will also be asked to name the database if you create a new one. **Figure 8-3** shows the opening screen in Access.

The Access Ribbon

Because you will be working with a simple database in the exercises in this chapter, all the tabs on the ribbon will not be used. Explained here are the four tabs in Access, two of which you will use in the exercises (the other two are beyond the scope of a basic chapter on Access). Many contextual tabs will also appear as you work in the table (Table Tools), generate queries (Query Tools: Design), and work with forms and reports (Form and Report Layout Tools: Arrange, Format, and so forth). See **Figure 8-4**.

Home	This tab contains the Views, Font, Rich Text, Records, Sort & Filter, and Find groups.
Create	Use this tab to create tables, forms, reports, and queries.

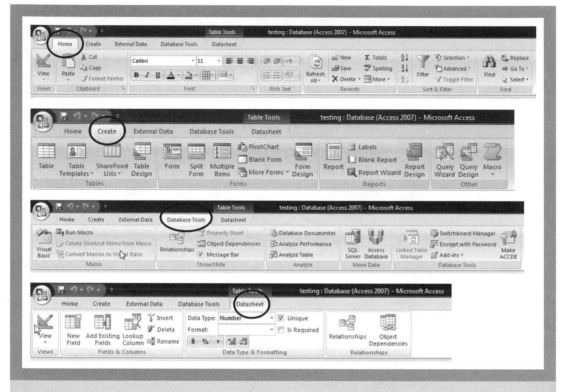

Figure 8-4 Ribbon Tabs in Access

External Data	Use this tab to import or export data, collect email data, and work with SharePoint lists. You will not be using this tab for your basic functions.
Database Tools	This tab contains the Macro, Show/Hide, Analyze, Move Data, and Database tools. You will also not be using this tab for your basic functions.

Basic Access Functions

To open a new database:

1. Start **Access**.
2. **Click** the **Blank Database icon** to create a new database.
3. When the Blank Database task pane appears (see **Figure 8-5**) on the right of the screen, **select** the **Database 1** text in the **FileName** text box and **type a name** for the database.

4. **Click** the **folder** next to the text box field to select the location for the file. Be sure to indicate the correct storage device.

5. **Click** the **Create** button [Create] to create the database. Now you are ready to create the table structures.

To open an existing database:

1. Start **Access**.

2. On the Open Recent Database task pane, **click** an existing **database file**. If the correct database file is not listed, click the **More** link to see additional database files that are stored at other locations. See **Figure 8-6**.

3. Select the **location** and **name** of the database to open.

Figure 8-7 shows the two possible screens once you open the database. Note the database name in the title bar. Additional steps are described later to create a database table. The newly created database screen now expects you to create the table structure for storing the data. The already-created database expects you to add records, generate reports, create new tables, query the tables, and so forth.

Saving and Closing the Database

Each database created is stored as a separate file with an extension of .accdb and contains the structure (tables), data, reports, forms, macros, and queries. Once the database is opened, the ribbon is available to assist in working with the database. Again, there are many contextual tabs in Access.

Once a database has been created and used, it needs to be closed before exiting the program. The records entered into the database are immediately stored in the database; the table structures are not saved until you save the table. Query and report results are not stored in the database; only the design structure of each is stored.

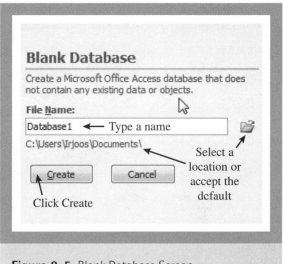

Figure 8-5 Blank Database Screen

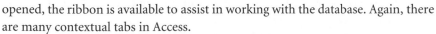

Figure 8-6 Open an Existing Database

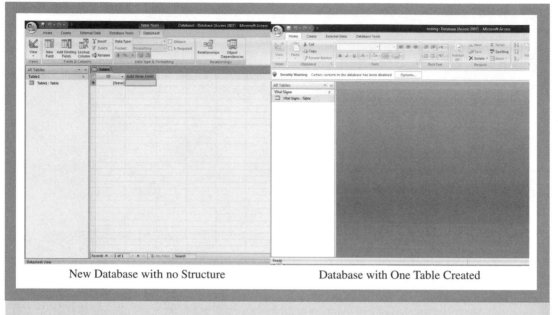

New Database with no Structure   Database with One Table Created

Figure 8-7 Main Screen When the Database Is Opened

To close the database:

1. **Click** the **Database close** button **X**.
2. Respond to any prompts regarding saving any unsaved data, forms, and reports.

To create the table structure:

1. Make sure you have a blank database opened and named.
2. If you are adding tables, **click** the **Create** tab and then **click Table**.

To enter the field names:

1. **Click** the appropriate **Tables** tab in the main window if it is not selected.
2. **Right-click** the **ID column**, then **click Rename column**; alternatively, **click Table Tools** tab, **Datasheet** tab, and in the **Fields and Columns** group, **click** the **Rename** button 🖉 Rename .
3. **Type** the **field name**, and **press Enter** or **Tab** to go to the next field name.
4. Continue typing the field names until you are finished.

Table structures may also be created in table design view, where more options for customizing the structure and each field are available. **Figure 8-8** shows a screen in design view.

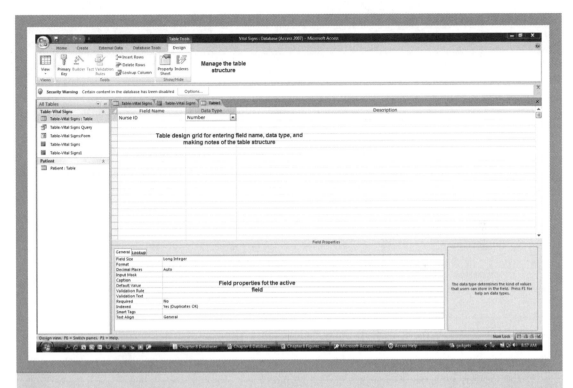

Figure 8-8 Table Design View

To set the data types for each field:

1. **Click** the **Datasheet** tab under the Table Tools contextual tab. Make sure you are in Datasheet view.
2. **Click** the **field name**.
3. In the Data Type and Formatting group (see **Figure 8-9**), **click** the **down arrow** for Data Type and **select** the correct **data type**. You may also select a format for the data and decide which field or fields will be the primary key or unique ID. **Table 8-3** shows the types of data permitted in Access.
4. Continue selecting data types until you are finished.
5. **Select** the **field** that will serve as a unique identifier for the record and

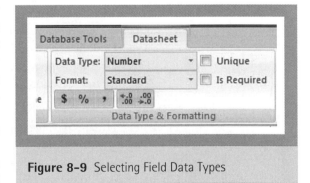

Figure 8-9 Selecting Field Data Types

TABLE 8-3 DATA TYPES IN ACCESS

Data Type	Description
Text	Text, numbers, spaces, and special characters up to 255 characters.
Memo	Use for long comments; can contain the same data type as the text field; holds a maximum of 2 GB of data.
Number	Use if the data will be used for calculations; it can contain both positive and negative numbers as well as commas and decimal points. This data type is automatically rounded up.
Date/Time	Use to store dates and times.
Currency	Use to store financial data and when you don't want automatic rounding of values.
Yes/No	Use for the presence or absence of a condition such as true and false, yes and no, or paid and unpaid.
Hyperlink	Use to link to Web sites or files.
OLE Object	Use to attach an OLE (object linking and embedding) object to a record; use to attach a file created in other programs.
Attachment	Use to attach multiple files such as images to the database.

click the **Primary Key** button in Design view or the **Unique Identifier** button Unique in Datasheet view. **Close** the table design window.

Entering and Editing Data

To enter data:

1. **Double-click** the **table name** in the All Tables task pane to open the table.
2. **Type** the **data** in each of the appropriate fields.
3. **Press** the **Tab** key to move to the next field.
4. When all fields are complete, **press** the **Tab** key to start a new record.

If you make a mistake while entering the data, use the backspace key to erase the error and then retype the data. Another way to edit the mistake is to place the cursor in the field and click. Use the cursor keys to move to the place of the mistake. Type the correction, and delete the extra letters with the Delete key. Use the Tab key to move to the next field.

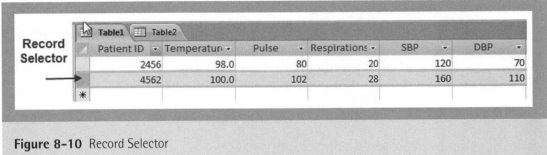

Record Selector		Patient ID ▾	Temperature ▾	Pulse ▾	Respirations ▾	SBP ▾	DBP ▾
		2456	98.0	80	20	120	70
→		4562	100.0	102	28	160	110
	*						

Figure 8-10 Record Selector

To add another record in an already-created database:

1. **Double-click** the **table name** in the open database.
2. **Click** the **first** blank row.
3. **Type** the **new data** in the appropriate fields.

To change the contents of a field:

1. **Highlight** the **data** to be replaced.
2. **Type** the **new data**.

To delete a record from a table:

1. **Click** the **record selector** for the record to be deleted. See **Figure 8-10**.
2. **Press** the **Delete** key. **Click Yes** to confirm the deletion of this record.

An alternative approach is to **click** the **Delete Record** icon on the **Home** tab, **Records** group.

Saving a Table and Exiting the Database

After creating and adding records to the database, you must save the table's design. Records are saved as they are entered, but table structures are not saved automatically. The name for the table should reflect the entity that it describes. Tables take the name of Table1, Table2, and so forth until named and saved.

To save a table:

1. **Click** the **Save** button on the Quick Access toolbar.
2. In the table dialog box, **type** the **name for the table**.
3. **Click OK**.

To exit the database:

1. Make sure all changes are saved.
2. **Click** the **Close** button.

Database View: Simple Form

There are two main views for working with a database: Datasheet and Form Views. When opening an existing database, the data are displayed in Datasheet view. That is, they are in rows and columns just like a spreadsheet. To view the data one record at a time, you must first create a simple form and then display the records in it.

To create a simple form using the Form Wizard:

1. **Click** the **Create** tab.
2. **Click** the **More Forms** button ⊞ More Forms ⸱ in the **Forms** group and **select** the **Form Wizard** ⊠ Form Wizard from the menu.
3. **Click** the **double chevron** button ⟩⟩ to place all the fields in the form, and then **click Next**.
4. Accept the defaults by **clicking Next**, **Next**, and then **Finish. Figure 8-11** shows one record displayed in Form view.

To switch from one view to the other:

1. **Click** the **Table** tab to move to the Datasheet view as noted by a table symbol on the tab.
2. **Click** the **Form** tab to move to the Form view as noted by a form symbol on the tab.

Use the following keys or buttons to move through tables in Datasheet and Form views:

Tab	To go to the next field in the record
Shift+Tab	To go to the previous field in that record
Click Next Record	To go to the next record in the database
Click Previous Record	To go to the previous record in the database
Last Record	To go to the last record in the database
First Record	To go to the first record in the database
Double-Click Specific Record, Type Record Number	To go to a specific record in the database

Sorting and Finding Records

When using a database and opening a table, the records may not be in the order that is desired for viewing. For example, you may want to review the records by job position or by patient diagnosis or by date. It is easier to sort the records than it is to scroll through them to find the ones for which you are looking. Records can be rearranged or sorted by using a sort button on the Home tab, Sort and Filter group.

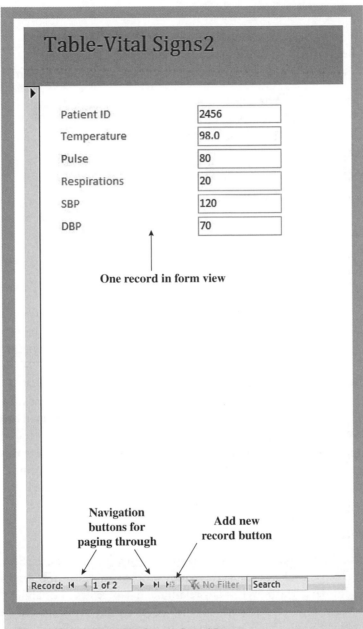

Figure 8-11 Record in Simple Form View

To sort records in a table:

1. Open the **database** and **table** to be sorted.
2. **Click** the **field** on which the sort will be based.
3. **Click** the **Sort Ascending** button or **Sort Descending** button .

Sometimes it does not matter what the order is, because the goal is to find a specific record to either verify some information or update the record. The Find feature searches only the field selected. It does not have the same power that the query feature does.

To find records:

1. Open the **database** and **table**.
2. **Click** in the **field** that has the data for the search. The field column does not need to be highlighted.
3. **Click** the **Find** button .
4. **Type** a value in the **Find What** box.
5. **Select** a **Search** option, and **select** a **Match** option.
6. **Click Find Next**.

Note that these Find and Find and Replace options work just like their counterparts in Word and Excel, except that in Access you are looking for specific information in records.

When you find the first record to be changed, click back to the table on that record field, and make the change. Then return to the Find dialog box, and click Find Next; repeat this process until all records are found and updated. When all changes are made, click the Close button. If you need to make multiple changes involving the replacement of all or one value with the same different value, use the Replace feature (accessible from the same group as the Find command) to make multiple changes at one time. Heed the warning that when the Replace feature is used, it is not possible to undo the operation.

Searching or Querying the Database

Databases allow you to search for specific information or records. Searching, however, is an exacting process and requires some knowledge of both the database and the data. The power of any relational database lies in its ability to link multiple tables together and pull only the data needed from each table. Save the query only if it is one that is repeated often; do not save queries if they are one-time searches.

Several types of searches are possible. For example, you can search all records but display only selected fields from one or more tables. Alternatively, you can combine two or more tables and display selected fields from them. Directions for creating a simple query follow.

To search one table with selected fields using the Query Wizard:

1. Open the **database** and select the **table**.
2. **Click** the **Create** tab on the ribbon.
3. **Click** the **Query Wizard** button in the other group.
4. **Select Simple Query Wizard** and then **click OK**.
5. **Click** a **field** to display in the query results and **click** the **chevron** button to place it in the results table. You may also click the **double chevron** button to place all of the fields in the **Selected Fields** text box. Only those fields in that text box will appear in the query results.
6. Continue until all fields desired appear in the Selected Fields text box, and then **click Next**.
7. Accept the defaults and **click Next** and then **Finish**.

To search two tables with selected fields:

1. Open the **database**.
2. **Click** the **Create** tab on the ribbon and then the **Query Design** button in the **Other** group.
3. **Click** the **correct** tab for the data source—a table, a query, or both.
4. **Click correct table or query** to add the table or query to the upper part of the query screen.
5. **Click** the **Add** button. Repeat this process until all tables and queries are added. **Figure 8-12** shows an example.
6. **Double-click** the **fields** from the table and/or query in the upper screen to place them in the design grid on the bottom of the window. These fields will appear in the results of the query.
7. **Type** any **criteria** for the query in the appropriate criteria row in the appropriate field column.
8. **Click** the **Run** button in the **Results** group of the Query Tools, Design tab to see the results.
9. **Save** and/or **print** the results as needed.

In Figure 8-12, the query was looking for patients whose temperature is greater than 100 degrees Fahrenheit. The results yielded two patients with slightly elevated temperatures. See **Figure 8-13**.

This feature allows you to create a subset of records that meets specific criteria. It is possible to use a single criterion, such as the city, or multiple criteria, such as the city and ZIP code or, as in this case, temperature. The criterion is set by typing the condition in the Criteria cell for the field to which the criterion applies. See the example in Figure 8-12.

To limit a search to a specific group of records, you can use comparison operators, such as equal to (=), less than (<), greater than (>), less than or equal to (<=), greater than or equal to (>=), and not equal to (<>). It is also possible to use wild

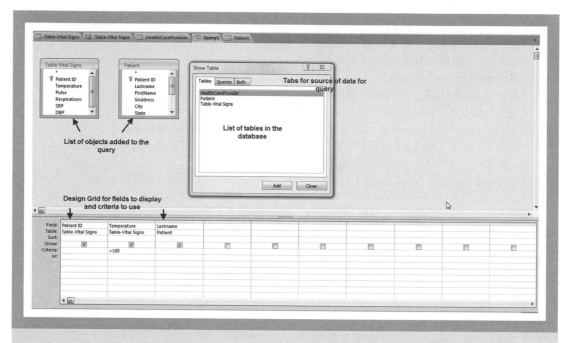

Figure 8-12 Sample Query Design Screen

card characters such as the asterisk (*) to substitute for any number of characters and a question mark (?) to substitute for one character. The Boolean operators AND and OR may also be used to construct queries.

Generating a Report

One of the primary reasons for creating and maintaining a database is the reporting feature. It is possible to report the total contents of a table or to generate

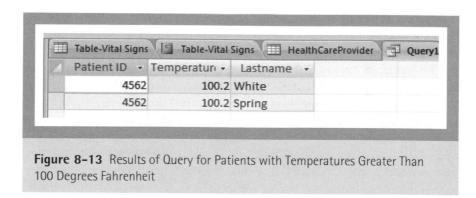

Figure 8-13 Results of Query for Patients with Temperatures Greater Than 100 Degrees Fahrenheit

multiple reports for each table, with each report providing a different view of the data. Creating a report of the results of queries allows them to be displayed in formats that are pleasing to read. Access has both an AutoReport feature and a Report Wizard feature to help create reports. The AutoReport feature creates a simple report showing all the fields in the table.

The major difference between forms and reports is that reports are intended for printing and not for display in a window. In contrast, forms are meant to be displayed in a window on the screen. Reports are designed to report some result, whereas forms are used for entering or changing values of fields.

Several types of Access reports are available: single column, tabular, stacked layout, mixed, justified, mailing labels, and unbound reports. Which report type you select depends on the data and the way in which they are to be displayed. This section covers the process of creating simple column and grouped reports. The process for designing any type of report involves thinking about how the report should look, identifying the data needed to generate the report, and identifying how detailed data will be presented.

To create a simple, single table report:

1. Open the **database** and select a **table**.
2. **Click** the **Create** tab.
3. **Click** the **Report** button in the **Reports** group.
4. **Click** the **Save** button to save the report.
5. **Type** a **name** for the report.

These steps generate a simple report showing all fields in a column and all records in a row. You can make changes to the report by selecting an object and then deleting, moving, or adjusting the look of that object. For example, you can select the time object and press Delete to remove it if a time isn't needed on the report.

To print a report:

1. Once the report is generated, **click** the **View down arrow** button on the **Home** tab.
2. **Click Print Preview** from the View options area on the ribbon. If this is a long report that spans multiple pages, use the **Next** ▸ and **Last page** ▸| buttons to move through it.
3. Make sure the report looks correct before sending it to the printer.
4. **Click** the **Print** button in the Print Preview screen or the **Office** button, **Print**, and **Quick Print**.

Grouped reports allow organization of data in a particular fashion by grouping like records together. For example, a healthcare worker might group records by department or diagnosis or healthcare provider. The example here uses the Report Wizard to help design and lay out a report.

To create a grouped report:

1. **Select** the **table** or **query** for the report.
2. **Click Report Wizard** in the **Create** tab, **Reports** group.
3. **Add** the **fields** wanted in the report, and then **click Next**.
4. **Select** the **field to group the report by**, and then **click Next**.
5. **Set** the **Sort** order, and then **click Next**.
6. **Select** a **layout** and **orientation**, and then **click Next**.
7. **Select** a **style** for the report, and then **click Next**.
8. **Click Finish**.
9. **Click** the **Save** button on the Quick Access toolbar or the **Office** button, **Save**.

Using Databases with Other Office Applications

Just as there are functions within other Office products that allow interaction among the various Office applications, so data from Access can be exported for use in Word and in Excel. For example, databases with information about customers and their addresses can be used in mail-merged letters and address labels. The specifics of these functions are beyond this basic text, but help is available within the applications or in other books about their use.

Summary

This chapter presented basic database concepts necessary for understanding the world of databases, including information about the database structure and related terms. Specific directions for using Access as an example of one database then followed. Learning how to use databases increases your ability to retrieve and use information in them, and the results produced in this way can facilitate the decision-making process.

EXERCISE 1 Searching an Online Database

This exercise was developed for readers who don't have access to the Access database program. It will give you a feel for querying a database to find information and will introduce you to the database functions offered by Excel.

■ **Objectives**
1. Use data from online databases to answer selected questions.
2. Identify knowledge needed to find the data.
3. List fields available for searching.
4. Use the data to create an Excel chart.

■ **Activity**
1. Obtain data from the Centers for Disease Control and Prevention.
   a. Go to **http://wonder.cdc.gov/Welcome.html**.
   b. **Click** the **Mortality—Underlying Cause of Death** link.
   c. **Click** the **ICD10 Code**.
   d. Complete the form to answer this question: What is the leading cause of death for 20- to 24-year-old persons in your state? Choose the latest year in which data are available.
   e. What was the leading cause of death for 20- to 24-year-olds in your state? (You may have to sort the results in descending order.)
   f. How would you classify the top few leading causes?
   g. Which fields are searchable in this database?
   h. What did you think of the way in which results were displayed?
2. Obtain U.S. Census data.
   a. Go to **http://www.census.gov/**.
   b. **Click Statistical Abstracts** at the bottom of the page.
   c. **Click Health and Nutrition** on the left-side pane.
   d. **Click Health Insurance** on the pop-up window.
   e. **Click Excel** format for **147—People With and Without Health Insurance Coverage By State:2006.**
   f. **Save** the file to your USB storage device.
   g. Go back and look around this site. What do you need to know to use it? See if you can answer these questions from the data at this site:
      ■ What is the population and rank of your state?
      ■ How many people per square mile are there in your state?
      ■ What is the average income of your state?
   h. How does this site compare to the CDC site visited in activity 1?
3. Create two Excel charts.
   a. Open the Excel file (**09s0147.xls**) downloaded in activity 2.
   b. Select the appropriate data to **create a column** chart of **all** states and the percentage (**%**) of people who don't have health insurance. Place these

data on their own chart sheet in Excel. Do NOT sort the data first. Make sure you only select cells needed to produce the chart. Press and hold down the Ctrl key while selecting noncontiguous cells.

c. **Create a second chart** of the **total number** of people in each state without insurance. Place those data on their own chart sheet in Excel.

d. What are the top three states with the largest number and largest percentage of people without health insurance?

4. Place the answers to the questions in this activity in this document in *italics* at the end of the question. If you don't have an electronic version of this exercise, create a Word document with the answers.

5. Copy the two Excel charts into the Word document by placing them at the end of the document, with each chart appearing on its own page.

6. Save the Word document as **Chap8-Ex1-Lastname**.

EXERCISE 2 Create a Table and Enter Data

■ **Objectives**

1. Create two tables with a linked field.
2. Enter and save the data.
3. Edit fields and add records.

Although most readers of this book will not be responsible for developing a database for use in a healthcare setting, this exercise was developed to give you an appreciation of the task. You may, however, serve on a committee responsible for assisting the IT department in developing a database for a specific project.

■ **Activity**

1. Start Access.
   a. **Insert** your USB storage device into a USB port. *Tables in the database will be created on the removable storage device.*
   b. **Double-click** the **Access icon**. You may need to access the program by selecting **Start, All Programs**, and **Microsoft Office, Microsoft Access** *or* by using the **Microsoft Office desktop shortcut** or the **Access icon** on the Quick Launch area of the taskbar.

2. Create the table structure.
   a. **Select** the **Blank Database** icon
   b. In the Blank Database task pane on the right side of the screen, **type Staff Insurance** in the **File name** text box.
   c. **Click** the **Folder icon** next to the database name to select a location for the database.
   d. Navigate to the **USB storage device** and the **correct folder** and **click OK**. The new location appears under the file name. See **Figure 8-14**.

e. **Click** the **Create** button Create . A new window opens, ready for you to create the first table structure in the new database. Now you are ready to enter the fields for the first table.

f. **Click** the **View button down arrow** in the **Home** tab, **View** group. **Click Design View**.

g. **Type** the table name: **Table-Staff**. **Click OK**. The Design view window appears.

h. **Type Employee ID Number** in the first cell under Field name. **Press** the **Tab** key. **Click** the **Down arrow** in Data Type and **select Number**.

i. **Press F6** to change the length of the field (field size) in the bottom half of the window.

j. **Type Double**; alternatively, use the down arrow on the far right and select **Double**.

k. **Click** the **Description** column in the top half of the screen or **Press F6** to go back to the top half of the screen. **Press** the **Tab** key to go to the next column or click the appropriate cell in the Description Column.

l. **Type Unique Identifier, Whole number**.

m. **Click** the **Key** button in the **Tools** group of the **Table Tools Design** tab, and then **press** the **Tab** key.

n. Continue typing the field names, sizes, and descriptions as outlined here. When you are finished, your screen should look like **Figure 8-15**.

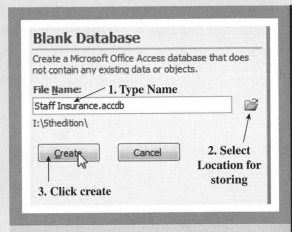

Blank Database

Create a Microsoft Office Access database that does not contain any existing data or objects.

File **N**ame: — 1. Type Name
Staff Insurance.accdb
I:\5thedition\

Create   Cancel   2. Select Location for storing

3. Click create

Figure 8-14 Blank Database Task Pane

Field Name	Data Type	Field Size	Description
Last_Name	Text	8	Staff person's last name with first letter capitalized
First_Name	Text	10	Staff person's first name
Street_Name	Text	20	Street address
City	Text	15	City
State	Text	2	State; use the two-letter, all-capitalized abbreviation

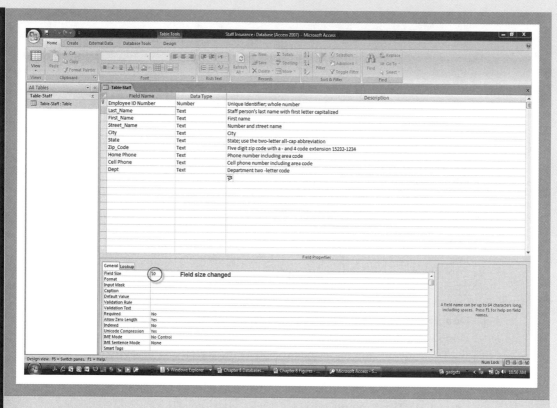

Figure 8-15 Staff Table Structure

Field Name	Data Type	Field Size	Description
Zip_code	Text	10	Five-digit ZIP code plus a hyphen (-) and the four-digit extension
Home_Phone	Text	12	Phone number, including area code
Cell_Phone	Text	12	Phone number, including area code
Dept	Text	2	Department two-letter code

o. **Click** the **Save** button in the Quick Access toolbar or use the **Office** button, **Save**.

p. Which type of data does the program accept in the field Zip_code?

q. What other data types can you use in Access?

r. Where can you find this information?

3. Create a second table.

a. Use the directions mentioned previously to create the new table; call the new table **Table:Insur**. Enter the following field names and data types:

Field Name	Data Type	Field Size	Description
Employee_ID Number	nNumber	Double	Unique identifier, whole number
Carrier	Text	30	Insurance carrier
Policy_#	Text	11	Individual's policy number
Amount	Currency		Policy value amount
Exp_Date	Date/Time		Expiration date of policy

b. Make sure to save this structure.

4. Enter data.

   Enter data into both of the tables created previously. If you make a mistake while entering the data, use the Backspace key to erase the error and then retype the data. Another way to edit a mistake is to place the cursor in the field, click the field, and use the cursor keys to go to the place of the mistake. Type the correction, and delete the extra letters with the Delete key. Use the Tab key to move to the next field.

a. **Double-click** the **Staff** table to open it.

b. **Type** the following data into the appropriate fields.

TABLE: STAFF		
20342314	21345678	97564378
Lisa Smith	Mary Jones	Robert Kiminsky
34 Terry Blvd.	5997 Irish Place	99 Moonlight Lane
Pittsburgh	Bethel Park	Forest Hills
PA 15267-2345	PA 15102-1267	PA 15343-8934
412-333-3333	412-111-7659	412-999-3557
412-555-7934	724-666-3412	724-444-3290
PT	4W	6S

TABLE: STAFF		
41235690	23534561	12454556
Pat Holmes	Jan Wish	Anna Quinn
45 White St.	7886 Center Ave.	912 Modern St
Carnegie	Greentree	Moon City
PA 15106-3421	PA 15106-3421	PA 15111-6754
412-719-1122	412-719-5195	412-719-3227
724-100-3421	724-100-5609	412-100-5681
4W	OR	ER

c. **Click** the **Save** button to save your work. **Click** the **Close** button for the datasheet window.

d. **Select Table:Insur**, and repeat the process to enter the data for the Insurance table.

TABLE: INSUR		
20342314	21345678	97564378
Allstate	Statewide	Mutual Care Provider
A20034231	2345612	M197564378
2,000,000	500,000	2,000,000
2/12/10	6/20/13	4/10/12
41235690	23534561	12454556
Statewide	Fireman's	Statewide
4562340	F345612	8976002
4,000,000	1,500,000	5,000,000
10/1/14	12/5/10	11/18/11

5. Edit records.

Add Another Record to the Staff Table.
a. **Double-click** the **Staff** table to open it.
b. Go to the end of the records and **click** in a **blank row**.
c. Type the following data: **55577722, Mains, John, 123 Irish Place, Whitefish, PA, 15261-0123, 724-333-1234, 724-536-5782, ER.**
d. **Click** the **Save** button.
e. **Close** the Staff table.

Add Another Record to the Insur Table.
a. **Double-click** the **Insur** table to open it.
b. Go to the end of the records and **click** in a **blank row**.
c. Type the following data: **55577722, Statewide, 8976100, 5,000,000, 9/28/12.**
d. **Click** the **Save** button.
e. **Close** the Insur table.

Change the Contents of One Record.
a. Open the **Staff** table.
b. Highlight **333-1234** in the phone number field of the **John Mains** record.
c. **Type 345-1234**, and **click** the **Close** button. The change is automatically saved.
6. Close **Access**.
a. **Click** the **Close** button to close the application.
b. Remember to remove your USB storage device.
7. If required by your professor, submit your file or prints of the data in the tables.

EXERCISE 3 Create, Search, Sort, and Generate a Report

■ **Objectives**
1. Search (query) the database using one table, two tables, all fields, and selected fields.
2. Sort the database.
3. Prepare and print a report.

■ **Activity**
1. Search for data.
    Open the **Staff Insurance** database located on your USB storage device.

    Basic Search for Specific Criteria in One Table
    First you want to know the answer to the following question: "Do any of the staff have an insurance policy with Statewide?" If the answer is yes, how many staff members have such a policy?
    a. **Click** the **Create** tab and **select Query Wizard** .
    b. **Click Simple Query Wizard** and **click OK**.
    c. **Click** the **Insur** table from the **Tables/Queries down arrow** at the top of the window.

d. **Click** the **chevron** >> to display all the fields in the selected text box, and then **click Next**.

e. Accept the defaults for the next screen, and then **click Next**.

f. **Type** the table name **Employees with Statewide** for the title of the query.

g. **Click** the **circle** next to Modify Query Design and **click Finish**. The query design screen appears.

h. **Type Statewide** in the cell that is at the intersection of the carrier column and the criteria row.

i. **Click** the **Run** button ❗.

j. Answer these questions but do not close the application:

  ▪ Do any of the staff use Statewide as their insurance carrier?

  ▪ If so, how many staff use Statewide as their insurance carrier?

This was an example of a simple search displaying all of the fields from a single table that meet a specific criterion. Notice this information isn't too helpful, as you don't know *which* staff members have their insurance with Statewide. All you know is the number of individuals who meet this criterion, the expiration date for the policy, and the amount of the insurance.

Search of Two Tables

To make the results more meaningful, add the **Staff** table to the search.

a. **Click** the **View** button on the **Home** tab.

b. **Select** the **Design View** option. The design view screen appears.

c. **Right-click** the top blank area of the window and **select Show table** from the shortcut menu.

d. **Select** the **Staff** table and **click Add**. The Staff table now appears at the top of the screen.

e. **Click Close** to close the **Show Table** dialog box.

f. **Double-click** the **Last name** and **First name** fields in the Staff table to add them to the results table.

g. The last thing you have to do before running the query is to connect the two tables. Drag the **Employee ID Number** from the Staff table onto the Insur table's **Employee ID Number** field. A line is drawn connecting the two tables.

h. **Click** the **Run** button ❗ to see the results.

i. Now you decide that you don't need to see the employee ID number or the policy number. Go back (**Click View** icon on the Home tab) to **Design view** and remove the checks in the **Show row** for those two fields.

j. **Run** the query again. **Click** the **Save** button.

Displaying All Records But Only Selected Fields

a. **Click** the **Create** tab.
b. **Click** the **Query Design** button.
c. Select **Table:Staff. Click** the **Add** button, and then **click** the **Close** button on the Show table dialog box.
d. **Double-click** the **Employee ID Number, Last_Name, First_Name,** and **Dept** fields listed in the Table:Staff to display the field in the query table. You may need to enlarge the Table Staff window to see all the fields.
e. **Click** the **Run** button. Only fields selected are displayed in the results.
f. **Click** the **Printer** button on the Quick Access toolbar to print a copy of this query or go to the **Office** button, **Print,** and **choose Quick Print.**
g. **Click** the **Close** button for the query window.
h. **Click No** to not save this query.

More Complex Search on Two Tables with Additional Criteria

This query answers the following question: Which staff members have liability policies due to expire in January, February, or March 2010? Based on the query results, a reminder to renew and provide current information on their policies can be sent.

a. **Click** the **Create** tab.
b. **Click** the **Query Design** button.
c. **Select Table:Insur. Click** the **Add** button.
d. **Select Table:Staff. Click** the **Add** button, and then **click** the **Close** button on the Show Table dialog box.
e. **Double-click** the **Employee ID Number, Last_Name, First_Name,** and **Dept** fields listed in the Staff table to display the field in the query table.
f. **Double-click** the **Exp_Date** field of the Insur table.
g. **Drag** the **Employee ID Number** from the Staff table on top of the **Employee ID Number** on the Insur table to relate the two tables.
h. **Type > =1/1/10 AND <2/28/10** in the cell found at the intersection of the Criteria and Exp_Date fields.
i. **Click** the **Run** button.
j. **Print** the results.
k. Answer the following questions:
   - How many staff members have insurance policies that are about to expire?
   - Which departments have staff members with soon-to-expire insurance policies?
l. **Click** the **Close** button for the query window.
m. **Click Yes** to save this query. **Type Query:expdate. Press Enter** or **click OK.**

2. Sort the data.

Sometimes you want to place the records in a different order from the one in which they are displayed.

   a. Open **Table:Staff**.

   b. **Click** the **Last_Name** column heading. That is, click over the words **Last-Name**. The total column is now highlighted.

   c. **Click** the **Sort Ascending** button .

   d. **Click** the **Printer** button on the Quick Access toolbar to print a copy of the data in this order or use the **Office** button and **select Print**.

   e. **Click** the **Close** button of the table window.

   f. **Click No** to not save the sort changes.

3. Find a specific record.

To Find a Specific Record for the Purpose of Checking Some Information in It

   a. Open **Table:Staff**.

   b. **Click** in the **City** field. The field column does not need to be highlighted.

   c. **Click** the **Find** button .

   d. **Type Carnegie** in the **Find What** text box.

   e. **Select All** as the **Search** option, and **select Whole Field** as the **Match** option.

   f. **Click Find Next** twice, and **click OK** to the prompt for no more records found.

   g. **Click** the **Close** button in the Find and Replace dialog box.

To Find a Record to Update It

   a. **Click** in the **Last_Name** field. The field column does not need to be highlighted.

   b. **Click** the **Find** button .

   c. **Type Smith** in the **Find What** text box.

   d. **Select All** as the **Search** option, and **select Whole Field** as the **Match** option.

   e. **Click Find Next**, and then **click** the **Close** button to close the Find and Replace dialog box.

   f. **Press** the **Tab** key until you are at the home phone number field.

   g. **Highlight 3333**, and **type 1234**. **Click** the **Close** button and then **click Yes** to save the change.

4. Generate reports.

AutoReport

   a. **Double-click** the **Query:expdate** result table.

   b. **Click** the **Create** tab, and then **click** the **Report** button . The report appears.

   c. **Close** the **Report**, click **Yes** to save it, and name it **Report:ExpIns**.

Report Wizard

a. **Double-click** the **Staff** table.
b. **Click** the **Create** tab and the **Report Wizard** button Report Wizard .
c. **Click** the **Add all fields chevron** >> and then **click Next**.
d. **Select Dept** for the grouping, **click** the **single chevron** > , and then **click Next**.
e. **Click Next** to accept the default.
f. **Select Block** and **landscape** and **click Next**. Note that the report is automatically saved in the database unlike queries that need to be saved if needed repeatedly.
g. **Select Concourse** and **click Next**.
h. **Type Staff Report**, and **click Finish**.
i. **Click** the **Printer** button on the Quick Access toolbar or **select** the **Office** button, **Print**.
j. **Click** the **Close** button, and exit Access.

EXERCISE 4 Design a Small Clinical Database

■ **Objectives**

1. Examine the problem in the Vital Signs table used in the chapter.
2. Design a record structure to use to generate a reminder or work list for caring for a group of patients.
3. Enter data for 10 patients.
4. Print a report.

■ **Activity**

1. Look at the structure for the Vital Signs table. What is the major problem with this table? See Figure 8-10 for the fields in the table. How would you correct the major design flaw? HINT: Since Patient ID is a unique identifier, how will you accommodate multiple entries for vital signs?
2. Create a new database by creating the table shown here. Add at least five additional rows with appropriate data for a patient record to provide the information that you would need to deliver patient care. Consult a reminder sheet, worksheets, and patient plans or progress notes from your clinical facility for ideas of which data to include.

Field Name	Field Type	Field Size	Description Data
Last Name	text	20	Patient's last name
First Name	text	15	Patient's first name
Room Number	number	4	Four-digit room number

Field Name	Field Type	Field Size	Description Data
Gender	text	1	F for female or M for male
Primary Dx	text	25	Main reason for hospitalization
Secondary Dx	text	25	Secondary reason for hospitalization, if any

3. Enter the data for eight patients.
4. Which problems, if any, did you encounter?
5. Save the data.
6. Search for an individual patient.
7. Search for all patients with a specific diagnosis.
8. Add two more records.
9. Generate a work list or reminder sheet for a group of patients.

ASSIGNMENT 1 Clinical Experience Database

■ **Directions**

1. Construct a table structure(s) to use for monitoring your clinical experiences. Use a table similar to the one in Exercise 4 that identifies the fields, data type, and field size. Use a Word table for the planning.
2. At the bottom of your table(s) (or on the next page), explain the rationale behind the table(s). Which questions were you trying to answer? Which experiences were you trying to monitor?
3. Open Access, and create the table(s). Then enter records for 10 of your experiences. Provide a printout of the table structure as created and the data in the table.
4. Conduct a search to answer one of your questions. Print the results.

ASSIGNMENT 2 Data Classification, Taxonomy, and Data Sets

■ **Directions**

1. Use a browser and go to http://www.nursingworld.org/MainMenu Categories/ANAMarketplace/ANAPeriodicals/OJIN/FunctionalMenu/ AboutOJIN.aspx. **Type standard languages** in the search text box. Select two articles to read. Define the following terms: *classification systems, taxonomies, standard languages,* and *data sets.*

2. In your browser, type **http://nursingworld.org/npii/terminologies.htm**.
   - Which content is covered in the ANA-recognized data element sets?
   - Are any of these used in your clinical sites?
3. Here are some sites to learn a little about SNOMED:
   http://www.ihtsdo.org/snomed-ct/who-is-using-snomed-ct/
   http://www.ihtsdo.org/snomed-ct/
   After looking at the information from these sites, why is SNOMED so important in the United States?
4. Go to the following site: http://healthit.ahrq.gov/portal/server.pt?open=514&objID=5554&mode=2&holderDisplayURL=http://prodportallb.ahrq.gov:7087/publishedcontent/publish/communities/k_o/knowledge_library/key_topics/health_briefing_01232006100413/standards.html.
   - What are the major advantages and disadvantages of doing this type of work?
   - What are the database and automation implications of this work?
   - Describe in a short paragraph which of these standards are being used in your clinical facility.

Using the World Wide Web

Objectives

1. Describe the Internet and the World Wide Web.
2. Define related Internet terms.
3. Explain the components of a World Wide Web address.
4. Identify the hardware and software that are needed to connect to the Internet.
5. Use browsers to explore the World Wide Web.
6. Download files from the Internet.
7. Describe the Web page creation process and the healthcare professional's role in it.

This chapter focuses on the Internet. People access the Internet for the purpose of communicating with others, obtaining information and files, and accessing Web servers so as to purchase products or services, watch movies, play games, and so forth. This chapter begins with a brief definition and description of the Internet and World Wide Web. This information is followed by a discussion of Internet services, means of connecting to the Internet, addressing, browsing and locating information, use of search engines, and downloading files. A brief description of the process of creating Web pages is also included. Additional information on Internet communication (e.g., email, newsgroups, list services, video chats) and informational resources (searching and search strategies) appears in Chapters 10 and 12, respectively.

The Internet

Most of us think of the World Wide Web (WWW) as the Internet. In fact, the Internet is more encompassing than the WWW. Any function such as communications (email, listservs, and so forth) and file downloading (FTP) that uses the Internet networking protocols is part of the Internet, even when the Hypertext Transfer Protocol (HTTP) is not used.

The Internet, sometimes referred to as the information or global superhighway, is a loose association of millions of networks and billions of computers around the world, all of which work together to share information. It is a truly global network that provides people with quick access to information and services from all over the world.

Structure

No one source foots the bill for the Internet; everyone pays for his or her part. For example, colleges and universities pay for their connections to some regional network. This regional network, in turn, pays a national provider for access.

Many institutions and companies donate their computer resources in the form of servers and computer technicians to hold up some part of the Internet. Other companies own and operate components of the Internet in the form of communication lines and related switching equipment. The main lines that carry the bulk of the traffic are collectively known as the **Internet backbone**. In the United States, they were called network access points (NAPs; each owned by a different company) and metropolitan access exchanges (MAEs). These designations are changing, such that in many parts of the world they are now referred to as Internet eXchange Points (IXPs).

Some of the major players in this system are MCI, Sprint, and WorldCom. These companies sell access to Internet service providers (ISPs) and other large businesses (sometimes called commerce service providers [CSPs]). The ISPs and CSPs, in turn, sell access to the Internet to other large businesses, organizations, and smaller ISPs. The smaller ISPs then sell access to smaller businesses, organizations, and finally individuals. Through their interconnection, these networks create high-speed communication lines that crisscross the United States. These high-speed communication lines extend communication to the United Kingdom and the rest of Europe, Australia, Japan, Asia, and the rest of the world. Some of these countries provide Internet speeds much higher than found in the United States. It is important to note that not all points along the route are well developed. In the United States, the backbone has many intersecting points. If one point fails or slows, data are quickly rerouted over another part. This redundancy was one of the key points in the Internet's development. In some parts of the world, the network may have less redundancy, making it more vulnerable to slowdowns or breakdowns. In addition, governments in some countries control the backbone in their country, which means they dictate who gets access to the rest of the world.

Control

No one organization governs the Internet. Instead, this massive network relies on a group of organizations to form a check and balance system to make sure things work. Here are a few of the key players:

- The Internet Society (ISOC) is a supervisory organization that is made up of individuals, corporations, nonprofit organizations, and government agencies from the Internet community. It holds the ultimate authority for the direction of the Internet and provides a home for several organizations that deal with Internet issues and standards (http://www.isoc.org).
- The Internet Architecture Board (IAB) is responsible for defining the overall architecture of the Internet (the backbone) and all of the networks attached to it. It approves standards and the allocation of resources such as Internet addresses (http://iab.org).
- The Internet Engineering Task Force (IETF) focuses on operational and technical issues related to keeping the Internet running smoothly as a whole (http://www.ietf.org).
- The World Wide Web Consortium (W3C) manages the Hypertext Mark-up Language (HTML) standard, other Web-related standards (e.g., SHTML, SML, and CSS), and other specifics as they relate to the Web part of the Internet. This organization promotes interoperability for the various Web components (http://www.w3.org).
- Backbone ISPs, cable and satellite companies, regional and long-distance phone companies, and various agencies of the U.S. and other countries' governments contribute to the Internet telecommunications infrastructure.
- The Internet Assigned Numbers Authority (IANA) and the Internet Network Information Center (InterNIC) are the two organizations responsible for assigning IP addresses and domain names, respectively (http://www.iana .org and http://www.internic.org).

Protocols

Communicating with other computers, many of which don't share the same structure or operating systems, requires a means for all of the computers to "talk" to each other—that is, to speak the same language. For the Internet, this base protocol (set of rules) is called Transmission Control Protocol/Internet Protocol (TCP/IP). Every computer on the Internet must use and understand this protocol for sending and receiving data. TCP/IP uses a "packet-switched network" that minimizes the chance that data will be lost when the packets are sent over the transmission medium.

The TCP part of the protocol breaks every piece of data into small chunks called packets. Each packet is wrapped in an electronic envelope that contains the Web addresses for both the sender and the recipient. Once the packets are created, the IP part of the protocol determines the best route for getting the packet from one point to another point. Each packet may arrive at its destination by a different route. Routers examine the destination address and then send the packet to one router after another, until it reaches its final destination. Each router sends the packet by the best route available at that time. When the packet arrives at its destination, TCP takes over. Its function is to identify each packet, make sure that it is intact, and then reassemble the packets to reconstruct the original data.

In addition to these protocols, some others might be encountered—for example, FTP for transferring files, telnet for remote logging in, and mail protocols such as POP3 (Post Office Protocol 3), SMTP (Simple Mail Transfer Protocol), and IMAP (Internet Message Access Protocol). Most of the time, these protocols operate seamlessly from the perspective of the typical Internet user.

The World Wide Web

Some consider the World Wide Web (WWW, also known more simply as the Web) the easiest of the Internet services to use. This part of the Internet is the graphical portion that stores electronic files, called Web pages, on servers that are accessed from the user's computer. Keywords (**hyperlinks**) in a document are highlighted. Selecting a keyword takes the reader to another part of that document related to that word, to another document at that site, or to another site. In addition, some graphics and buttons are hyperlinked, permitting the user to go to different sites or to obtain more information at the current site. The protocol used on the Web is HTTP.

Presented here are terms related to the World Wide Web.

Client–Server	Client–server computing is the de facto model for network-oriented computing. Servers and clients interact with one another while exchanging information. Servers provide the information—in this case, Web pages—and clients consume it. The client is the computer that knows how to communicate with a Web server.
Hyperlinks	Hyperlinks are text or graphics that are linked to other parts of a file or to other files at the same site or other sites. When the pointer of a mouse rests over a hyperlink, it turns into a hand (🖑).
HTML	Hypertext Markup Language is the tagging that is used to code the Web page files so that they can be displayed in a browser on a variety of computers. Included in these tags are commands for linking text and graphics.

HTTP	Hypertext Transfer Protocol is the communications protocol that is used for accessing and working with the World Wide Web. Do not confuse it with HTML, which is the tagging language.
Web Browser	Web browser software is used to access Web pages on the Internet and to interpret HTML code and turn it into readable form. Two of the major browsers are Internet Explorer and Firefox. Safari is the default browser that comes with the Mac OS.

Services on the Internet

Many services are available on the Internet. Most people, when using the term "Internet," use it to mean the World Wide Web. In fact, the Web is just one part of the Internet, albeit the most heavily used portion. Basically, the services available can be classified into four categories: electronic communications, information services, information retrieval, and entertainment.

Electronic Communications	These services permit you to communicate with other people on the Internet via electronic mail, bulletin boards, chat rooms, instant messages, blogs, list or discussion services (such as listservs), news groups, and social networks such as Facebook and MySpace. In addition, electronic communications media include video sharing services such as YouTube and photo sharing services such as Flickr and Photobucket; these services are discussed in Chapter 10.
Information Services	Information services are commonly referred to as remote login, or information access. These services permit you to log in to other computers from your computer for the purpose of obtaining information. The two main services in this area are telnet (used by many librarians) and the Web (used by all). Growing in use are streaming applications, which permit users to view videos and podcasts of educational materials and to interact with one another in real time. The focus here, however, is information access.

Information Retrieval	These services permit users to obtain files from other sites and bring them to their own computers, a process commonly referred to as file transfer. File Transfer Protocol (FTP) is the most commonly used protocol for transferring files from one computer to another. Since the development of the Web, the interface for transferring files has become more user friendly and not command driven.
Entertainment	These services consist of listening to the radio, watching TV programs and movies, and playing games interactively over the Internet.

All of these services have evolved so that they are easier to use now than they were a few years ago. For example, when transferring a file, you do not need to know all of the commands for downloading files or for activating FTP—knowledge that was essential for completing these operations in the past. Most of the time today, file transfer is a matter of clicking on a download hyperlink and responding to prompts. Graphics may even be downloaded by right-clicking the image and selecting "Save picture as" from the shortcut menu. In this way, the user is isolated from the background commands necessary to use these services.

Another trend in Internet services is that some sites that use protocols such as telnet and gopher are closing as the Web part continues to grow. Telnet sites permitted the user to log in to a computer and access another site to view the other site's information. Many of these sites permit anyone to use them. Librarians continue to use telnet services, but most of the general public does not. Gopher sites were hierarchically based menus for accessing information available on the Internet; the user selected from the menu and a submenu until the information was found. Now Web and search sites make it much easier to find and access this information by using search engines, directories, and hyperlinks. Thus many of the services once provided by telnet and gopher sites are being replaced by Web sites and searching facilities.

Connecting to the Internet

This section outlines the equipment and software needed to access the Internet. The services desired determine the equipment needed to access the Internet. For example, using the Web to access and play multimedia files requires a higher-level computer than accessing a text-based email program on a UNIX computer. In addition, software is needed for each type of service accessed. To make things easier software-wise, most ISPs and browser programs now come with many features bundled into one easy-to-install program.

Computer

Although the computer requirements for accessing the Internet are not very demanding, the computer must have sufficient RAM, a fast processor, and free hard drive space. Each provider lists the minimum hardware and operating system requirements needed to use its services. The level of computer required really depends on what you want to do on the Internet. If you expect full multimedia information to appear on the computer instantly, you will need a higher-level computer with higher-speed connections and full multimedia capabilities—sound cards, speakers, and good graphics. If the expectation is to use primarily email, a basic computer or smart phone will do. For example, a student might want to pull up the video podcast of a demonstration missed in class or view a required DVD used in an online course. That individual could use an iPod for the video podcast but will need a computer of much greater capacity to view the DVD. These requirements are greater than those for simply accessing email or downloading text documents.

Network Connection

From home, the computer needs to have a connection to the server or host computer. This is generally accomplished through a phone line, a digital subscriber line (DSL) line, satellite dish, cable, or fiber-optic connection. On campus, connection is done through the campus network connections, which can be either wired or wireless. **Broadband** connections such as DSL and cable, which are faster than dial-up access, can provide an ongoing connection to the Internet. Unfortunately, this nonstop access also means that the end user is more vulnerable to hackers. To protect against hacker incursion into their computers, broadband users should install a personal firewall as well as antivirus and antispam software. Chapter 13 provides more details about security.

Modems

A modem is used to provide an interface between the computer and the transmission channel for converting the data into a form that can be transmitted via the selected transmission line. At home, this can be a dial-up modem, a DSL modem, a cable modem, a satellite modem, or a wireless router/modem.

Dial-up modems are still in use in many parts of the United States because of the costs and unavailability of other types of connectivity. They are the slowest means of connecting, and they tie up the phone line; however, they are readily available and are relatively inexpensive.

DSL modems provide connectivity by using the digital portion of the regular copper telephone line. This type of access is faster than a dial-up connection, does not tie up the phone line, is a little more expensive, and can be always "connected" unless you turn it off which most people do not do. The downside is the lack of availability in some areas and the inherent security issues that arise because the computer when turned on is always connected to the Internet.

Cable modems are designed to work with a cable TV line and are specified by the cable provider. They provide faster access to the Internet than traditional phone and DSL modems. A cable modem typically has two connections, one to the cable wall outlet and the other to the computer via an Ethernet card. Costs vary greatly depending on location and cable provider; speed fluctuates based on how many people are sharing the bandwidth at the same time. Security issues exist with cable as well.

A **satellite** Internet connection uses a satellite dish antenna and a transceiver (transmitter/receiver) that operates in the microwave portion of the radio spectrum. The installer generally provides and configures the modem, sets up the dish, and brings the system to a wall jack. These connections are subjected to weather interference and latency, but provide an option for fast Internet connections in rural areas not reached by DSL or cable.

Fiber-optic connections (such as the Verizon Fios service) rely on a **wireless router** to provide the connectivity between the computer, phone wire, and fiber-optic panel. This option provides for faster connection speeds than DSL or cable, but is a little more expensive. Many ISPs now bundle this option with TV and phone service.

Cards and Adapters

A special device is needed to move the data from the computer or mobile device through the transmission media (e.g., phone lines, cables, radio waves) to the access provider. Some computers (i.e., laptops) have wireless and network cards built into them instead of using modems.

A **wireless card** is used to provide connectivity via mobile computers. It converts the data into radio signals. This type of connection can be very fast and may be available in areas not serviced by cable or DSL. The downside is that the device must be within a 10- to 20-mile radius of a hot spot or access point. The number of wireless access points is increasing daily with free WiFi (Wireless Fidelity) available in many cafes, airports, and bookstores.

A **network card**, which is installed into a computer, enables a direct connection to a network. It is the typical connection found in college dormitories, laboratories, and offices. This type of access does not need a modem but does require a special cable and an active network port.

USB cellular modem is a wireless adapter that connects a laptop to a cellular telephone system for data access and transfer. The adapter plugs into a USB port, although some models use the PC card slot. Some cell phones can also be used as the wireless point for access and transmission of data.

Access Providers

Access providers are organizations that provide access to an Internet host computer. They often supply the software needed to connect to the Internet as well as the appropriate connection equipment. Because several types of access providers exist, users need to choose the type of access that is appropriate for them.

Internet Service Providers

ISPs provide access to the Internet and email. Many also provide special services such as news, data storage, Web hosting, and specialized databases. Examples include America Online (AOL), Verizon, Comcast, DirectTV, and a host of others depending on your geographic location. There is a great deal of competition among ISP providers.

Here are some considerations for selecting an ISP:

- Is the cost for unlimited connecting time or per hour? Is there a setup fee?
- What is used to connect to the Internet?
- Is the connectivity fast and reliable at *all* times of the day? In other words, what is the ratio of subscribers to bandwidth?
- Is there reliable and responsive technical support on a 24/7 basis?
- Is there space on the server for personal home pages?
- Are all of the desirable services available, such as email, instant messaging, Web and related multimedia files, FTP, newsreader, and telnet?
- What is the maximum size for file attachments and for the email account?
- What is available for privacy and security? Does the ISP offer a firewall? Parental controls? Free virus protection?
- For dial-up connections, are there local access phone numbers or toll-free numbers with national access?
- Do you get to choose your account logins and passwords? How many users can you have on one account?
- Does the ISP provide secure backup services so that you can store your personal data?

Free Internet Access

Some community-based computer networks are designed to help local citizens access and share information and resources without cost; others are free ISPs that make their money from paid sponsors or advertisers. Funding to support community-based access is generally made available through local libraries, government agencies, or interested local businesses such as airports. This type of service is generally restricted to people who live in or are temporarily visiting the community. Many of these networks rely on a group of volunteers to assist in developing and maintaining the system. In many cases these free services have limited security. As a result users should use caution accessing personal information such as financial data over these networks.

Temporary Access for a Fee

Internet access may also be provided through local businesses such as hotels, coffee shops, or delis, which are sometimes referred to as cybercafes. Some of these providers have time restrictions; others charge varying fees for temporary access. Some hotels provide free access in the lobby or bar area, but charge for access from guests' rooms.

Company or Institutional Access

Access to the Internet may be provided to an employee or student in an institution through the organization's computer and connection facilities. Once connected to the company's network, the user has access to all of the capabilities provided by the company, including Internet access and email. Some companies provide mobile users with cards to plug into their laptops that give them access to the corporation's network through a cellular connection; others require a physical presence at the facilities or connection to the network from a home connection. The user must remain an employee or student to continue to use the access, and he or she is subject to the policies of that organization or institution (acceptable use policies).

Software

The software needed to access the Internet depends on how it is being accessed and who provides the connection service. Communication protocols that coordinate data transfer to and from the local computer and the Internet (e.g., TCP/IP) and protocols for the various services (such as email, Web, and FTP) are needed. If access comes through a university or corporate network, often special software is needed to access the internal network. This software is generally obtained from the company and works behind the scenes once installed. Most information technology (IT) departments provide easy-to-use instructions for installing programs. Other companies provide Web-based interfaces to their mail clients.

The Internet front-end software is the software with which the user interacts (the browser). It might be a comprehensive program, such as Firefox or Internet Explorer, or a program provided by the service provider. Usually this software is provided free of charge when the user becomes a subscriber (AOL), is available for free downloading (Firefox), or comes with the operating system (Internet Explorer).

User IDs and Passwords

You must have a user ID (name) and password to use the services of the ISP. The user ID and password may be chosen by the user or assigned by the institution using its naming standards. For example, some institutions use the user's last name, first letter of first name, and middle initial; others use the last name, first letter of first name, and a number; thus a user ID might be irjoos, joosir, or joosil. Many ISPs let users choose their own IDs as long as someone else on the system does not have that ID; the ID could then be ngtcrawler, nurseJane, or hojo.

What is important is that each user on that system must be uniquely identified in the system. No two system users can have the same user ID on that system. Some ISPs and institutions handle duplicate IDs by assigning numbers to the end; thus ngtcrawler becomes ngtcrawler2, and nurseJane becomes nurseJane2.

If you are selecting an ID on your own, it is wise to select a neutral ID as opposed to a provocative ID. For example, sexyme, drugpusher, and partyanimal are not appropriate ID names for a professional healthcare worker.

Although the user ID is public knowledge, the password is private. Passwords should be safeguarded just like a personal identification number (PIN) for a bank (ATM) account. They should not be given to anyone or written down where others can see them. In addition, each system has its own criteria for what are acceptable passwords. For example, many systems require a minimum number of characters and a combination of letters and numbers; thus the password bri8ll might be acceptable. Dictionary words and common-knowledge words such as a spouse's name or a pet's name should be avoided as passwords, because they are too easy for someone to break. Use nonsense combinations that make sense to you. An example might be gcle2009, where g = green, cle = Camry LE, and 2009 = year of the car. (Additional information on forming strong passwords appears later in this book, in Table 13-5.)

Understanding Addressing

While you must have a user ID to access the Internet, your computer must have a unique address when connecting to the Internet. This address allows the computer to get information from a Web server and, in turn, to receive information from other computers. Although humans use words and graphics to communicate, computers prefer to use numbers.

This section discusses IP addresses, domain names, and URLs—all terms used to locate and differentiate one computer and its files from all other computers and files on the Internet.

IP Addresses

An Internet Protocol (IP) address is a unique identification number that distinguishes each computer on the Internet. The university or service provider assigns this number to the computer. To communicate effectively, no two computers can have the same number at the same time. A computer may be assigned a fixed or static address or a dynamic address that changes each time the user accesses the Internet.

The IP address uses a number from 0 to 255 for each part of its four-part number. For example, this number may be something like 208.34.242.17. Because the number of computers connected to the Internet is fast approaching the 4.2 billion mark in terms of possible addresses for the IP system, work is proceeding on finding alternative numbering systems that do not require major hardware or software changes. This new scheme, which is called CIDR (Classless Inter-Domain Routing), replaces the older system. A CIDR IP address looks like a normal IP address except that it ends with a slash followed by a number, called the IP network prefix; an example is 123.231.1.123/16.

Current addresses sometimes include a subnetting feature that uses reserved IP addresses within a local area network. These addresses cannot travel on the Internet and require a network address translation (NAT) device to convert their data packets when they move to the Internet.

What is important for you to understand is that your computer needs an IP address when it is connected to the Internet for things to work.

Domain Names

A domain name is an address, similar to that used by the postal service, that points to a computer with a specific IP address. It is a description of a computer's location on the Internet. Domain names create a single identity for a series of computers used by a company. A special Domain Name System (DNS) computer looks up the name and matches it with its assigned number. Examples of domain names are www.adobe.com and intranet.school.edu.

The domain name contains a few components that are separated by a period (**Figure 9-1**). On the left is the more specific name for the computer; to the right is the category that describes the nature of the organization. The first item is the name of the host itself (www or online). The next item, which consists of the second-level domain name (google or school), is registered with an organization

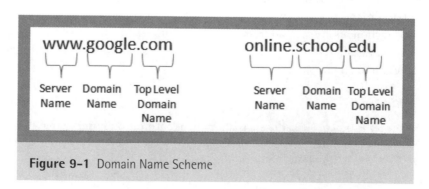

Figure 9-1 Domain Name Scheme

or entity like the Internet Network Information Center (InterNIC) registration services. The last item (e.g., com or edu) is the top-level domain name and describes the purpose of the organization or entity that owns the second-level name. It is assigned by nature of the organization.

Here are a few of the common top-level domain names. For a more complete listing and description, consult http://www.iana.org/gtld/gtld.htm. Additional top-level domain names are always being proposed.

aero   Air transportation industry
com   Business or other commercial enterprises
edu   Postsecondary institutions
gov   Government agencies or departments
mil   Military
net   Network service providers or resources
org   Organizations, usually nonprofit or charitable
pro   Professionals or other licensed people

All of these top-level domain names are used in the United States. There are also country top-level domain names such as "ca" for Canada and "nz" for New Zealand.

A domain may also contain other components between the host (Web server) and the second-level domain; these are called subdomains. Subdomain names are used by large organizations that support many Internet servers. For example, the U.S. government and its many agencies differentiate one agency from another through use of the subdomains. An educational institution may have subdomains for each school or department. For example, in the address www.nursing.school.edu, "nursing" might represent the nursing school's or department's Web server (www). Also, other countries sometimes use a similar naming system; for example, in Virginia.co.uk, "co" is the equivalent of .com and "uk" represents the United Kingdom.

Anyone can register with the InterNIC to obtain a second-level domain name. However, there is a fee for having one's own second-level domain name. To see who owns specific domain names, go to http://www.internic.net/whois.html. Some enterprising people have registered a variety of names of big corporations and now make money selling the rights to these second-level domain names to those organizations.

Understanding the domain names will help you identify the type of information likely to be obtained from a certain site. Knowing that the site is a government agency, such as the IRS (http://www.irs.gov), means that the forms and their instructions provided there are legitimate. Sites such as those operated by the National Library of Medicine (http://www.nlm.nih.gov) and the Centers for Disease Control and Prevention (http://www.cdc.gov) are very likely to provide current and reliable information. However, information from someone's personal home page may or may not be accurate or reliable. However, be careful. Note the difference between the Web sites for http://www.irs.gov and http://www.irs.com or http://www.cdc.gov and http://www.cdc.org where the only difference is the domain name. The same thing happens with slight variations in second domain names. Note the difference in the Web sites between http://www.webmd.com and http://www.mdweb.com.

URLs

URLs help a computer locate a Web page's exact location on the Web server. Although IP addresses and domain names locate the computer, they do not locate the Web documents on the server. The URL helps the computer find the actual Web pages. See **Figure 9-2** for an example.

Consider the following URL: http://www.nursing.pst.edu/foundations/courses/nsg412.html. The first part, http://, identifies the communications protocol that the computers are using to communicate with one another. Other examples are FTP and telnet. Most URLs today start with http:// because most users are accessing the World Wide Web. Some will start with http:// because it is a secure server connection.

The second part of the URL, www.nursing.pst.edu, identifies the Web server or host computer where the page is located. Recall that the first part of this address describes the local host site, and the second part describes the domain name that is registered to that institution. The institution can decide how it wants to set up its local host. For example, the local host might be named as www or www .healthschools, or www.dept.

The third part, /foundations/courses/, tells the server where the file is found. The slashes represent folders, just like those on your computer. This part of the URL provides the computer with the information about the location of a Web page file.

The last part, nsg412.html, is the actual file name for the browser to display. Most of the time it will be an HTML or HTM file. HTML files are static Web pages in which the content is created at the time the page is created. The trend

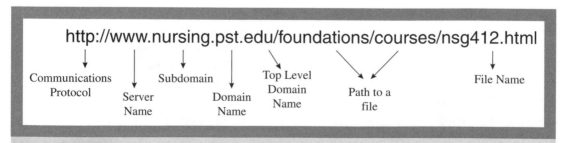

Figure 9-2 URLs

today is for Web pages to be dynamic, meaning that they are interactive. Such a Web page can accept and retrieve information from and for a user. These Web pages generally require some form of HTML and either a program or script. Programs and scripts are instructions that tell the computer how to perform a task; examples include CGI (Common Gateway Interface), ASP (Active Server Pages), DHTML (Dynamic Hypertext Markup Language), and Java applets.

When URLs are typed in the location or address box in a Web browser, no spaces can appear between their parts; the URLs must have forward slashes and be typed exactly as given. If the numeral one (1) is typed for the lowercase letter "L" (1), the computer will not be able to find the site and will return an error message. If the URL appears in an electronic form, you can highlight it and use the copy-and-paste feature to place the URL in the address text box to avoid typing errors. Note that most current browsers do not require you to type the "http" part of the URL; it is the default used if nothing is typed. If you access a secure site such as that operated by ADP (Automatic Data Processing), which is a business that processes payroll data, you would be required to type https://.

Using Web Browsers

A Web browser is the software program that is used to display Web pages on the World Wide Web. Although many different browsers are available, currently the two most frequently used browsers are Microsoft's Internet Explorer and Mozilla's Firefox. (This information changes over time, with current statistics being maintained at http://www.w3schools.com/browsers/browsers_stats.asp). Internet Explorer comes on a Windows PC, and Safari is bundled with any Apple computer. Many users download and use Firefox on either a Mac or a PC. Internet Explorer is no longer available for the Mac. Although these browsers are in competition with one another, they are very similar in how you interact with them. Other browsers are also available that allow you to surf the Internet without leaving traces on the computer of where you have been. Browzar (http://www.browzar.com) is one such example. Some people prefer to use these types of browsers on public computers. Some Web sites are browser specific and do not display their pages well if not using the correct browser. In those cases, there will be a notice on the Web page, something like "best viewed with" and the name and version of the browser.

Because browsers, like most software, are constantly being revised, you need to check and install the updated version of your browser on a regular basis. Frequently the IT department will update computers at work and in school labs, but you are responsible for performing this task on your own personal computer. Many universities provide a CD-ROM and/or Web site that provides updated browsers, virus checkers, and other utilities. These tools are usually updated at the beginning of the academic year and should be used every year—not just the first year you are a student. However, be cautious when updating your browser.

Beta versions may include unacceptable bugs. In addition, you must still check regularly for security updates for your broswers.

To check for the version of Internet Explorer on the computer:

1. **Open** the browser.
2. **Click** the **chevron** » on the right of the toolbar. See **Figure 9-3**.
3. **Click Help** and then **About Internet Explorer**. A window appears with the version number. Note that you may also click **Help** on the menu bar if it is displaying.

To check for the version of Firefox on the computer:

1. **Open** the browser.
2. **Click Help** on the menu bar. See Figure 9-3.
3. **Click About Mozilla Firefox** on the menu. A window appears with the version number.

To check for updates for Internet Explorer:

1. **Open** the browser.
2. **Click Tools** or **Tools** on the toolbar and then **Windows Updates**. Because Internet Explorer is part of the operating system, any updates that are needed will be shown.
3. Windows will now check for updates. Make sure you have a live Internet connection.
4. A window displays the updates needed.
5. Follow the directions provided to get the updates.

To check for updates for Firefox:

1. **Open** the browser.
2. **Click Help** on the menu bar.
3. **Click Check for updates**. A window appears listing the updates needed.
4. Follow the directions to get the updates.

Internet Explorer will automatically be updated if the operating system is set to perform this task. All the user has to do is say "yes" to the message that appears asking if it is okay to do this. If the system is not set up for automatic updates, you can change that setting. Go to the **Control Panel**, click **Automatic updates** under the **Security** area, and then click **Change settings**. Make the changes desired on the screen that appears (**Figure 9-4**).

Firefox can also be set up to perform automatic updates. Go to **Tools**, **Options**, Advanced, and **Update** tab. When the screen shown in Figure 9-4 appears, make the desired changes.

To update the program to a newer version, you can go to the appropriate Web site and select the new version for download. With each new version, more

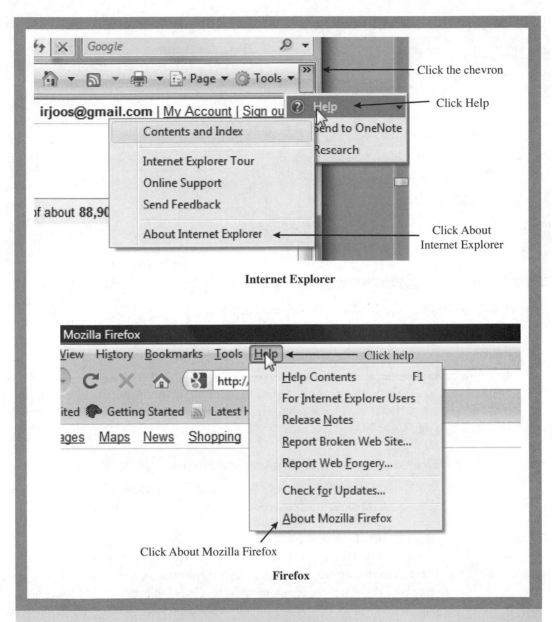

Figure 9-3 Obtaining Version Information for Internet Explorer and Firefox

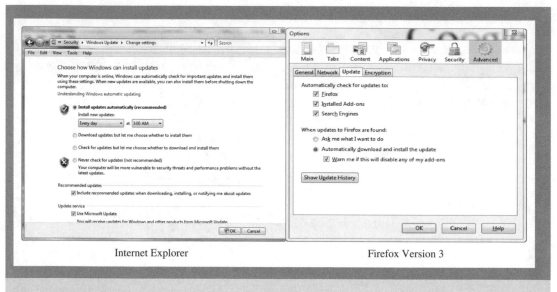

Figure 9-4 Changing Settings to Check for Automatic Updates

capabilities are built into the browser. However, the basic functions—the ability to use the back, forward, stop, search, print, and home buttons—remain constant. Newer versions will build in your current settings and retain items such as your bookmarks or favorites.

Orientation to Internet Explorer and Firefox

While the Internet Explorer and Firefox browsers have many similarities, there are enough dissimilarities between the two to warrant describing both here.

Main Elements of a Browser

Like the applications in the Microsoft Office suite, Web browsers have similar main elements—title, menu bars, toolbars, scroll bars, status information, and page tabs. Because these components were covered in previous chapters, only the additional features of browsers are discussed here. Page tabs, sometimes referred to as tabbed browsing, permit you to open a new Web site in a separate tab for quick access when you are working in multiple Web sites.

The Toolbar

Figure 9-5 shows the basic layout of the screens for both Internet Explorer and Firefox. Both browser versions change frequently, so the screen shots may look slightly different from the actual screen that you see on your own computer, but the same functionality should be present.

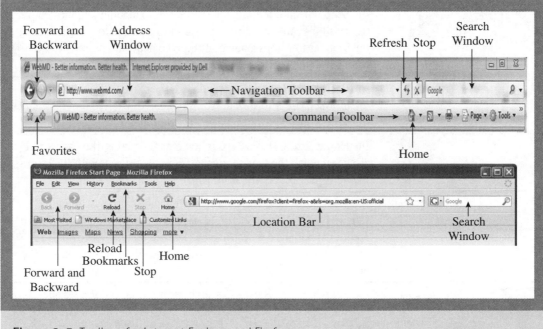

Figure 9-5 Toolbars for Internet Explorer and Firefox

The functions of browser buttons are described below. If no image for that function appears in a column, then the browser doesn't have one. Instead, you will need to use the menu bar to access this functionality.

Internet Explorer	Firefox	Functions of Browser Buttons
		The **Back** button retrieves the last page viewed in this session. It permits you to retrace your steps backward, one Web page at a time. This button becomes active only after you have visited another site. **Back history** (called Recent Pages) provides quicker access to sites visited this session because it allows you to skip clicking the Back button multiple times. Click the down arrow to the right of the Back button to view these sites and then choose the desired site.
		The **Forward** button retrieves the previous page viewed this session. It allows you to retrace your steps forward, one Web page at a time. This button becomes active only after the Back button has been used. **Forward history** (also called Recent Pages) provides quicker access to sites visited during the current session because it allows you to skip clicking the forward button multiple times. Click the down arrow to the right of the Forward button to view these sites and then choose the desired site.

		The **Stop** button interrupts the browser from loading a requested page. Use this function if it is taking too long to connect to a page. Clicking the Stop button stops loading of the Web page and permits you to continue doing something else or to go to another site.
		The **Refresh** or **Reload** button updates the current page displayed in the browser. Use it to view a site visited earlier whose contents change frequently, such as a stock market, sports event, or weather site.
		The **Home** button retrieves your home page—that is, the page displayed when the browser opens. Do not confuse it with the term "home page"—that is, the main page of a host's site.
		The **Print** button prints the current Web page or frame. In Internet Explorer, one copy of the current page is sent to the default printer. Additional options are available by clicking the down arrow to the right of the Print button. In Firefox, use the **File** menu and select the **print option** desired.
		The **Search** button is used to search for information on Web sites. Type the keyword in the search text box; then click the Search button or press the Enter key. The results of the search will be displayed in the search site window. Many browsers default to Google for searches.
		The **Favorites** and **Bookmarks** buttons allow you to mark favorite places so that they can be accessed quickly and easily. For Firefox, click the **Bookmark** option on the menu bar to obtain a list of options from which to choose. Both browsers also have a button for adding a current page to the list of favorites or bookmarks. Firefox also has a button for the most frequently visited sites that makes it easy to return to them without typing in a URL.
		The **History** button located in the favorites center or as a menu option permits you to revisit sites that were accessed during previous sessions. These sites stay in the history folder for a set number of days. By default, this period is 20 days for Internet Explorer and 90 days for Firefox. You can change the number of days if you like.

Starting the Browser

Chapter 4 described several ways to start programs. To start the browser, double-click the browser icon. If the browser is not on the desktop, click the **Internet Explorer** or **Firefox** option on the Quick Launch area of the taskbar. If that option is not available, use the **Start** button and **All Programs** to find the browser.

When the browser starts, a specific home page opens. This page might be the institution's or browser's Web page. You have the ability to change your home page by using the Tools, Internet Options feature that is found in both browsers.

To change the home page in Internet Explorer:

1. **Select Tools**, **Internet Options** from the toolbar.
2. Make sure that the **General** tab is selected.
3. If the home page desired is not selected, **select** the text in the **Address** text box of the home page options section of the window.
4. **Type** the new **URL**, and **click Apply** button. If you are on the page to be used as the home page, **click** the **Use Current** button and **click Apply** button.
5. **Click OK** to close the Internet Options dialog box.

To change the home page in Firefox:

1. Select **Tools**, **Options** and then click the **Main** icon.
2. Select the text in the **Location** text box of the home page section of the window and **type** the new **URL**. **Press Enter**. The next time you start Firefox, it will default to the new home page. If you are on the page you want to use as the home page, **click** the **Use Current Page** button.
3. **Click OK**.

Now when the browser starts, it will point to the new home page. This same process may be used to change how long sites stay in the history folder. For Internet Explorer, follow these steps: **Tools**, **Internet Options**, **General** tab, and **Setting** button under the Browsing history section. For Firefox, follow these steps: **Tools**, **Options**, and **Privacy** icon.

Browsing or Surfing the Net

Browsing or "surfing" the Net refers to the process of clicking hyperlinks to go to another part of a document, to a different document, or to another site. To use a hyperlink, click it. Most Web pages identify text hyperlinks by placing them in a different color and often by underlining them. The pointer changes to a hand (🖑) when it is placed over a hyperlink. Be patient: Sometimes it takes a significant amount of time to load a Web page. Graphic-intensive Web pages may come in faster through a broadband connection. Heavy traffic on the Internet slows the loading time.

If you have the URL for a site, you can simply type it in the address text box to access the site. Most current browsers do not require typing the http:// part of the address, but rather automatically insert that part. The computer requires the user to be exact; thus you must make sure that the address is correct.

To go to a site by typing the URL:

1. **Click** the **text** in the Address or Location text box to select the text.
2. **Type** the **URL** and **press Enter**.
3. **Click** any **hyperlink** objects or text to surf.

Using the History List

The history list keeps track of sites that have been visited over the past several days and offers a convenient means of redisplaying those pages. Unlike favorites or bookmark lists, which store page locations that you have specifically designated as candidates to be revisited, history items are saved automatically when visiting a site. Most browsers store all sites visited in this folder regardless of how you arrived at the site. Some locator or address drop-down lists store sites only where the URL was explicitly typed.

To use the history list in Internet Explorer 7:

1. **Click** the **Favorites** button and then the **History** button.
2. **Click** the **day of the week** that the site was visited.
3. **Click** the **site** and/or related **actual pages** at the site.

To use the history list in Firefox 3:

1. **Click View**, **Sidebar**, and then **History**. The history sidebar appears on the left. Alternatively, you can **click** the **History** option on the menu, although it won't show sites by days of the week.
2. **Click** the **day** when the site was visited.
3. **Click** the **site**.

Printing a Web Page

There are some subtle differences between Internet Explorer and Firefox when it comes to printing. When the printer icon is clicked, Internet Explorer sends one copy of the current document to the default printer. When the printer down arrow is clicked, the user has the option to select what is printed. (See **Figure 9-6a**.) Firefox has no printer icon to click; instead, using the Print command brings up the Print dialog box for the user to choose a printer, select pages, select the number of copies, and determine whether to print the page as laid out or only selected frames from the page. (See **Figure 9-6b**.) When the computer prints a Web page as a result of the Print command, it will print both the graphics and the text.

To print a Web page from Internet Explorer:

1. Go to the **Web page** to be printed.
2. **Click** the **Printer** button. If you are printing a site with frames, the active frame will be printed.

To access print options from Internet Explorer:

1. **Click** the **down arrow** next to the printer icon on the toolbar and then **click Print**.

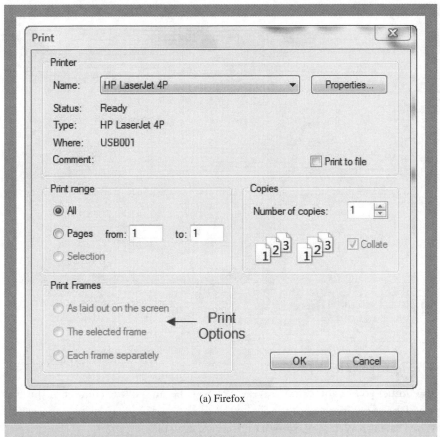

(a) Firefox

Figure 9-6a Print Options for Firefox

2. **Click** the **Options** tab.
3. Make the appropriate selections from the dialog box.

To print a Web page from Firefox:

1. Go to the **Web page** to be printed.
2. **Click File**, **Print** from the menu bar.
3. Make the appropriate selections in the printer dialog box, and press **Enter**.

Both browsers give you the option to preview the material before printing and to change the print setup. The print preview function can be very useful in helping you determine how many pages will print before you actually click the Print button.

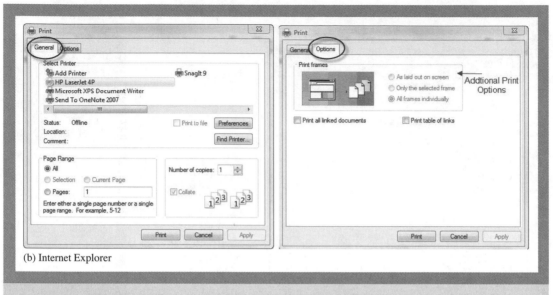

(b) Internet Explorer

Figure 9-6b Print Options for Internet Explorer

Saving a Web Page

Sometimes you might want to save a Web page because of the content or the tagging (the codes inserted in the file to tell the browser how to display the page). When saving a Web page, several options are available:

- **Web Page, Complete** saves all of the files that are needed to display the page in its original format. These data include graphics, frames, and style sheets.
- **Web Archive** saves a snapshot of the current page in a single archive-encoded file. This option is not available in earlier versions of Internet Explorer and Firefox and in some current browsers, and the file may not be readable by all browsers.
- **Web Page, HTML** saves only the code (tags) and text on the Web page; it does not save the graphics, sounds, or any other files displayed on the page but not embedded in the page.
- **Text Only** saves just the text from the current Web page in straight text format, permitting it to be imported into any word processor. It does not save the code.

To save a Web page in Internet Explorer:

1. **Select Page** and **Save as**.
2. **Select** the **location** and **file name** or accept the **defaults**.
3. **Select** one of the options for **file type**.
4. **Click** the **Save** button.

To save a Web page in Firefox:

1. **Select File** and **Save page as.**
2. **Select** the **location** and **file name** or accept the **defaults.**
3. **Select** one of the options for **file type.**
4. **Click** the **Save** button.

To save just a graphic from a Web page:

1. **Right-click** the **graphic.**
2. **Select Save Picture** or **Image** or **Target as.**
3. **Select** the **location** in which to download the graphic.
4. **Type** a **file name** or accept the **default.**
5. Under **Save as type**, **select** a **graphic file format** such as jpg or gif.
6. **Click** the **Save** button.

To copy information from a Web page into a document:

1. Select the information to be copied.
2. **Click** the **Page** button in Internet Explorer or **select** the **Edit** menu in Firefox and then **Copy.**
3. Go to the document, and **click Paste** when the cursor is at the appropriate spot.
4. Be very careful of copyright rules and plagiarism.

To create a desktop shortcut to a frequently accessed Web page:

1. **Right-click** somewhere in the Web page, but not on a graphic.
2. Select **Create Shortcut** from the shortcut menu, and **click OK.**

Two other saving features can be used with Web pages. First, you can save the file as a desktop background. Second, you can send a Web page to someone else through email. These features can be found on the shortcut menu once you are on the appropriate page.

Creating a Bookmark or Favorite

Bookmarks or favorites save the URLs of frequently visited sites. Use this feature to help organize a list of Web pages so that they can be easily found later. The basic functions needed to use this feature are found in all versions of both browsers, although the exact procedure for saving bookmarks or favorites varies between browsers.

The basic functions are as follows:

- Adding and removing bookmarks or favorites from your list
- Organizing the list of URLs into categories or folders
- Editing and arranging the bookmarks or favorites

A number of factors make it difficult to create bookmarks. For example, many computer facilities provide a prescribed set of bookmarks or favorites, such as those designated by a library or a computer lab. The facility may place limitations on what may be changed or added to this set. In addition, you may not have access to your bookmarks and favorites when you are using a different computer. For these reasons, it is recommended that you create a folder to hold these items on a removable storage device, rather than a folder on the hard drive. The procedure for doing so is described in Exercises 1 and 2 at the end of this chapter. If you are using a personal computer, the process of creating and managing bookmarks and favorites is similar to the procedure discussed in Chapter 3.

Managing Internet Files

Each Internet site visited sends temporary files to the computer. These files include cookies, temporary Internet files, and surfing history.

Cookies

Cookie files are designed to enhance the online experience by recognizing the visitor when he or she returns to a Web site and recording what was done at that site. For example, a cookie might remember what reservations were made the last time the visitor accessed hotels.com or which credit card number was used to order something from LLBean.com. Although cookies should be harmless when you are using a personal computer, it may pose a problem when you are using laboratory or work computers. Sites can only read cookie files they place on the hard disk; they cannot read files placed by other sites or other files on that computer.

Temporary Internet Files

Temporary Internet files are sent to the computer for the purpose of speeding the loading of graphics files when a Web site is visited multiple times. The problem with these files (and with cookie files) is that they take up space on the hard drive and are not deleted automatically. Therefore, you must periodically delete these files. How often this task needs to be performed depends on how many sites have been visited. Failure to purge these files periodically could lead to a full hard drive. These files also serve as a record of places visited on the Internet. You can manage these files through the browser interface or directly from the hard drive.

History Files

A history file keeps track of where you have been on the Web. If anyone else uses that computer, it may be wise to delete the history folder contents. For example, an abused client might search the Internet for resources about abuse. If the client doesn't know about deleting the history files, the abuser might become aware of this research. For this reason, the healthcare professional should make the client aware that the history files should be deleted before leaving the computer. Some laboratories set up their computers to automatically delete the content of this folder when the user logs off.

To delete cookie, temporary Internet, and history files through Internet Explorer:

1. Open **Internet Explorer.**
2. **Select Tools, Delete Browsing.**
3. **Click** the **Delete Temporary Internet Files, Delete Cookies,** and **Delete History** buttons. There are also two other options to delete form data and passwords.
4. **Click** the **Close** button.

To delete cookies and history files through Firefox:

1. Open **Firefox.**
2. **Select Tools, Clear Private Data options.**
3. Place checks in **History, Cache,** and **Cookies.** You also have a few other options.
4. **Click** the **Clear Private Data now** button.

Search Sites (Engines) and Searching

The Internet contains a vast amount of information. Unfortunately, there is no single source to index the Internet that is analogous to the Library of Congress, which indexes books. Instead, you have to search to find the information you want. You should design your search of the Internet to find relevant information in an effective and efficient manner (more on this topic in Chapter 12).

Search sites are places on the Internet where you go to find information. Search engines are software programs that are used to find and index information. Several hundred different search sites and engines are available on the Internet. Generally, they are divided into three main categories, although the differences between these categories are disappearing as each increases its functionality.

Directory	A directory is a hierarchical grouping of WWW links by subject and related concepts. Such directories are created by people who searched the Web and then group the links by subject. Therefore, they preselect the information appearing in the directory. The amount of irrelevant information found in directories is far less than that turned up by either keyword search sites or meta search engines. Not all search sites include directories.
	Directory sites are great choices for finding information quickly when one knows little about the topic and the topic is broad or common. They are not good for ferreting out obscure facts. Links to outdated or moved Web pages also pose another problem. Yahoo, Open Directory, and About are three popular directory sites.

Keyword Search Site	A keyword search site comprises a server or a collection of servers dedicated to indexing Internet pages, storing the results, and returning lists of links that match particular queries. They provide access to the largest portion of information on the Internet, but often return a lot of irrelevant information. The indexes are normally generated using spiders or bots. Sometimes the terms "search site" and "search engine" are used as synonyms; they are different, however. Most keyword search sites have advanced search features for narrowing the search, but the results set returned may still be very large. Google, Ask, and Live are three popular keyword search sites.
Meta Search Engines	Meta search engines are not really search engines. Rather, they work by taking the user's query and searching the Web by using several different keyword search sites at one time. These tools are gaining in popularity because they permit one-stop searching. Meta search engine sites provide a good picture of what is available because they use several different search engine sites and the information is not preselected as it is in directory sites. They may restrict some of the advanced search features, however. A few examples of these tools are Mamma, Clusty, DogPile, and Kart00.

Each of these search tools has a different interface or appearance, but all share several common features. Understanding how to use search sites begins by understanding a few relevant terms:

- **Hits** are a list of links that are returned as search results when a search engine is used.
- **Query** refers to the combination of terms that you enter into a search engine to conduct a search.
- **Ranking** is a process of indicating how relevant a hit may be. Many times a search engine will organize the search results by their ranking. Because the methods used by search engines to rank pages vary, ranks may not always be useful.
- **Robots** are used to create a database of links that are accessed when you conduct a search. These computer programs search the Web, locate links, and then index the links to create the results database. Indexing is usually done by using the words in the URL and title of the HTML file and by counting the frequency of words used at the Internet site. Some robots search the full text, whereas others review only a portion of the site. Robots are also called *spiders* and *crawlers*. The problem with this approach is that programmers can fool the robots by using little tricks in the coding; also, robots cannot access any pages that do not have links to them or require logging in.

Search Site Issues and the Invisible Web

Information on the Internet is being published faster than search sites can index it; that is, search sites cannot keep pace with the sheer volume of information being produced. Adding to the problem is the issue of *who* is publishing to the Internet. Early Web pages were published by government agencies, nonprofit institutions, and educational institutions. Today, however, more Web sites that market or sell products and services are publishing to the Internet.

Current search engines are limited in what they can index. This is creating an area of the Web referred to as the "invisible Web" (Bergman, 2001). In addition to the sheer volume of information to be indexed, other factors influence what a search site can index. Examples include the editorial policies of family-friendly sites and news sites; databases' practice of requiring users to type search strings, as in the scheme used by the CDC databases; sites' requirement that visitors log in to visit certain parts, as is the case with the *Chronicle of Higher Education* site; pages that contain only images; certain file types such as pdf and exe; dynamically generated pages; and placement of documents behind firewalls. Some search sites acknowledge these difficulties by providing for links to current news sites such as those operated by CNN or by having links to databases that index only images, videos, and so forth.

Rajaraman, co-founder of Kosmix (www.kosmix.com), states that the current technology is trying to find a needle in a haystack when what is needed is to explore the haystack (Wright, 2009). In other words, research is needed to analyze used search terms used and to try and match them with databases that are likely to contain the desired information.

Accessing Search Sites

Using a search engine begins by accessing the search engine site on the Internet. Open the browser and type the URL for the search site. Some users' default home page is a specific search site such as that operated by Google. To see other search sites available, type "search sites" or "search engines" in the Search text box and press **Enter**.

Portal-type directory structures (such as the Librarians' Index to the Internet) and clearinghouses or reference sites (such as Search Enginewatch, Search Engine Showdown, How Stuff Works, and Reference Desk) also provide links to the most popular search sites as well as a wealth of other reference sites. Likewise, many ISPs and college/university libraries provide links to search sites on their main pages. A good place to start when conducting an Internet search might be to check out what your library recommends as quality search sites.

Transferring Files

One of the functions that most Internet users want is the ability to transfer files from a server on the Internet to their own computers. Before the advent of the Web, using the FTP (File Transfer Protocol) communications protocol and program was the only way to transfer files from one computer to another over the Internet. To do this, the user had to access FTP and then type commands such as "fetch" and "put" to tell the computer what to do. By contrast, with today's Web browsers, transferring files is as simple as clicking a download button and telling the computer where to place the file. The FTP functions behind the scenes of the Web browser.

Because of the file limitations of certain email programs, some organizations give their employees access to the organization's own FTP server so that they can move files around from one place to another. This process is generally faster and considered more secure than working over the Internet. There are no graphics on the FTP server—just the files. There are also no file size limitations, so this approach is the preferred choice when transferring large files. If you need to transfer a variety of other types of files, such as compressed (zip), program (exe), and database (mdbx) files, use of FTP may be required because some firewalls block files with these extensions. In contrast, if you need to save the current Web page in HTML format or capture a graphic, follow the directions given earlier in this chapter. The browser works well for transferring these files.

To use FTP, the following items are needed:

- A local computer that is capable of running FTP with an Internet connection.
- A remote computer running FTP with an Internet connection.
- The Internet address for the remote server. This is usually ftp.same-second-domain.same-high-level-domain.
- An account on the remote server (perhaps). Some FTP sites are run as anonymous sites, which means a login is not needed or, if a login is needed, the user ID is something like "anonymous" and the password consists of the user's email address or even nothing.

To access FTP through a Web browser:

1. Start the **Web browser**.
2. In the Address or Location text box, **type ftp://ftp.domain.topdomain**.
3. Log in if required.
4. Browse to find the **file** to transfer and **right-click** it, **click Save target as**, or click the **Download** button if there is one.
5. **Select** a **location** in which to place the file and a **file name** if needed, and then **click Save**. The file is now being transferred.

Two commonly used terms regarding transferring files are *download* and *upload.* Downloading is moving a file from one computer (generally a server) to another (generally a local PC). This generic term does not specify how this task is accomplished, just that the files were transferred. Uploading is transferring a file from a local computer to a remote server (the reverse direction from downloading); this process is used when moving local HTML files to a Web server for publishing on the Internet. Although the telnet communications protocol can be used to run TCP/IP and remotely log in, the discussion here focuses on implementing FTP through Web browser facilities.

Here are some points to consider when retrieving files from the Internet:

- *Know what you want to download.* Some FTP sites are cryptic and assume that the user knows the file name and understands how the site is organized. When at an FTP site, look for a file that describes the site and its organization; this file is usually a text file titled "index," "read.me," or "files.lst." Select it, and read how things work at that site.
- *Keep security in mind.* Downloading files from the Internet can introduce a virus into your system. Most sites take precautions to prevent viruses from entering their files, so the chances are good that the files will be clean. However, to be on the safe side, it does not hurt to check the downloaded files (especially files with an .exe or .com extension) with an antivirus program before installing them on the computer. Many experts believe that there is a greater chance of getting a virus from email files than from FTP sites.
- *Know the system requirements for the file.* Many sites assume that users know which operating system—Windows Vista or XP, Linux, or Mac OSX—they are using, as different versions of files are typically provided for the different systems. Many sites will also tell the downloader how large the file is, how much space is needed on the hard drive to run the program, and how much memory the program requires. Make sure that the file is the correct one for the system you are using.
- *Obey copyright laws.* Several types of files are available for download. Freeware files are available without cost. For example, many free graphics files are available for use when you are creating Web pages. Although some are totally free for use, others have restrictions such as "free for use at nonprofit Web sites." If the file is used, some sites require acknowledgment of the developer or originating site on the Web site that uses the file. Shareware files can be tried for free; if users like the program, they pay a small fee to register the program. Many times the registered version is a later, better version than the shareware one. Finally, program or application files can be downloaded. Some of these programs provide a trial (limited) version; others require the user to buy the full program before downloading it. Trial versions usually last 30 days and then become unusable.

Failure to follow copyright laws can create serious legal problems for people who violate these laws.

Creating and Evaluating Web Pages

This section of the chapter provides an overview of creating Web pages and evaluating their design. It is not intended to make you a full-fledged Web designer, but rather focuses on providing some helpful information for design and evaluation. Material on evaluating the quality of the content of a Web site is covered in Chapter 12. After visiting various Web sites, most users begin to appreciate when a site is well designed and develop criteria for what they find most appealing in a site's design. In addition, while many healthcare professionals may not do the actual coding for Web pages, they may provide input into the content and layout as well as the means by which users move around the site. This sort of assessment becomes easier when the professional has some basic background in Web design issues.

Creating Web Pages

Although the first thing that most Web page creators want to do is start tagging the documents, there is, in fact, a structured process for designing Web pages. This process, which is outlined here, serves as a guide for things to consider when creating Web pages. Paying attention to these items at the beginning of the Web page development process will save time and energy in the long term.

- *Decide what is to be accomplished with this site.* Answer these questions: What is the intent of this site? What do I want to accomplish with this site? What are the purposes and goals of this site? Create a statement that reflects the answers to these questions to serve as a guide during the development and maintenance of the Web site.
- *Identify the target audience to help focus the design and content.* Many Web sites are created without identifying the *who*—that is, the intended users of the site. A design for teenagers, for example, may not be appropriate for professional audiences.
- *Develop a site map showing the relationship between the parts.* Which pages will be there? How will they link or relate to other pages? Keep in mind that users may access these pages in varying ways and may not always start at the beginning.
- *Develop criteria for inclusion of content.* How will decisions be made about which content to include? What are the criteria for inclusion? Keep in mind the intent of the site and the target audience.
- *Decide who will be responsible for maintaining each part of the site.* Consider how often the data may need to be updated, and then determine a schedule for reviewing and updating the parts. While the Webmaster is responsible for the design and coding of the Web site, others are generally responsible for filling in the content.
- *Decide on the design that best presents the content.* A consistent look to the site helps keep the user oriented as to place. It is helpful to place navigational aids consistently in the same place on each page that identify the *who, what, when,* and *where* of the content. Make these navigational aids, such as buttons, easy and clear to follow. Develop these standards at the beginning, and then use them consistently.

Once these guidelines are addressed, some specific things should be considered regarding design and layout. Although these points serve as a guide, good design is a matter of a person's own personal taste and style, not someone else's. Good design also keeps in mind the intent of the site and the target audience. Decide whether it is more important to have a flashy site, albeit one where some people may not be able to access all its features, or whether it is more important that all people who use the site can access its features.

- *Consider differences in user resources.* Remember that some people still access the Internet through dial-up modems and not the faster Ethernet, cable, DSL, or fiber-optic connections. Graphics take longer to load than text, and the audience will be lost if they have to wait too long for the graphics. Use the 10-second rule: The page should load from many different types of connections in 10 seconds. Also, consider that not everyone uses the latest technology, so some users may not have the latest version of a browser or the same size of monitor used by the developer during the design of the Web site. When in doubt about design, keep it simple.

- *Design a template or layout to use with most of the pages.* Make sure that each page has a descriptive title located in the same place on every page and that buttons and navigational aids are used to take the user back to the home page or to other pages at this site. Also include identifying information such as who created the page, when it was created or last revised, and how to contact the Webmaster with questions. Many pages also include relevant copyright information.

- *Use graphics and sound as appropriate.* Graphics and sounds should add to the content, not detract from it. Although it may be possible to place many graphics on the page, do not do so unless those images help convey the message of the page. Keep in mind two key rules: "Simpler is better" and "White space is good." Many users find graphics and sound distracting; other users may access the page in settings where sound is distracting to others. Pay attention to copyright requirements, especially when using graphics created by others.

- *Keep graphics reasonable in size.* Try to maintain a balance between size, resolution, color, and look. That means to try and keep the size between 25K and 30K with a resolution of 72 dpi. Use the appropriate graphic file format—gif for images and jpg for photos. Use thumbnail graphics (small, postage-stamp-sized pictures), and give the user the option to look at the graphic in a larger version. Keep in mind that what most users see when the page loads is the first 4 inches of a printed page.

- *Select colors carefully.* Make sure that the colors work together and are easy to read and pleasing to the eye. If the designer lacks color sense, someone else should select the color scheme; alternatively, the designer can use an already developed color scheme. Be especially careful with colors if users will be printing the Web pages.

HTML Files

Once the documents are designed in terms of layout and content, they need to be coded or tagged. The Hypertext Markup Language (HTML) provides a mechanism for displaying text- and graphics-based documents in Web browsers. *Tagging* describes the process of indicating the appearance of contents of a Web page by specifying fonts and font-related attributes as well as location or layout of the text and graphics. HTML code consists of a series of tags embedded in the Web document that tell the browser how to display the page. The tags look like the example here:

```
<HTML>

<HEAD>

<TITLE>Welcome to Healthcare Tips Online</TITLE>

</HEAD>

<BODY>The purpose of this Web site is to provide the general public with
some tips for working with healthcare providers and being intelligent con-
sumers of healthcare services.</BODY>

</HTML>
```

In this example, the first and last tags (<HTML> and </HTML>) tell the browser that this is an HTML file. Tags placed between the HEAD tags are for informational purposes and are not displayed in the browser window. The TITLE tag displays the Web page title in the title bar of the Web browser. All text between the BODY tags appears in the browser window.

When a browser locates a Web document by using the URL or by being sent there through a link, it interprets these tags regardless of which platform the user is using. As a consequence, Web pages can be displayed on Windows, UNIX, and Macintosh computers and basically look the same.

Many tools are available for creating HTML documents. They are divided into three main groups:

- ASCII editors require the document creator to type the tags and text directly into the document. Notepad, which comes with the Windows operating system, is an example of an ASCII editor.
- HTML converter programs take a document created in another program and convert it to an HTML file by adding the tags. The Microsoft Office suite is an example of this type of program. The user saves the file created as a Web page instead of a Word document.

■ HTML editors are software programs with a graphical user interface that helps the developer create HTML files without having to type the tags. Expression Web (the replacement for FrontPage), Dreamweaver, and GoLive are popular HTML editors.

Each of these tools has both advantages and disadvantages. For example, using a converter program such as Word results in documents appearing differently than they do in the word processor. The program has to interpret the formatting and convert it into HTML tags. Because this conversion is not always done cleanly, the creator may need to play with the tags to ensure that the document will be displayed correctly. ASCII editors are tedious to use but provide excellent control over the Web page. HTML editors are more powerful than converters, but the creator gives up some control over the Web page design. Exercises 4 and 5 provide experience with creating a simple Web page.

Summary

This chapter covered the basics of using the Internet—specifically, terminology and concepts such as Web, URL, FTP, and hyperlinks. An introduction to connecting to the Internet and the related requirements followed. A brief orientation to the two most commonly used browsers, Microsoft Internet Explorer and Mozilla Firefox, was presented, showing both their similarities and differences. The chapter concluded with a brief discussion of the creation of Web pages and the evaluation of Web page design.

References

Bergman, M. (2001). The deep web: Surfacing hidden value. *Journal of Electronic Publishing* 7(1). Retrieved January, 22, 2009, from http://quod.lib.umich.edu/cgi/t/text/text-idx?c=jep;view=text;rgn=main;idno=3336451.0007.104

Wright, A. (2009). Exploring a deepweb that Google can't grasp. Retrieved February 23, 2009, from http://www.nytimes.com/2009/02/23/technology/internet/23search.html?_r=2

Additional Resources

Bare Bones (http://www.sc.edu/beaufort/library/pages/bones/bones.shtml): This site is a great tutorial site for learning about searching and search sites.

Health Information on the Web (http://websearch.about.com/od/invisibleweb/a/medical.htm): This site is a good starting point.

Search Engine Showdown (http://searchengineshowdown.com): This site has some interesting statistics about search engines. It also includes some tutorials.

Search Engine Watch (http://searchenginewatch.com/): This site has excellent descriptions of searching and search engines. It tries to keep up-to-date with what is happening in the world of Internet searching. It is a good reference source.

EXERCISE 1 Introduction to Microsoft Internet Explorer and Browsing

---

Check the book's Web site for a similar exercise using Firefox or for these exercise files in electronic format.

■ **Objectives**

1. Define selected words related to a Web site.
2. Identify different types of Web addressing.
3. Use Internet Explorer to access the World Wide Web and to connect to different sites.
4. Organize favorites and add sites to a favorites folder.
5. Print a document from the World Wide Web.
6. Transfer both a home page and a graphic file from the Web.

■ **Activity**

If this file is provided to you in electronic format, place your answer in *italics* in this document. If no file is provided, open a blank Word document and place your answers there, along with the appropriate question number and letter.

1. Define the following words and answer the related questions.
   a. Home page. (Hint: there are two different meanings.)
   b. Which home page is opened when you connect to the college computer laboratory or your workplace computer?
   c. What is a link or hyperlink?

2. Understand Web page addresses.

   a. What is the difference between an email address and a Web address or URL?

   b. Here are some addresses. Decide which type of address (email, user, IP, URL) each is.

      43.134.020.12

      cdc.gov

      Nancy_Drew

      FNightingale@crimea.com

   c. What might be the host name for a computer at the National Library of Medicine?

   d. Nancy works in the Nursing Department at the University of Pennsylvania. What might be the full Internet address of that department?

   e. Do you want to find out who owns a particular domain name?

- **Double-click** the **Internet Explorer** icon. The browser opens.
- **Click** the **Address** text box to highlight the text.
- Type **www.networksolutions.com/** in the address text box, and **press Enter**. The Network Solutions Web site opens.
- Mouse over the **Domain Name** tab at the top of the screen. A menu appears.
- **Click** the **WHOIS Search** option. A new Web page appears with a search text box.
- **Type upmc.edu** in the search text box, and **press Enter**.
- Scroll down and answer this question: Who owns this domain name, and what is the primary IP address?
- **Click** the **Back** button on the browser toolbar. The Search window appears.
- **Highlight** the text in the search box.
- **Type WebMD.com** in the query text box, and **press Enter**.
- Answer this question: Who owns this domain name, and what is the primary IP address?
- **Click** the **Back** button on the browser toolbar. The Search window appears.
- **Highlight** the text in the search box.
- **Type nursing.com** in the query box, and **press Enter**.
- Answer this question: Who owns this domain name, and what is the primary IP address?
- **Click** the **Back** button on the browser toolbar. The Search window appears.
- **Highlight** the text in the search box.
- Type the **name of your local healthcare facility or school** in the query text box, and **press Enter**.

- Answer this question: Who owns this domain name, and what is the primary IP address?

3. Use Internet Explorer 7 to connect to sites.

   a. **Click** the **text** in the Address text box in Internet Explorer to highlight it.

   b. **Type http://www.mapquest.com** and **press Enter**.

   c. **Click** the **MAPS** button 🌐, and type your **address**, **city**, **state**, and **ZIP code** in the correct text boxes.

   d. **Click** the **Search** button. A map of your location appears.

   e. How accurate is your map?

   f. Why might this information be helpful to a home care health professional?

   g. **Click** the **text** in the Address text box in Internet Explorer to highlight it.

   h. **Type weather.com** and press **Enter**.

   i. **Type** your **ZIP code** (your actual ZIP code, not the words) in the Zip text box and **click Search** or **press Enter**.

   j. Look around the site.

   k. What is the forecast for the next 10 days in your city?

   l. Why might this information be important to a home care health professional? To a patient?

4. Create and work with favorites.

NOTE: It may not be possible to complete this exercise on a public computer, as the system may prevent you from creating or customizing the system. Also note these directions are written for IE 7 running in Vista. Directions may be different for another version or operating system.

Organize Favorites

   a. **Click** the **Favorite** button ✦. It has the plus sign with the star. Alternatively you can select Favorites from the menu bar. A menu appears.

   b. **Click Organize Favorites** from the menu. The Organize dialog box appears.

   c. **Click** the **New Folder** button at the lower-left corner of the dialog box. A new folder appears in the upper window pane, waiting for a name to be typed.

   d. **Type Informatics Resources** and **press Enter**. The new folder appears in the top window pane.

   e. Repeat the process and create a second folder titled **PDA Resources**. The new folder appears in the top window pane. See **Figure 9-7** for the added folders.

   f. **Click** the **Close** button.

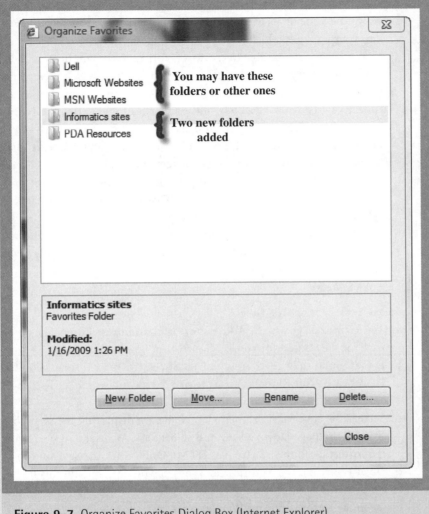

Figure 9-7 Organize Favorites Dialog Box (Internet Explorer)

Add Some Sites to the Correct Folder

a. Go to **www.pepid.com/** (type this address in the Address box of Internet Explorer). The home page of PEPID appears.

b. **Click** the **Favorites** button 🔖 or **select Favorites** from the menu bar. A menu appears.

c. **Click Add to favorites**. The Add to favorites dialog box appears.

d. Select **PDA Resources** from the **Create in** drop-down list (**click** the **down arrow** and **click PDA Resources**).

e. **Click** the **Add** button.

f. Go to **www.rnpalm.com/** and add this site to the PDA Resources folder.

g. Go to **www.ania.org/** and add this site to the Informatics Resources folder.

h. Now, find a site of an area of interest to you in your profession, and add it to your favorites folder.

While you may be able to create a favorites folder on the hard drive in the laboratory, most labs refresh the computers, which means that the results will be lost or that you must use the same computer in the lab each time. To make a copy of the favorites folder, **click** the **Favorites** button, **click** the **Import and Export** option, **click Next**, **select Export favorites**, **click Next**, **click** the **Favorites** folder, **click Next**, **click Browse**, locate your **USB storage device**, and **click Save**. The reverse process may be used to import your favorites into another computer.

You may also locate the folder in the **Favorites list** and **right-click** it. **Select Send to** and then the **USB storage device**. This file may then be imported into a browser using the process outlined previously; alternatively, you may be able to access the site by double-clicking the file in the folder on the USB storage device.

5. Save Web pages.

Save Web Page as HTML Only

a. **Type www.cdc.gov** in the Address text box, and **press Enter**. The home page for the Centers for Disease Control and Prevention opens.

b. Look around the site to find the **Fact Sheet: Anthrax Information for Healthcare Professionals** or use the search box and search for Fact sheet anthrax.

c. **Select File**, **Save** from the menu bar if you are displaying the menu bar or **click** the **Page Down arrow** and select **Save As**. Make sure to select the correct location and save it as **HTML Only**. **Click** the **Save** button.

d. Open **Word** and the **Anthrax** file. What do you notice about this file?

e. Close **Word**.

f. Open the **Anthrax** file in a Web browser. What is missing?

Save a Graphic from a Web Page

a. Type **google.com** in a browser and press **Enter**.

b. **Click** the **images** text under the browser tab (found at the upper-left corner of the window).

c. Type **health care** in the search box and **click** the **search images** button.

d. Look around at the images. **Right-click** on an image of your choice and select **Save picture as**.

e. Select the location and file name (if it needs to be changed). The file is now on your USB storage device.

6. Follow the directions provided by the professor for submitting this work and the electronic files.

EXERCISE 2 Searching Using Several Different Search Sites

■ **Objectives**

1. Identify three strategies used to construct a search query and the rationale for them.
2. Use the information from a tutorial to write a brief description of three different types of search sites and then compare the results of the search.
3. Find a site that compares different search sites and evaluate its quality.
4. Examine a Web site for an approach to finding information.

Make sure you have an Internet connection and a browser open. If an electronic copy of this exercise is provided, use *italics* to indicate your answers. If none is provided, place the answers in a new Word document using the same numbering and lettering system.

■ **Activity**

1. Check out this tutorial at http://www.brightplanet.com/. **Click** the **tutorials** link on the right side under **resources**. **Select Guide to Effective Searching**. Read the 10 guides for constructing your query under the Executive Summary. List three of the rules that you use frequently and your rationale for them.
2. Go to http://www.sc.edu/beaufort/library/pages/bones/bones.shtml. Complete the tutorials 11, 13, and 17. These tutorials are very short and to the point.
   a. How many lessons are in the Bare Bones tutorial?
   b. Write a short description of the three search sites in the tutorials you just completed.
   c. Access **Ask.com. Type robots surgery** in the Search text field and **Press Enter**. Note the number of hits. **Click** the **advanced search** button and **type edu** in the Domain text box. **Click Advanced Search** button or **press Enter**. Complete the table below with the results.

Search Site	Robots Surgery	Robots Surgery: Only edu	Sponsored Links?	Sample Topics
Ask				
Clusty				
Yahoo				

   d. Access **Clusty.com**. Repeat the same search as in part c except type **edu** in the Host text box. Add your results to the table.

    e. Access **Yahoo.com**. Repeat the same search as in part c except access the advanced search by clicking the **options down arrow**. Add your results to the table.

3. Compare search sites or search tools

    One of the hard parts about Web searching is learning the requirements for searching with each search site or tool.

    a. Conduct a search for a **comparison** of search engine features; in other words, find a site where multiple search sites are discussed and compared. Type the search strategy used here: _____.

    b. How effective was it?

    c. Type the URL of a good site you found here: _____.

    d. What did you like about this comparison of search sites?

    e. How up-to-date is it?

    f. Who is responsible for it?

    g. What are their credentials?

4. Go to http://www.noodletools.com/debbie/literacies/information/5locate/adviceengine.html.

    a. How is this site different from the others visited during this exercise?

5. Save this work and turn it in as directed.

EXERCISE 3 Downloading Files from the Web

■ **Objectives**

1. Define the term *downloading* and explain the process of downloading, including what needs to be done before and after the downloading.

2. Find out what is required to download files from specific sites in terms of file name, file size, requirements to run the application, precautions before using the downloaded file, and restrictions on using the downloaded file.

3. Use the browser interface FTP protocol to download files.

4. Identify the differences between downloading files using the browser interface and downloading files using FTP.

■ **Activity**

1. Answer the following questions:

    a. What is downloading?

    b. Which factors affect how long it takes to download a file?

    c. Of what does the user need to be careful when downloading files?

    d. Which information is needed *before* downloading?

    e. What are some common file types used when downloading?

    f. What needs to be done with many of these files before they will work?

2. Obtain a file through a browser from a Web site.
   a. In the Location or Address text box, **type www.download.com** and **press Enter.**
   b. **Click** the **Browse Utilities and Operating Systems** option under the Windows area on the left side of the window.
   c. **Click** the **File Compression** option in the left side of the window under the area called **Utilities and Operating Systems**.
   d. **Click** the **WinZip** file.
   e. **Select Version 12 or 11.1.**
   f. **Click** the **Download** button. **Click Save** to save this program to a disk.
   g. **Select** a **location**, and **click Save**. The file is now downloading.
   h. Answer the following questions:
      ■ What is the operating system requirement?
      ■ How long can you use it before paying for it?
      ■ What is the name of the downloaded file?
      ■ How much space does it need?
      ■ Which protocol is being used to download it? See **Figure 9-8**. Note that your screen may look different depending on your browser and its version.

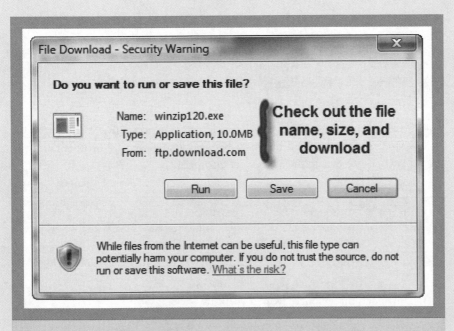

Figure 9-8 Downloading Screen

NOTE: Some Download buttons, such as the ones in Adobe Reader, do not give you a choice as to where to place the file on your system. If you use such a program, you will have to accept where the program places the downloaded file.

3. Obtain a file through a browser from an FTP site using the right-click technique.
   a. **Type ftp://ftp.irs.ustreas.gov** in the Location or Address text box.
   b. **Double-click Pub** directory, **Irs-pdf** directory.
   c. **Right-click f1040ez.pdf**, and select **Save copy as** or **Save target as**.
   d. **Select** the **correct storage device**, and **click** the **Save** button. The file is now downloading to your USB storage device.
   e. Close the **browser**.
   f. **Double-click** the **f1040ez.pdf** file that was just downloaded.
   g. Answer the following questions:
      - What happened?
      - What did you need to know to use this interface?
   h. Go back to the site, but instead of right-clicking the file to download the f1040cz.pdf file, **double-click** it.
      - What happened now?
      - How can you now save this file?

NOTE: To display PDF files, the system must have Acrobat Reader installed. Some files require special programs to read and display them. Most sites that use pdf files have a link to a free copy of the Acrobat Reader software.

4. After completing this exercise and Exercise 1 on saving Web pages and graphics, describe the differences between using the FTP protocol and the browser interface to the access FTP protocol.

EXERCISE 4 Creating a Simple Web Page with HTML

■ Objectives
   1. Define two additional tagging languages used for Web pages.
   2. Create folders in which to place your work.
   3. Download three images from a Web site.
   4. Use a text editor to enter HTML tags in two documents.
   5. Add a graphic and links tags.
   6. Save and print files.

NOTE: While tagging is very tedious, a little experience in doing it will help most health-care professionals communicate more effectively with the staff who do the tagging. A brief exposure to tagging provides a basis for understanding a few of the many issues that arise in creating Web pages.

■ Activity

Many languages besides HTML are used to create Web pages for more interactive sites and to enable sites to display data. When working through this exercise, either place your answers in this document (if provided in electronic form) or create a new blank Word document, place your name on it, identify the question being answered, and place your answers in that document in *italics*.

1. Explore Web tagging languages.
   a. Go to http://www.htmlgoodies.com/primers/html/. Look around the site. Besides HTML tutorials, which other Web tagging programs are covered at this site?
   b. Describe how two of these Web tagging languages are used. For example, XML (Extensible Markup Language) describes the content in terms of which data are being described, whereas HTML describes how those data are displayed.
2. Create folders to store HTML and image files.
   a. Create a folder called **HTML** and one subfolder in the HTML folder called **images** on your USB storage device. If you don't remember how to do this, review the material in Chapter 3 on creating folders.
3. Download images to use in the file.
   a. Open **Internet Explorer** or any other browser. Make sure you have an active Internet connection.
   b. **Type http://www.pdclipart.org/** in the address bar of the browser. The Public Domain Clip Art site opens. See **Figure 9-9**.
   c. **Click Food A to C**. Click the **apple delicious golden red** image.
   d. **Right-click** the image and select **Save picture as**. Place the file in the **images** folder created in part 2.
   e. **Click** the **Back** button on the browser **twice**.
   f. Scroll down until you find the **medical** grouping and **click** on it.
   g. **Click** the **page 2 tab** and repeat the process to download the **jog** clip art to the **images** folder.
   h. **Click** the **page 4 tab** and repeat the process to download the **weight** clip art to the **images** folder. Close the **browser**.
4. Create an HTML page with an ASCII editor.
   a. **Click** the **Start** button, **All Programs, Accessories, Notepad**.
   b. **Type <HTML>** and **press Enter. Type <HEAD>** and **press Enter**.

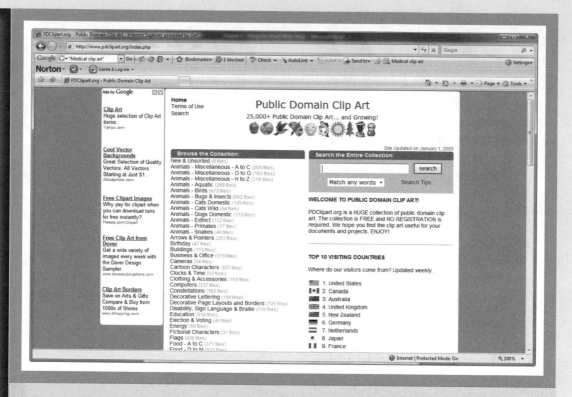

Figure 9-9 Main Page of the Public Domain Clip Art Site

c. **Type <TITLE>Living Healthy—Your Name </TITLE>** and **press Enter** (type your name in place of "Your Name"—for example, Irene's Home Page). This text will be displayed in the title bar of the browser.

d. **Type </HEAD>** and **press Enter**. This tag turns off the header tag.

e. **Type <BODY>** and **press Enter**. This tag turns on the body text that is displayed in the browser window

f. **Type <H1>Homepage of the Living Healthy Consulting Services </H1>** and **press Enter**. This tag enlarges the font to a Heading 1 level.

g. **Type Welcome to our Web site <P>** and **press Enter**. This is the first line of the text; the "P" places the next line of text on the next line.

h. **Type We are pleased that you are here to learn a little about living healthy. <P>** and **press Enter**.

i. **Type </BODY>** and **press Enter**. Type **</HTML>**. These tags turn off the BODY and HTML tags.

j. Save the file in the **HTML** folder on your USB removable storage device. Call the file **Home.html** and make sure the file type is **text**. A Web page icon entitled Home appears in the folder.

k. **Double-click** the **Home.html** file in the HTML folder. The Web page should be displayed.

> NOTE: If nothing is displayed, click the file in Notepad on the taskbar. Confirm that everything is exactly as specified in the exercise. There can be no missing slashes (/) to turn a tag off, no misspelled tags, and so forth. Correct the problems. Save the file and try opening it again.

5. Add images and a link to the file.
   a. Go back to **Notepad** and open the file if you closed it.
   b. Create a **blank line** before the </BODY> tag toward the end of the document.
   c. **Type Here are three things to keep yourself healthy. <P>**
   d. **Type Eat right!<IMG SRC= "images/apple_delicious_golden_red. png"> <P>** and **press Enter**. This tag will put the apple image in the file.
   e. **Type Keep your weight under control. <IMG SRC= "images/thumb_ weight.png"> <P>** and **press Enter**. This tag will place the scale in the file.
   f. **Type Get plenty of exercise. <IMG SRC= "images/jog.png"> <P>** and **press Enter**. This tag places the jog image in the file.
   g. **Save** the file and take another look at it.

Add a Link
   a. Go back to **Notepad** and open the file if you closed it.
   b. Create a **blank line** before the </BODY> tag toward the end of the document.
   c. **Type <A HREF= "http://www.cdc.gov/healthyliving/">Click here for the CDC's web site on healthy living! </A><P>**.
   d. Save the file and view it in the browser. A hyperlink should appear at the bottom of the page. Refresh the browser before you check the hyperlink to make sure it uses the new html file.

Link to Another File at the Same Web Site
   a. **Type <A HREF= "smoking_cessation.html">Smoking cessation</A>**.
   b. **Save** the file. Note the link won't work until you create the second file called smoking cessation.
   c. Create a second file like the home (index.html) file but save it as **smoking_cessation.html** in the HTML folder.
   d. Add your **own content** here—one or two sentences, a picture, and a link back to the home page (index.html file).

> HINT: To save typing time, save the home file using the Save as feature after changing the name to smoking_cessation.html. Now you can replace the content as needed without having to retype all the tags.

6. Save and print the files.
   a. Test your two files to make sure the links work and you can go back and forth between them. See **Figure 9-10** for what the first page looks like.
   b. Open the **browser** and **print** the two files. This shows what they look like in a browser.
   c. Open each file in **Notepad** and **print** them. This shows the code.
      - Did everything work?
      - Did you have any problems with it? If so, how did you solve them?

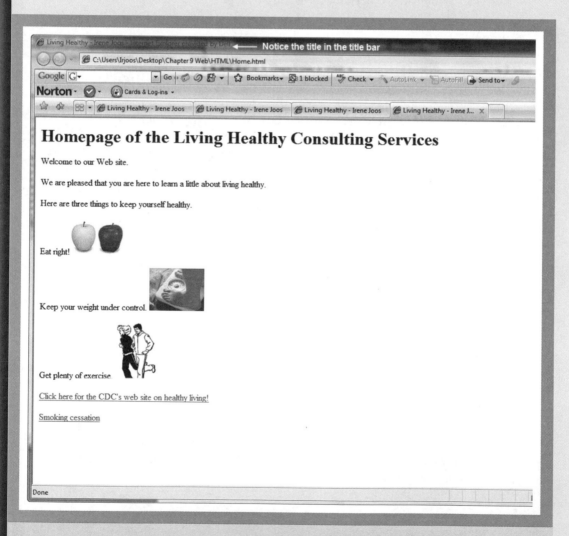

Figure 9-10 Home Page with HTML Tagging

That is all there is to it. Most people who do not tag HTML documents frequently refer to references when looking for the appropriate tags or use the source code from other sites when they find something they like. However, to do so, you have to have some basic understanding of the codes.

EXERCISE 5 Creating a Simple Web Page Using Microsoft Word

■ **Objectives**
1. Create the appropriate folders in which to place the Web pages.
2. Create two simple Web pages using Microsoft Word.
3. Edit the pages.
4. Add graphics and links.

■ **Activity**
1. Plan. In this exercise, you will create two Web pages—one will be the index page or home page, and the other will be the favorites page that will teach you how to link to and from the home page.
2. Create a folder to hold all of the HTML files created for this exercise. Call it **WordHTML**. In that folder, place a subfolder called **graphics**.
3. Create an HTML file.
   a. Start the page and save it as a Web page.
   b. Start **Word**. Word opens.
   c. **Click** the **Office** button, **New**, and the **Create** button (found in the lower-right corner of the screen). You may also **double-click** the **New blank document icon.**
   d. **Click** the **Office** button and then **Save as**. The Save as dialog box appears.
   e. Select the **location** in which to save the file—in this case, the **WordHTML** folder created on your removable storage device.
   f. **Type Index** in the File name text box.
   g. **Click** the **Save as type arrow** and then **click Web Page**.
   h. **Click** the **Change Title** button and **type Healthy Living** by clicking the **Change Title** button on the Save as dialog box. This will be the Web page title that appears in the browser title bar.
   i. **Click OK** and then the **Save** button to save this file as a Web page.

   Add Content to the Web Page
   a. Type the following content, pressing the **Enter** key after each line.
   Healthy Living Tips
   Welcome to our Healthy Living Web site.
   This site provides health tips and links to great healthy living sites.
   Each week features a different healthy living tip.

b. Click the **bullet button** on the **Home** tab, **Paragraph** group and then type the following content, pressing the **Enter** key after each item.
Exercise
Eating
Stress Reduction and Time Management
Regular Checkups and Immunizations

Format the Text

a. **Select Healthy Living Tips** and apply the **Heading 1** style from the Styles group.
b. **Select Welcome to our Healthy Living Web site** and apply the **Subtitle** style.
c. **Select both lines** of the next text and apply **center** justification.
d. Place an **extra line** between the second and third lines, and between the fourth and fifth lines.

Apply a Theme and Add a Graphic Line

a. Go to the **Page Layout** tab, **Themes** group and apply the **Foundry** theme.
b. Change the font of the body text to **Rockwell body 12 points** for all text except the title and subtitle.
c. Place the insertion point between the subtitle and the third line of text.
d. **Click Insert, clipart.**
e. **Type lines** in the Clipart search box and then **click Go.**
f. **Click** the **green line** that has shades of green going from dark to light.
g. If necessary, size the line to go from left to right margins.
h. **Click** the **Save** button to save the file.
i. Open the file **Food.docx** that was either supplied to you by the professor or was downloaded from the Web site.
j. Save it as a Web page (Food.html) after applying the same theme as the index page. Give the web page the title **Healthy Eating** by clicking the **Change Title** button on the **Save as** dialog box.
k. Add a Heading 1 to the beginning of the page: **Healthy Eating Tips**.
l. Add the same **green line** between the title of the page and the body text.
m. Change the body text to **Rockwell body 12 points**.

4. Edit the documents created in part 3.

a. Make sure the **food** file is open.
b. Go to the bottom of the food page and **type: For a good site about the food pyramid, try Inside the Pyramid sponsored by the U.S. Department of Agriculture.**
c. **Select** the **Inside the Pyramid** text and **click** the **Insert** tab, **Hyperlink** in the **Links** group.

    d. In the Address text box at the bottom of the dialog box, **type http://mypyramid.gov/pyramid/index.html**. The text to make a hyperlink should appear in the top text box because you selected it.

    e. **Click** the **Save** button to update the file.

    f. Open the **Index** file.

    g. **Type** at the bottom of the page **Please direct questions to the Webmaster.**

    h. Select the text **Webmaster** and **click** the **Insert** tab, **Hyperlink, Email address** button in the left pane.

    i. In the Email text box, **type your email address**. The text to display should appear in the top text box because you selected it. **Click OK.**

    j. **Press** the **Enter** key twice, **type Last updated on**, and insert **today's date**.

    k. Change the font size of the entry in j to **8 points**.

    l. **Click** the **Save** button to update this file.

5. Insert graphics and link the pages.

    a. Open the **Food** file.

    b. Using a browser, search for an image of the **food pyramid**.

    c. Download the image to the **graphics** folder in the HTMLWord folder after making sure you aren't violating any copyrights.

    d. Insert a **two-column, one-row table** after the bulleted list.

    e. **Click** in the first column of the table. **Select Insert, Picture**, and locate the picture in the graphics folder.

    f. **Press** the **Tab** key and **type** the following text in the second column: **Here is a picture of the recommended food pyramid that might be helpful as you select food.**

    g. **Remove** the lines from the table.

    h. **Resize** the image.

    i. **Center** the text in the cell of the second column.

    j. Go to the bottom of the page and **type Home**.

    k. **Highlight** the text **Home** and **click Insert, Hyperlink.**

    l. **Click** the **Existing File or Web Page** button.

    m. Select the **Index.-** file from the list and **click OK.**

    n. Go to the **Index** file and highlight the word **Eating**.

    o. Repeat the process to **insert a link** back to the Food page.

    p. **Save** the files.

    q. Open the **browser**.

    r. **Select File, Open**, and **Browse**.

    s. **Select** the **Index.html** file on the removable storage medium.

    t. **Click** the **Eating** hyperlink to go to that file.

    u. **Click** the **Home** linked text to go back to the index file.

    v. **Print** each document. They should resemble **Figure 9-11**.

Healthy Living Tips
Welcome to our Healthy Living Web site.

This site provides health tips and links to great healthy living sites.
Each week features a different healthy living tip.

- Exercise
- Eating
- Stress Reduction and Time Management
- Regular checkups and immunizations

Please direct questions to the webmaster.

Last updated on 1/19/2009.

Index File

Healthy Eating Tips

Having lots of energy, feeling good, and being healthy is the essence of healthy living. It is not about being pencil thin, depriving yourself of that sugar treat, or fallowing such a strict diet that you can't possibly be successful. It's about balancing your intake with a variety of delicious and health food with some "treats" that may not be as good for you.

Here are some healthy eating strategies.

- Eat a variety of foods that include groups like vegetables, whole grains, and fruits as well as those that you might east more often like breads, meat, and potatoes.

- Use a smaller dish to keep your proportions in line. Do not "SUPERSIZE" anything. Sometimes starting with a soup or salad helps make you feel full without adding a lot more calories.

- Drink plenty of water and stay away from all the sodas. Sodas add nothing but empty calories. If needed, limit the intake of sodas to once a week or month. You will be amazed at how quickly you no longer "need" the soda.

- Eat enough calories and try to balance your intake with your exercise. If you have a lot of calories one day, try and limit your caloric intake the next day. Keep the range between 1400 and 2500.

- Buy and eat locally grown fresh vegetables and fruit.

- Limit your treats to once a week.

- Limit but don't eliminate sugar and salt

- Listen to your body as to when to eat and when to stop.

- Sit down and eat. Chew your food slowly.

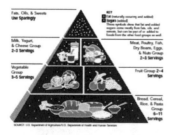

Here is a picture of the recommended food pyramid that might be helpful as you select food.

For a good site about the food pyramid try Inside the Pyramid sponsored by the U.S. Department of Agriculture.

Home

Food File

Figure 9-11 Sample Web Pages Created Using Word

ASSIGNMENT 1 Searching the Internet

■ Directions

Use a search engine or site to answer these questions.

1. What are streaming applications?
2. What is the difference between downloaded and streaming audio and video?
3. What is the current problem with streaming audio/video on campus or from a modem connection?
4. What is the advantage of Web radio? Find a Web radio station and describe it here.

ASSIGNMENT 2 Searching for Information

■ Directions

1. Go to Clusty.com and answer these questions.
   a. Where did Clusty get its start?
   b. What is Vivisimo?
2. Find the site that is entitled **NoodleTools** and the page that helps you find the best strategy for the information needed.
   a. List the URL: _____.
   b. List the sites suggested if you need to refine and narrow your topic:
      _____.
   c. List the sites suggested if you need to find quality sites for health and life sciences: _____.
   d. Who are the two people responsible for this site? _____
3. Use an image database to find a picture of your city and a landmark in your city.
   a. Which image search site did you use?
   b. Place the URL here: _____.
   c. Type your search string here: _____.
   d. How many images (jpg files) did the search return?
4. Download one of the images to your USB storage device.
   a. What is the size and name of the file?
   b. Paste the image in a Word document and submit it with this assignment.
5. Do a search for "cookies" as it applies to the Internet (not food that we eat).
   a. What is a cookie?
   b. What is the potential problem with cookies?

   c. What is the relationship of the cookie file to the temp and temporary Internet folders?

   d. How do you go about deleting information from the temp and temporary Internet folders and the cookies files?

   e. How often should you delete this information?

6. Complete a search using a directory site, a keyword search site, and a meta search site.

   a. Construct a table (4 × 3) in Word listing the three sites you used.

   b. Construct a search for some health-related topic that you are currently studying.

   c. List the search sites (e.g., Yahoo) in column 1 of the table; your search strings in column 2; and the results (e.g., how many hits, examples of the types of sites returned) in column 3.

   d. Which site provided the best results?

ASSIGNMENT 3 Creating a Personal Home Page

■ **Directions**

1. For this assignment, you will create a personal home page. You may use whatever software you prefer to create it (anything from an ASCII editor to an HTML converter to an HTML editor).

2. This home page should meet these criteria:
   - Follow the guidelines given in class and the references for good design.
   - Include at least one of each of the following:
     - A button
     - A graphic or image found on the Web
     - A colored background
     - A picture (make sure that you are not violating someone's copyright; it is easier if you use a picture that you have taken and scan it)
   - Include a link to your biographical sketch.
   - Include a link to a Web page at another site.
   - Include a link to your college or university home page.
   - Use only graphics that are appropriate for the content.
   - Have at least four HTML files linked together.

3. Part of your grade will be assessed based on your presentation of your home page to your classmates. Be prepared to show your home page and talk about its development. This means that you need to make sure that all of your graphics and HTML files are on your removable storage device in the proper places.

ASSIGNMENT 4 Adding to Your E-Portfolio

■ **Directions**
1. Think about exercises or assignments completed in this chapter.
2. Select two exercises or assignments that demonstrate your ability to find relevant information on a topic or skill in using the Internet.
3. Write a one-page summary explaining what you learned from the activity and how it might help you in your profession.
4. Add the summary and the documents to your e-portfolio as directed by your faculty member. This task may require access to Web sites or specific software that is provided by your school. If your school has no e-portfolio process, create a PowerPoint presentation highlighting the material and that follows the guidelines on creating quality presentations found in Chapter 6. You may also use OneNote to add the information and start a e-portfolio.

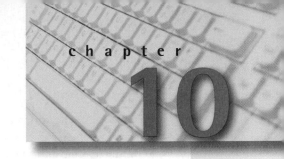

Computer–Assisted Communication

Objectives

1. Identify the components needed to establish computer-assisted communication.
2. Describe computer communication modalities: email, electronic discussion groups, bulletin boards, chat rooms, blogs, and Internet conferencing.
3. Identify security threats when using email.
4. Send email messages and attachments.
5. Join an electronic discussion group.
6. Access newsgroups, bulletin boards, chat rooms, and online social networking communities.

Communication is the process and structure of sending and receiving messages by a variety of means. In computer-assisted communication, the computer enhances the communication process by either structuring the message or providing a channel through which to send and receive messages. This chapter focuses on the use of a computer system as a channel for communicating messages over both short and long distances. Messages sent by a computer system take many forms; two examples are a short email note and an extensive personal profile created in an online community. The focus here is on two-way communication, rather than on one-way or broadcast communications such as podcasts or videos.

Terms Related to Computer-Assisted Communication

The following terms are important to understand when examining different computer-assisted communication modalities. They are introduced here, and more specific information about some of these terms appear later in the chapter.

Aggregator	A software application or program that collects information from various online sources such as blogs, podcasts, and Web sites so that this information can be shown together in a single view.
Attachment	A file that accompanies an email message but is not included in the body of the message itself.
Blog	A self-published Web site containing dated material, usually written in a journal format. Blogs may contain text, pictures, video, audio, and URLs of other relevant sites. They usually include a process for readers to post their comments and reactions. Miniblogs called tweets are growing in popularity using a social networking service called Twitter. They are restricted to 140 characters.
Bounce	Failure of a message to be delivered promptly. Emails can bounce for more than 30 reasons: The email address is incorrect or has been closed; the recipient's mailbox is full, the mail server is down, the system detects spam or offensive content, and so on (EEC, 2009).
Bulletin Board	A public area for messages; it is similar to its counterpart that hangs on a wall. Bulletin boards are typically organized around specific topics and may be part of an online service and accessed through Internet search engines. Bulletin boards may be open to everyone, or they may be restricted to members of certain groups and accessed through passwords. Several examples of bulletin boards can be found at http://www.healthboards.com/.
Chat	Real-time communication between two or more users via a computer. Most Internet services have built-in chat features.
Chat Room	A designated area or "room" where individuals gather simultaneously and "talk" to one another by typing messages. Everyone who is online usually sees the messages. Some students may "visit" their professor in a chat room during virtual office hours when taking online courses.

Electronic Discussion Group	An email service in which individual members post messages for all group members to read.
Email	A message that is composed and sent over a computer network to a person or group of people who have an electronic mail address. Email can be sent over a local area network or over the Internet.
Emoticon	A way to show an emotion via text on the computer. These symbols or combinations of symbols substitute for facial expressions, body language, and voice inflections.
Filter	A tool that automatically moves incoming emails into separate folders according to criteria that either you or your Internet provider has specified. Filters can also be included in a virus checker or a software program used to manage your email. An example is the Junk Mail folder in Microsoft Outlook or the Spam folder on AOL.
Instant Messaging (IM)	A communication service that permits you to send real-time messages via a private chat room to other individuals who are online. This is considered real time communications between two people; you may however have several different IMs going at the same time with different friends who have been added to your buddy list. Because IM systems have not been standardized, individuals communicating with one another must use the same system and must be registered through the system to get an IM address. Many readers will be familiar with this concept in the form of text messaging on a cell phone.
Internet Conferencing	A type of communication in which two or more persons interact over the Internet in real time, receiving more or less immediate replies. This communication can involve interaction via text, audio, or video.
ListServ	The trade name of a software program that manages automated discussion lists. This term is commonly used to refer to all mailing lists (just as "Xerox" was extended to refer to all photocopiers, not just those manufactured by Xerox). When someone posts a message to a discussion list, everyone on the mailing list receives the message via email. The official list of ListServ lists can be found at http://www.lsoft.com/lists/listref.html.

Newsgroup	Informational material and articles organized around a particular topic, such as Alzheimer's disease or child abuse. Newsreaders can post a message to the newsgroup for all to read and respond. To participate in a newsgroup, you need to have newsreader software. A newsreader is provided in Microsoft Outlook but you will need to add the News Command and subscribe to a newsgroup.
PGP (Pretty Good Privacy)	Software that is used to encrypt and protect email as it moves from one computer to another. PGP can be used to verify a sender's identity (EEC, 2009).
Phishing	Fraudulent email that solicits private information such as passwords or credit card numbers. It can result in identify theft.
RSS (Really Simple Syndication)	A scheme that makes it possible for users to subscribe to and receive information about a specific topic that has been published on blogs, podcasts, and other social networking applications. This aggregated information is delivered back through a feed, and the content may then be read through a feed reader or email message.
Spam	Electronic junk mail. This type of email is unsolicited and/or not from an identifiable source. As well as being irritating, it may be deceptive.
Spim	The spam of instant messaging. Part spam and part instant messaging, it is being used by an increasing number of advertisers.
Tags	Terms that function as keywords associated with online content such as blog postings, bookmarks, and Web sites. Tags make it possible for an aggregator to effectively search the Internet and group together related information.
Web 2.0	The second generation of Web utilization. This term does not refer to a change in technology, but rather a change in how Web technology and applications are now being creatively used to enhance and expand information sharing, communication, and collaboration. Examples of Web 2.0 include the evolution of Web-culture communities, social networking sites, video-sharing sites, and blogs.
Webinar	An interactive presentation, lecture, workshop, or seminar delivered over the Internet. In many cases,

	the participants ask questions or offer comments via a chat or voice application.
Wiki	A Web page or a collection of Web pages that can be viewed and modified by anyone who has access to a browser and the Internet. Wikis are proving to be robust, open-ended collaborative group sites. One of the most commonly used wikis is Wikipedia, an online editable encyclopedia (Educause, 2005). Because of the ability to edit the web page, many faculty do not accept Wikipedia as a reliable source for information.

Components Needed for Computer-Assisted Communication

Both the sender and the receiver of an email message must have the appropriate hardware, software, and a connection to the network if they are to communicate successfully. The basics of computer-assisted communication require a sender, channel, medium, and receiver, as illustrated in **Figure 10-1**. In computer-assisted communication, the sender is the person creating the message. He or she interacts with the specific application on a computer; this application can be used to send an email, contribute to a blog, or participate in a chat. The software program working as an application within the hardware and software of the computer will code the message for transmission across the channel. The channel includes equipment such as telephone wires, twisted pair, fiber-optic cables, radio

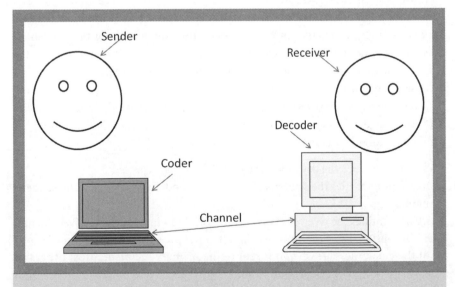

Figure 10-1 Communication Model

waves, or satellites as well as the software that actually transmits the message to the decoder. The computer must be connected to the communications channel by either a modem, a network card, or a wireless card in the computer. The computer that receives the message must then decode or translate the message back into a format that can be understood by the receiver. It is essential that both computers, as well as the channel, support the same communications protocol and standards if they are to "talk" to each other.

Obviously, most computers do not have a direct channel as pictured in Figure 10-1, but rather send messages through a network. Most universities and hospitals are networked. A network consists of all computers and related devices that are connected together for the purpose of sharing devices, programs, and data. Refer to Chapter 2 for additional information on networks and to Chapter 9 for additional information on the Internet.

Electronic Mail

Electronic mail (email) is a way to send messages to others in electronic form. Users write email just like they would write a letter with word processing software. However, instead of printing the message and sending it via the postal system, email users typically click a Send button in the email program. The email message arrives at its destination within a matter of seconds or minutes, depending on where it is going and the traffic on the network. Just as there are many different word processing, graphics, and spreadsheet programs, so there are many different email programs.

Many search sites and Internet service providers offer free email services. Almost all email programs share a common set of functions, as outlined in **Table 10-1**. Although this chapter provides general information about using email, it does not provide step-by-step procedures for using a specific program. Check the help information online or the documentation for the system in your institution for assistance in using your specific email system.

Email messages consist of two parts: the header and the body. The body is the actual message. The header has at least four (and sometimes five) sections that provide useful information:

Date: This includes the date and time that the message was sent.
From: This identifies the sender's email address and, in many cases, the sender's name.
To: This identifies the receiver's email address and can include the receiver's name.
CC: This optional section identifies the other people who will also receive a copy of the email message when it is sent to the primary recipient. Most programs also provide an optional blind carbon copy (BCC). When the BCC function is used, a copy of the email will be sent to one or more additional receivers; their names will not appear in the header seen by the other receivers, however, so only the sender will know that these individuals have received a copy of the

TABLE 10-1   EMAIL APPLICATION FUNCTIONS

Functions	Description
Configure email settings	When you set up your email program you will make several decisions, such as the way in which your name is displayed, your incoming and outgoing mail server names, and your password. Some of this information you will need to obtain from your Internet service provider; in other cases your institution will make these decisions for you.
Compose and send an email message	There are significant variations in the type of formatting available when composing an email message. Some applications permit you to use all of the same text formatting available in your word processing package; others accept only plain text with no formatting.
Reply to an email	When replying to an email, check whether you are replying to everyone who received the original email or just to the author of that email message.
Forward an email	Never send an email that you are not willing to have published. All emails can be forwarded to another person or even several people whom you may not intend to read your words. They may also be printed without your consent or knowledge.
Maintain an address book	An address book is a list of your contacts and their email addresses. It is also possible to maintain distribution lists in your address book.
Attach files to a message	Any type of file can be attached to an email message, including word processing, graphics, spreadsheet, audio, and even video files. The receiver will need the appropriate software to be able to open these files. Note that some institutions also restrict certain types of file attachments like .exe and .accdb files.
Create and attach a signature to an email	Your signature file includes your name and contact information that you want to share in your emails. This information can be attached automatically to all of your emails.
Organize and save email	Most email programs allow you to create folders in which you can categorize and save emails. For example, you may want to save all of the emails related to a course in a folder with the name of the course.

message. Using the BCC option also avoids sending an email with a large distribution list in the header.

Subject: This is the topic discussed in the email. This field will be blank if the sender omitted this information. Some university email systems will not accept email if the subject field is blank. Always include one to three words in this section.

Email users are given a certain amount of space to store email messages on the server of their email provider. If email messages are never deleted, eventually the space allotted will become filled and other messages will be returned to the senders. Thus people with email accounts should read their email often and delete messages that are no longer needed. By moving previously read messages to folders, the inbox of the email system is kept uncluttered and new messages are more readily visible when the email program is started. In addition, some organizations have policies where they will automatically delete email sitting in the inbox, sent folder, or delete folder after a set time. Moving them to folders will avoid critical email from being deleted. It is possible, however, to occupy all of your allocated space with email messages that have been moved to folders. Most programs allow users to systematically store the messages that they wish to keep in folders located off the mail server, either on the local drive or on another network server. Note that storing on the local drive means you won't have access to those messages if not using that computer.

Email Addresses

All email systems provide users with individual addresses. On a local area network (LAN), an email address operates much like an interoffice mail address; that is, the user's local email address usually consists of the user's ID only. In contrast, email sent over a wide area network (WAN) is like mail sent via the postal service, in that a full Internet address is needed. In an email address, an "at" symbol (@) always separates the user ID from the rest of the address. There are three parts to an Internet email address. Suppose the address is ramonanelson@comcast.net.

- The **user ID** is the name of the individual on the computer system where he or she receives email. No one else on that system has the same user ID. The user's ID in the previous example is ramonanelson.
- The "at" symbol (@) is always typed between the user's ID and the user's email system address.
- The **user's domain** is the location address for everyone who uses that email system. This part of the address functions like the home address of a person in postal service mail delivery; that is, everyone in the same family uses the same apartment or house address. In the previous example, the location address is comcast.net.

One of the email application functions that is especially useful when sending a message to a group of people is the creation of a **distribution list** (also called an **alias** or **mailing list**). The distribution ID is the name assigned to the list. Each time the sender addresses an email message using the distribution ID, each person whose email address is included on that list receives the message. For example, a list called ClassN402 might contain the addresses of all students in a healthcare informatics class. When a message is sent to the ClassN402 distribution address, the message is sent to everyone on that list.

Email Etiquette (Netiquette)

Just as there are rules governing what is acceptable to say and do during social interactions, guidelines exist for acceptable ways of communicating using email. Many of these rules can also be applied to other forms of online communication. *Netiquette* is the name given to electronic communication conventions. Some of the main rules of netiquette include the following:

1. Start the message with a greeting, just like with any communication, and make it specific to the recipient(s): "Hi, Kurt," "Mary," or "Greetings, Colleagues." With email, there is a tendency to be less formal than is common in a face-to-face communication. However, when dealing with faculty and medical personnel, it is better to use formal titles. It is also important to be correct in which title is used. For example, do not refer to a PhD-prepared professor or a physician as Mr. or Mrs.; use Dr. instead.

2. Include in the message only what is appropriate for others to read. Never assume the message is private.

3. Be clear and concise. Email messages include only words. When people communicate face to face, they use intonation and body language as well as words to send the message. With email, no observation of the recipient is possible, so no immediate feedback or the ability to adjust the message midway is available. As a general rule, if a message can be misinterpreted, it will be. "Emoticons," like the smiley face, have been developed to signify feelings. Standard emoticons include the following:

    :-) Basic smiley
    ;-) Winking smiley—means "just kidding"
    :-(Sad face
    8-) Smiley with sunglasses
    -o : Surprised

    There are several other emoticons, and several Web sites that list these symbols. As with all communication tools, however, the symbol must be known to both the sender and the receiver to be effective in supporting communication. Text messaging abbreviations are not considered acceptable in most email messages. For example, do not use the letter "U" to stand in for "you."

4. Keep it short. Do not quote huge amounts of material. When replying, put the reply early in the message body so that readers do not have to wade through material to get to the response. If a longer message is needed, attach a file with the message.

5. Always specify the content of the message in the subject line so that readers know what to expect. This information can also help readers discriminate between what might be a legitimate message from someone known and what might be a message containing a virus.

6. Never type in all capital letters. THIS IS CONSIDERED SHOUTING.

7. Make the message one that is well presented. Check the spelling and grammar.

8. Respect copyright. Always give credit to others for their work, and follow copyright rules for using material (see Chapter 12 for guidelines related to copyright).

9. Avoid flaming, which is voicing very strong antagonistic opinions or attacking someone. Never respond when you are angry. It is hard to look professional or explain your thinking if you are in the middle of a "cat fight" or "flaming war."

10. Sign the message. The signature should include at least the sender's name and email address. It can also include the sender's postal mail address, telephone number, title, and professional affiliation. It is possible to create a "signature" file ahead of time and use it as a standard addition to all email.

11. Do not send chain letters. A chain letter is an email that ends with the suggestion that the message be forwarded to several other people. One of the best ways to stop this type of junk email is not to forward it. If there is a specific email with a message you do want to share with a specific person, delete that part of the email suggesting that person forward the email before sending it forward.

Email Attachments

A file sent along with an email message is called an attachment. Any type of file can be sent via email, including text files (Word files), graphics (PowerPoint files), spreadsheets (Excel files), audio (.wav files), and even video. Be certain that the recipient of the file has the appropriate software to open and run the file being sent. For example, if you send an Excel document, the recipient will need to have the Excel software or a plug-in to access that document. Some email systems limit attachment sizes. If the receiver's email system does not accept your attachment because it is too large, it will be bounced back to you. Some email systems also do not accept files with certain extensions, such as .exe or .accdb.

Inserting Attachments

Most email applications have a menu command or a tab that starts a separate dialog screen in which you can insert an attachment to a message. In that dialog screen, users can browse the computer and point to and click the file to be added. Some email programs provide the ability to attach multiple attachments at once; however, most email applications will limit the number of attachments that can be included with one email message. Once a file is attached, you should be able to determine this fact by looking at the screen.

Reading Attachments

Most programs use an icon on the email message list screen that indicates an attachment is present. For example, Microsoft Outlook uses a paper clip image to indicate that an email has an attachment. To open and view the attachment, the receiver must have the same software or something that will interpret the original file and allow it to be read. Typically, clicking the attachment indicator either opens the file or opens a dialog box that allows the viewer to save the attachment to a file or to open the attachment. Sometimes you will need to right-click to see these options.

Safe Email Practices

To protect the computer, it is wise not to open attachments without checking them for a virus. Most virus-checking software will give you the option of setting up your virus checker so that all attachments are scanned automatically as they come into your email program. However, no virus checker will catch every virus. Malicious computer hackers have developed systems that enable them to access a user's address file and send messages to everyone in the list, making it appear as if the message is from that user. Thus it is prudent not to open attachments, even from known individuals, unless they are expected.

While all attachments can include malicious applications, executable (.exe) attachments are highly suspect. Once opened, these attachments may create a variety of problems on the computer.

Some systems routinely check all attachments before permitting the user to open them. Nevertheless, the best course of action is to save the attachment to a file—just be sure to note in which folder the file is being saved—and then explicitly check it with an antivirus program such as Norton Utilities or McAfee Antivirus software before opening the file. If a file with a virus is found, delete the file from both your email list and the computer's delete folder without opening it.

Today, at least 80% of the U.S. population has Internet access in the home, and email is becoming a primary tool for communication, sometimes rivaling even the telephone (Duffy, 2008). Along with its advantages, however, has come the irritating problem of unsolicited messages—that is, spam. Spam has become so problematic that a federal law regulating junk mail went into effect in 2004. To date, the Controlling the Assault of Non-Solicited Pornography and Marketing (Can Spam) Act, although resulting in a few prosecutions, has not greatly reduced the volume of spam (Federal Trade Commission, n.d.).

Many Internet providers offer spam-blocking products for their customers, and some email programs have filters that may be set to block spam related to specified subjects or from specified addresses. It is wise to never open messages from anyone or any company that you do not know. Never respond to spam because this reply can confirm that your email address is active and you are reading these emails. Always report spam to your Internet service provider. Most ISPs that provide email functionality make sending such reports easy, through an option on the email menu. In an attempt to prevent advertising spam from coming into email accounts, some individuals set up a separate account for electronic discussion groups, ordering online, and registering warranties to control the number of advertisements coming to their personal email account.

No matter how an email is addressed or which trademarks appear on the email, you should never provide personal information such as your password, account number, or Social Security number in response to an email message. Some emails fraudulently represent commercial companies by including the company's headers or logos on the email message and then request personal information. Your bank and any other company that you do business with will never request this type of information by email.

These so-called phishing scams can lead to identity theft. A common phishing scam on campus is to send emails offering part-time work. The email will look like it is coming from a campus email address. However, when students apply for the job by providing all of their personal information, including their Social Security number, they have just been caught in a phishing scam. If you receive such an email job offer, call the university's human resources department by phone and ask if the message is legitimate.

Online Tools for Collaboration

As the Web has evolved, a number of tools and applications have been developed to support online collaboration and creativity. Just as people communicate for a variety of purposes, so these tools can be used to support a variety of activities. Healthcare professionals should consider how these tools can be used to support their professional communication as well as how patients and healthcare consumers might use these tools to deal with health and other personal issues.

Electronic Discussion Groups

People with common interests frequently join with like-minded individuals to form an organization. The types of interests and the structures of these organizations vary widely. The joining of people with common interests also occurs in the virtual world of the Internet. Online discussion groups are often referred to in terms of the applications that are used to manage these groups. One of the most common examples of such a term is "listserv," which comes from one of the software programs used to support this process. It is often used in place of the term "online discussion group." Examples of online discussion group software programs include Listproc, ListServ, and Majordomo.

Electronic discussion groups may be either moderated or unmoderated. On a moderated list, each email message is reviewed and approved by someone before it is posted. On an unmoderated list, no one reviews posts before they are sent to members. Most lists are unmoderated. The discussion group relies on the integrity of its members as well as online peer pressure to encourage participants to abide by the list rules. An unmoderated list will develop its own culture, so not all of the rules will necessarily be written. For example, on some discussion groups, announcements of job opportunities are welcome. On others, these messages are considered off topic and not welcome.

A discussion group software application maintains the mailing list for a group of people with common interests. The membership list includes the group of people who have joined together by subscribing to the same list. The discussion group will have a computer name that reflects the interest of the group. For example, snurs-1 is the name of an electronic discussion group for undergraduate nursing students. To communicate with other people on the list, participants send messages to the discussion group's email address. The message will then be sent as an individual email message to each person on the list. When the message is distributed to each member on the list, it is referred to as being "posted to the group."

To join the group (to subscribe), individuals send an email message to the application email address. This email address is different from the one used to post messages to the discussion group. Because the subscription request will be read and answered by a computer program, the message must follow the specific format required by that application. If the discussion group is moderated, your request will also be read by a person. In either case, you will receive a response to your email letting you know you are subscribed. The commands employed for communication with the discussion group application software and the address to use when posting a message will be included in this response. Be sure to save these directions for later use after subscribing. With most discussion groups, the specific procedures for joining and posting messages can also be accessed either through email or on the Web site that introduces the electronic discussion group.

Joining an Electronic Discussion Group

Procedures for joining electronic discussion groups are similar. The following steps represent the typical approach to joining a list:

1. Address the email message to the appropriate email address for subscribing, not the list's email address for posting to the discussion board. For example, listserv@listserv.arizona.edu is the address of an electronic discussion group for subscribing. A complete list of the online discussion groups hosted at Listserv.Arizona.edu can be seen at http://www.lsoft.com/scripts/wl.exe?XH=LISTSERV.ARIZONA.EDU.

2. Put no other information in the header. Leave the subject line blank.

3. In the body of the message, type the following: **Subscribe \<list name\>** **\<firstname lastname\>** (for example, subscribe nursenet Nancy Smith). Some online discussion group software programs accept the word "sub" in place of the word "subscribe," whereas others require the word "join." Some online discussion group software programs require your email address rather than the first and last names.

4. Put no other information in the body of the email message. Do not sign your name or thank the online discussion group. Remember that this message is *not* a communication with a person but is rather a set of commands being sent to a computer.

5. If the attempt to subscribe is unsuccessful, an error message from the computer will be emailed back. This message will try to indicate the type of mistake made. If the message is not meaningful, get help at the local site.

6. If the attempt to subscribe is successful, a welcome message from the online discussion group will arrive. It may contain a great deal of information that is not entirely meaningful initially. Even so, save this message!

7. If there is a time when participation in the online discussion group will be decreased and email will not be read, send a message to the online discussion group suspending the email service. To stop receiving email from the list, send an "unsubscribe" message to the correct electronic discussion list address. The specific directions for stopping email or for unsubscribing can be found in the welcome message from the list. Failing to stop online discussion group email may result in a full mailbox, with messages being bounced back to the online discussion group. This is very poor list etiquette. Some lists, however, permit archiving messages while on vacation.

Posting an Email Message to a List

It is wise to read several postings on a list before posting a message. Each list has its own culture. It is helpful to know the list and the nature of the list before posting.

1. Send the appropriate message to the list's address. For example, NURSENET is a global forum on nursing issues. Note the difference in the list's address for posting message (nursenet@listserv.arizona.edu) and the discussion board's address for subscribing to the list (listserv@listserv.arizona.edu). In both cases, the domain part of the address is the same, but the user ID part of the address is different. When posting a message to the list, users are communicating with people and not a computer. For this reason, many lists require users to type an ID and password before the messages can be posted.

2. Put the topic of the message in the subject line. This information is very helpful to receivers when they are reading their email directory. If the posting is a response to another person's email, use the same words to identify the subject topic as the previous sender used. Many email programs will insert the

subject and address automatically if the reply function is selected. If selecting the reply function with an email message from online discussion group software, confirm that the email program inserted the correct list address before posting the message. For example, if you only want to respond to the person who posted the initial message you want to be sure you are not replying to the list. Messages are sometimes posted with a request that the response is "offline." This means the poster is requesting you respond directly to them and not to the full list.

3. When typing the message, use appropriate Netiquette.
4. Because some email programs clip off the header on incoming messages, always sign the message with your name and email address at the end of the message.

Usenet Newsgroups

Usenet is a form of an online bulletin board system. With this service, users read and post messages or articles in categories called newsgroups. There is no central server but rather a large, constantly changing group of servers that store and forward messages. Newsgroups are organized by topics in a hierarchical tree structure. The first part of the topic identification is general, but each successive part becomes more specific. For example, the newsgroup related to nursing has the following name: sci.med.nursing. The newsgroup for nurse practitioners is named alt.npractitioners.

To read these messages and interact with the group, users must use a software program called a newsreader. Today, most Web browsers have newsreaders built into them, which has allowed more people to become involved in newsgroups.

Google has added another layer to the newsgroup concept. It provides a service that maintains a list of newsgroups and allows Web access using its Groups functionality. With this approach, you do not need a newsreader. The archives from the newsgroups can be searched in the same way that the Web is searched. In addition, Groups can be used to post comments to an existing Usenet newsgroup (Google, 2009).

Internet Conferencing

Internet conferencing involves two or more people interacting with one another over the Internet; they engage in a real-time conversation and receive more or less immediate replies, depending on the speed of their connections. Chat, or text-based interaction, was the original form of this type of communication. Now audio and video conferencing via the Internet is commonplace. Rather than calling a meeting or phoning colleagues, participants in Internet conferencing use a software program and the appropriate audio and video accessories that allow them to speak to and see colleagues over the Internet.

Chat

Although some chat rooms support graphics and voice, the basic chat interface is text. In text chat, two or more people communicate by typing messages that appear in a text window, which is visible to the other people in the same chat room. People use chat to communicate about specific topics because it offers a more rapid response than email. Many online vendors use chat to answer questions when you are shopping, for example. Chat rooms are one of the most commonly used resources on the Internet. However, as with chatting in a crowded room, often many simultaneous conversations are taking place. In text chat, the participant will see all of the messages that are part of those different conversations in the order that they were entered into the system. Thus following the sequence of a particular line of the conversation may be confusing at first.

Most chat systems allow participants to send private messages to individuals in the chat room as well as to participate with the group. Some chat programs, such as ICQ (http://www.icq.com), allow users to compile a "buddy list" of friends on the Internet. Using these programs, you can set up personal chat rooms and chat privately with friends. Most course management applications, such as Blackboard, include a chat function for use within a specific course. These programs follow a common protocol:

1. Register as required by the chat room before you can log in. As part of that process, you will select your user name, which is the name that everyone else in the chat room will see. In public chat rooms, nicknames are recommended to ensure better privacy. As with other user IDs, each name must be unique. In Blackboard or other course management programs, there is no additional registration required; once you log in to the course management program, you have access to the chat feature.

2. Log in and read the messages in the current chat session. Messages from those participating in the chat session as well as system messages and information about people entering and leaving the room will appear in a box on the screen. Each message is preceded by the user name of the person who submitted the message, thereby ensuring that each participant can tell who said what.

3. When you are ready to participate, type your message into the text entry box, and press Enter.

Using one of the many search engines on the Internet, it is possible to find a chat room of interest. Indeed, most search engines support chat rooms. Chat rooms are usually organized around topics of interest, age, or other categories. There are also topic-specific chat rooms located on many Web sites. For example, a list of chat rooms related to nursing issues can be found at http://www.nursingdiscussions.com/.

Chatiquette is similar to Netiquette in terms of the words and behavior acceptable while participating in a chat room. For more information about chatiquette,

visit http://www.ker95.com/chat101/html/chatiquette.html. Information on chatiquette as it applies to an online class can be found at http://ed.fnal.gov/lincon/
act/intro/chatiquette.shtml. Chat room safe behavior is also important, and safety
tips can be found at http://www.wiredsafety.org/safety/chat_safety/chatrooms/
index.html.

Wikis

In 2003, the Institute of Medicine identified five core competencies required of
all health professionals. Working as part of interdisciplinary teams is one of these
five core competencies (IOM, 2003). Today one can expect to find group projects required in most, if not all, educational programs for health professionals.
The flexibility inherent in using wikis makes them an excellent tool for developing asynchronous communication and group collaboration skills. Users can
add, edit, and delete text, movies, pictures, and sounds with very limited technical
knowledge. Because anyone with access can modify the content and format, in
academia access is often limited to the group members. However, if these group
members are going to produce a coherent product, they must learn to work
together in a non-face-to-face environment.

The following general rules can be helpful in establishing a culture of produc-
tivity when working with a wiki:

1. Select a group coordinator. This person will be expected to coordinate the
   activities of the other group members, so he or she should have less responsibility for contributing content to the overall project.
2. Establish clear rules for when and how materials can be added, modified, and
   deleted, including a procedure for informing others that changes were made.
3. Keep a copy of all deleted materials. You may need these materials later.
4. Establish clear rules for deadlines and the implications if these milestones
   are not met. For example, if one student does not contribute material that
   is useful in a timely manner, he or she might be removed from the group.
5. Have a backup plan if something should happen to your Web site or to any
   of the group members.
6. Once the group members have established their working rules and procedures, be sure the professor is comfortable with these procedures.

VoIP

VoIP is an acronym standing for Voice over Internet Protocol, which is the technology that makes it possible to transmit voice or sound via the Internet. With this
protocol, your voice is converted into a digital signal that travels over the Internet. If
you are calling a regular phone number, the signal is converted to a telephone signal
before it reaches the destination. VoIP can allow you to make a call directly from
a computer, from a special VoIP phone, or from a traditional phone connected to

a special adapter (Federal Communications Commission, n.d.). Several vendors offer VoIP-based services. In some cases, the software can be downloaded and used for free to contact others who have also installed this same software. For example, Skype.com offers free computer-to-computer calls when you use the software located at http://www.skype.com/download/skype/windows/.

Document Sharing

Online document sharing makes it possible for groups to work together on a common document even when the group members are separated in space. These applications let you upload files to a Web site where the group can work together in real time, for example, to edit a document. The person who establishes the document can control who has access to it by controlling who can join the group. The necessary files can be stored on the site so that asynchronous work can also occur. When you are finished, the final file can be downloaded to your PC. An example of this application can be seen at docs.google.com. The Google version of this application can be used for free.

Online Social Networking

Social networking sites are Web-based services that allow users to construct a profile, identify a list of other users with whom they share a personal connection, and traverse that list of connections (Boyd & Ellison, 2007). These sites offer a variety of services that serve to create online communities. For example, they include a process for building a profile that can include text, pictures, video, and audio files that can be shared with others. In addition, they provide a means of finding and connecting with others who are already in the community of users, such as leaving a message on the "wall" of another user.

The nature and purpose of the connections and the interactions will vary from site to site. For example, both MySpace and Facebook have a general purpose, whereas Linkedin focuses on building professional relationships. A list of social networking sites, along with each site's focus, can be found at http://en.wikipedia .org/wiki/List_of_social_networking_websites.

Summary

The Internet is changing where, when, and how individuals, businesses, organizations, groups, and communities communicate. This chapter reviewed several of the more common tools that are driving this change. The challenge for healthcare students is to use these tools to improve the effectiveness and efficiency of both their professional and personal communication.

References

Boyd, D. M., & Ellison, N. B. (2007). Social network sites: Definition, history, and scholarship. *Journal of Computer-Mediated Communication, 1*(1), article 11. Retrieved February 3, 2009, from http://jcmc.indiana.edu/vol13/issue1/boyd.ellison.html.

Duffy, J. (2008). 20% of the U.S. has never sent an email. *PC World.* Retrieved February 2, 2009, from http://www.pcworld.com/businesscenter/article/146019/20_of_us_has_never_sent_email.html.

Educause. (2005). 7 things you should know about wikis. Retrieved February 6, 2009, from http://net.educause.edu/ir/library/pdf/ELI7004.pdf.

Email Experience Council (EEC). (2009). Glossary. Retrieved February 1, 2009, from http://www.emailexperience.org/resources/email-glossary/.

Federal Communications Commission. (n.d.). Voice over Internet Protocol. Retrieved February 3, 2009, from http://www.fcc.gov/voip/.

Federal Trade Commission. (n.d.). Spam: Acts and regulations. Retrieved February 2, 2009, from http://www.ftc.gov/bcp/conline/edcams/spam/rules.htm.

Google. (2009). What is a Usenet newsgroup? Retrieved February 3, 2009, from http://groups.google.com/support/bin/answer.py?answer=46854&src=top5&lev=index.

Institute of Medicine (IOM), Committee on the Health Professions Education Summit Board of Health Care Services, Greiner, A. C., & Knebel, E, (Eds.). (2003). *Health professions education: A bridge to quality.* Washington, DC: National Academies Press. Retrieved February 6, 2009, from http://www.iom.edu/CMS/3809/4634/5914.aspx.

EXERCISE 1 Using Email

■ **Objectives**
   1. Access an email system.
   2. Change the password for an email account.
   3. Read, save, and delete email.

■ **Activity**
   1. If you do not already have an email account, obtain an account from the university computer center. An account gives you permission to use the system. This permission comes in the form of a user ID and a unique password. If the instructor or school has not provided you with an account, you need to set up a computer account before doing this exercise. If you have a user ID and password, you are ready to begin this exercise. If your university does not provide email accounts, use an Internet search engine to find one of the free online services to obtain an account.
   2. Find the documentation. Most institutions have documentation for computer programs available to users. Short handouts are usually available for free either in print or at the institution's Web site. More detailed documentation may be sold through the computer center and/or bookstore. Find

out where and how you can obtain documentation in your institution. Obtain a copy of the documentation for signing on to the system and for using email. With an account, you may also be able to access online help.

3. Sign on. Follow the directions for signing on to the computer system. Typically, you will **type** the **user ID**, and **press** the **Tab** key to go to the next text field. **Type** the **password**, and then either **press Enter** or **click OK**.

Remember that the password will not appear on the screen. In most email programs, it appears as a series of asterisks (******) in the Password text box.

If a message appears on the screen saying **Invalid password**, **Login incorrect**, or something similar, try typing the user ID and password again. Some systems are case sensitive; thus you need to note whether you should or should not use capitals in either the user ID or the password. Most systems give you at least three tries to get in before the account is locked out; you will then need to see the account administrator or call the Help Desk to have it unlocked.

4. Change the password. When signing on for the first time, some computer systems require you to change the password before proceeding. If the system does not require you to change the password, this should be your first action after signing on. Check the documentation for the specific process for changing a password.

In email programs:

a. **Click** the **Password icon**, *or* **select** an option on a **menu**, *or* **click** a **hypertext** link.

b. When prompted for the current password, **type** the **current password**, and then either **press Enter** or **click OK**.

c. When prompted, **type** the **new password**, and either **press Enter** or **click OK**.

d. When prompted, **type** the **new password** a second time, and either **press Enter** or **click OK**.

When you are typing passwords throughout this procedure, the passwords will not appear on the screen. The change is usually processed immediately, although on some systems, there may be a time lag before the new password takes effect. Check the system documentation.

5. Access the email system. Start the email program by **clicking** the **icon**.

6. Open and read each message.

a. **Double-click** or highlight the email **message**, and **press Enter**.

b. If this approach does not work, look at the screen for directions, and read the written documentation for the system. After you read each email message, look at how the email directory changed.

7. Send a message. Find the **email address** of a friend. Asking the friend for his or her address is the easiest way to do this. In college settings, there may be a faculty, staff, and student directory online that contains listings of addresses. One way to test your understanding of the correct procedure at the location is to practice by sending yourself a message. Once you master the procedure, practice sending messages to a friend.

   a. Start the **email** program.
   b. **Type** the **email address** of the friend in the **To** text box. Many programs permit you to select the address from the email address book by double-clicking it.
   c. **Press** the **Tab** key or **click** in the **Subject** text box.
   d. **Type** in the **subject**, and **press** the **Tab** key or **click** in the **Message** text box. Most likely you do not need to CC yourself. Most email programs automatically place a copy of all email sent out in your Sent folder.
   e. **Type** and **format** the **message**.
   f. **Click** the **Send** icon.

   The procedure for composing an email message varies greatly from one system to another. The previous information outlines the general process used by many of today's email programs. If this procedure does not work, read the local documentation for the following information:

   - How do you initiate the function to compose a message?
   - How do you enter the address of the person who will receive this message?
   - How do you enter the email message?
   - When the email message is ready, how do you give the send command?

8. Reply to a message.

   a. Open an email **message** (double-click it).
   b. **Click** the **Reply to Sender** button. The program inserts the sender's address and subject in the appropriate text boxes. The Subject text box uses the same subject and adds the prefix "RE:" to it. Note the option Reply to All versus simply Reply.
   c. In some email programs, you will need to type the **Reply** command. If you have received a message as part of a distribution list, find out how to reply to the author and how to reply to everyone on the list.
   d. Compose the **response**, and **click** the **Send** button.

9. Save or delete each message.

   a. Highlight the **message**.
   b. **Press** the **Delete** key or **click** the **Delete** button. In some Web-based email programs, you delete messages by clicking in the square box next to the message, and then clicking the Delete button.
   c. Read the local documentation for the delete procedure. In many email applications, you must "empty the trash" or "purge the Delete folder"

to remove a message. Once you have completed this step, you will not be able to recover deleted messages. If you do not delete messages, the mailbox will become full and eventually new messages will be bounced back to the sender. Most email programs automatically save a copy of all sent messages in a Sent folder. If these sent messages are left to accumulate, this folder will eventually take up too much space and new email sent to this mailbox will bounce. The sent message folder may also be automatically emptied by the system administrator after a set time period. Some email programs leave the undeleted messages in the inbox, whereas others move them to an older message folder. You will know the message is in the inbox if the message is listed in the message list each time you start the email program.

   d. Read the local documentation for the save procedure. Most systems permit you to move messages into online folders. Read the documentation for a procedure for saving messages in folders.

10. Exit the email program.

   In Windows-based email programs, follow one of these procedures:

   ■ **Click** the **Close** button in the upper-right corner of the screen.
   ■ Alternatively, select **File**, **Exit** from the menu bar.

   It is important to exit the email system with the computer still running. If you turn the computer off or just walk away without exiting email, someone else may be able to access your account without signing on. Once you exit the email program, complete the computer sequence for shutting down the computer as specified by the laboratory, library, or other locale.

ASSIGNMENT 1 Setting Up an Online Email Account

■ **Directions**

1. Use an Internet search engine to find a free email application. Which search strategy did you use to find a free application?
2. **Click** the **new user sign-in link**, and follow the instructions given. Read all of the privacy information. When given the choice, be sure that you select the free email service. How much storage space do you get for your email in this system?
3. Once you have registered, read the welcome message. How often do you need to use this system for your account to remain active?
4. Print this message to hand in, and answer the previous questions on the printout.

ASSIGNMENT 2 Accessing a Newsgroup

■ **Directions**
1. Access Google from a Web browser (**www.google.com**).
2. **Click More, Groups**, and then **Browse all Group Categories. Click Health** and repeat the clicking until you locate down to **Health Disabilities** or **Health and Fitness**.
3. Look at the groups listed across the page. Determine how active they have been by examining the number of posts. Select a group of interest. Print the Web page that contains the subject threads.
4. Select a subject thread that has at least eight articles, and follow that thread. In the frame on the left side of the page, select the discussion thread by clicking the first message; read that post, and then click the next message in the list; and so on.
5. Use the word processing application to answer the following questions:
    a. Which discussion topic did you select?
    b. What was the general theme of messages to this topic?
    c. What were your reactions to reading about this topic?
    d. Would you like to participate in a newsgroup? If so, which topics might be of interest? If not, what are your reasons?
6. Submit the responses to these questions and the Web page printout.

ASSIGNMENT 3 Electronic Discussion Group versus Literature Searches

■ **Directions**
1. Subscribe to a health-related electronic discussion group. Review the messages each week for the next four weeks. Make an annotated list of the topics discussed during that period. At the end of the four weeks, send a message to the application (*not* the list) to unsubscribe from the electronic discussion group. Turn in the list of the five top topics discussed.
2. Use an automated literature database to perform a literature search. Limit the search to the last two years. Search for articles related to the focus of the electronic discussion group. For example, if the discussion group relates to home health nursing, then use the term "home health nursing" as the keywords when doing the literature search.
3. Turn in an annotated list of the five topics most commonly discussed in the literature. Write a brief paper comparing and contrasting the two lists of topics.

ASSIGNMENT 4 Internet Resource Document

■ **Directions**

1. In this assignment, you will create an Internet resource document that can be used by other students. Resources on the Internet change frequently, so check each resource before adding it to the document. In other words, make sure the address is correct, the site is still available, and you have not misunderstood the focus of the site.

2. Work in small groups (three to five people) to create the resource document. The resource document should include the following information for specific topics of interest to the discipline or course:

   a. A list of chat rooms, including information on how to access them

   b. A list of electronic discussion groups, including directions for subscribing to them

   c. A list of newsgroups, including directions for how to access them

3. After each small group completes its document, the class will use docs.google.com to create a master document identifying all resources found by the class.

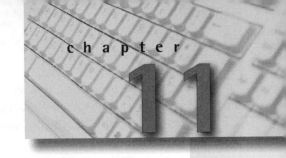

chapter 11

Distance Education:
A Student Perspective

Objectives

1. Conduct a self-assessment of your readiness for learning in a distance education environment.
2. Understand how the technology used to deliver distance education can influence your learning.
3. Develop appropriate learning skills for success in a distance learning course.
4. Identify distance education courses and programs that can meet your learning and career goals.

Introduction

This chapter, which focuses on distance education, is new with this edition of this book and was written in response to the major changes evolving from the integration of technology into the educational environment. Many students who were born after 1980 grew up using computers in their homes and their classrooms. High school students in many states are now required to take at least one online course before they graduate. With the growth of cyberschools, a significant number of students are now experienced distance education learners long before they ever take a college level course.

Other students in today's college classroom were introduced to computers long after they finished high school. These students may have limited or no exposure to learning in a distance education environment. Often, they may be intimidated by their more experienced classmates.

While there is significant variation in the learning experiences of the current college population, all students need to become comfortable using distance education technology. Much of future education will be delivered using these technologies. Health care is a fast-changing field in which competent healthcare providers are required to be lifelong learners. Increasingly, employers in healthcare settings are using distance education technology instead of face-to-face classes to deliver required training and updates. Many states also require healthcare professionals to obtain continuing education units (CEUs) for relicensure; in most cases, these CEUs are easily obtained through online learning.

This chapter focuses on those aspects of distance education that are important to you as a student and to your success with distance education. It is assumed that you are already enrolled in a higher education institution and understand the importance of continuing your education after you complete your current program. The content of this chapter includes a self-assessment tool to help you determine whether you can expect to successfully learn in a course or program offered through distance education; identifies the different technology options for distance education and their relationship to successful learning; outlines the study skills specific to successful learning in a Web-based distance education program; and suggests techniques for finding the best-fit distance education programs for your future learning.

Definitions of Terms Related to Distance Education

Several terms are used to refer to distance education learning itself, including *distributed education, online education, online learning, e-learning,* and *Web-based education* (Indiana University, Information Technology Service, 2003). The following terms related to distance education are used in this chapter:

Asynchronous	A communication exchange in which the people involved are communicating at different times. For example, email and discussion boards are asynchronous because the communicants do not need to be on the computer at the same time.
Chat	Real-time communication between two or more users via a computer.
Course Management Software or System (CMS)	A software application that is used by colleges and universities as well as corporations and government agencies to facilitate distance learning by centralizing the development, management, and distribution of instructional-related information and materials. A CMS provides faculty with a set of tools that allows the easy creation of course content—syllabi, course modules, lecture notes, assignments, tests and quizzes, and so forth—and is the framework faculty use to teach

and manage their class (eLearners.com, 2009). A CMS provides a portal for learners to access their course materials and activities. Two commonly used CMS programs are Blackboard and Moodle.

Distance Education
The delivery of education when the student and the instructor are in physically different locations. In today's learning environment, this type of education is often delivered over the Internet using a variety of technical tools such as a course management software package.

Synchronous Communication
Real time communicate between participants using their computers. Chat rooms and Internet meetings are examples of synchronous communication, because all of the individuals involved are on their computers at the same time.

Threaded Discussion
An online information exchange that is similar to a bulletin board, except that topics within each interest area are identified and organized together so that users can access and read only the discussions pertaining to a particular interest area.

Video Conferencing
A conference involving a computer, video camera, microphone, and speakers. Along with hearing audio, whatever images appear in front of the video camera are delivered to the participant's monitor. A "virtual" conference can involve two participants or many and is considered synchronous communication.

Virtual Classroom
A learning environment that exists solely online in the form of digital content and online communication. The content is stored, accessed, and exchanged through networked computer and information systems. Everything in a virtual classroom occurs in a nonphysical environment, and students "go to class" by connecting to the network rather than by traveling to a real, physical classroom.

Self-Assessment for Distance Education

Success in a distance education environment requires that you be motivated and interested in learning. Registering for a distance education course simply because you are late in registering and it is the only course that will fit in your schedule is not usually a good idea. Students who are ambivalent about being in school and have limited interest in their classes usually do very poorly early in the course in a distance education environment. However, if you are motivated, distance education provides great opportunities.

Some students take to distance education like ducks to water. From the beginning, they like the format and do well. Many other students go through an adjustment period and then do well in a distance education environment. These students discover how to learn in the new environment and then become successful. Unfortunately, a few students find distance education a constant frustration and never make the adjustment. The following questions will help you determine where you fit in this picture and where you may need to make adjustments.

What Are Your Literacy Skills and Background Knowledge?

Your literacy skills and background knowledge of the course content are important in ensuring a successful distance education experience. These skills include the following:

- Reading comprehension and the ability to express yourself in writing
- Basic computer literacy
- Knowledge of and aptitude for the specific subject being studied

If you prefer to hear new information rather than to read that content, if you prefer to talk rather than to write your ideas, or if you are uncomfortable with technology, distance education will be a major challenge for you.

Computer literacy is an important part of overall literacy. While you can succeed in a Web-based distance education course with minimal computer literacy, some comfort in working on the computer can be key to achieving success. In addition, if the course involves a field where you have little knowledge of the topic or lack the prerequisite background needed for that topic, distance education can be difficult. For example, if you have a weak math background or struggle with mathematical concepts and are taking a statistics course online, your lack of preparation or aptitude for mathematics can be a major challenge.

What Are Your Personal Attributes?

Some students appreciate the teacher reminding them of assignment due dates. Others have already noted the key dates in each of their courses. These students may hate to hear the same information repeated and feel that they are being nagged.

Some students like to have their work done early and do not like the sense of last-minute pressure. Other students feel they do their best work under pressure and will leave only enough time to barely get done.

Some students will set up a time and place to study and will resist distractions. For example, they can turn off distractions such as email and cell phones and check their email only after they have finished their project. Other students benefit from a traditional classroom where the distractions of daily life are eliminated.

As you think about these different personal attributes, are you organized, structured, not easily distracted, and a bit compulsive about meeting deadlines? If this description fits, you should do well in a distance education course.

How Important Are Social Interactions?

Is social interaction and getting to know your classmates on a personal level important to your education? Distance education courses usually encourage interaction between classmates and the teacher; however, that interaction focuses on the course subject. The informal interactions that occur between classes or within student organizations are often not part of the distance education experience. For some students, the lack of informal interactions proves too isolating so that they become less interested in the course. For these students, taking a distance education course can be similar to sitting at home reading the textbook.

Because the informal social relationships that occur on campus can lead to long-term professional relationships, some schools support online student organizations. Some schools focus on a virtual coffee house where students online go to chat. This practice can be effective, but requires the student to make that extra effort to sign on and become involved in the online community.

Several universities have designed self-assessment tools to help students determine whether they should participate in distance education. **Table 11-1** provides examples of these tools. As you look over these questions and do your own self-assessment, you will discover that you are stronger in some areas than in others. While your strengths will help you and your weak areas will challenge you, your motivation is the key factor. In many cases, the final outcome is determined by how badly you really want to complete the course or even the whole program.

TABLE 11-1   ONLINE SELF-ASSESSMENTS FOR DISTANCE EDUCATION

University	URL
Boise State University	http://www.boisestate.edu/distance/students/selfscreen.shtml
University of Illinois	http://www.ion.uillinois.edu/resources/tutorials/pedagogy/selfEval.asp
Bellevue Community College	http://bellevuecollege.edu/distance/WebAssess/
Washington State University	http://www.distance.wsu.edu/prospective/DDPquiz.asp
OnlineLearning.net	http://www.onlinelearning.net/OLE/holwselfassess.html?s=624.9050y691n.031y222s41

Along with your readiness for distance education, two other factors that determine your experience are (1) the amount of your total education delivered in this format and (2) the specific type of distance education technology used to deliver your education. Distance education technology can be classified into two major types: video conferencing and Web-based programs. Additional information about these two types of distance education technology is provided in the next section.

The technology used to deliver Web-based distance education is also an excellent tool for supplementing and supporting traditional classroom formats. As a result, the technology can be used to deliver part of a course, a complete course, or a complete program where graduates are never on campus. The degree of immersion in distance education can have a significant effect on your adjustment to the distance education experience. Taking a Web-based distance education course during the same term you are taking other classes at that school in the traditional format is a very different experience from taking all of your classes via Web-based distance education.

Distance Education Technology

The media and technology available to deliver distance education have moved through several generations (Bates, 2007). Initially, distance education used a print or paper format delivered by postal mail. This was followed by use of one-way broadcasting media such as television, radio, or mailed videocassettes.

The next major innovation involved two-way synchronous tele-learning, such as telephone-based conference calls and interactive video. The widespread acceptance of the Internet led to a fourth approach—asynchronous online learning usually delivered via course management software. A number of applications are now being added to this fourth option. These tools increase the degree of automation, interaction, and student control. Currently, all of these generations of technology remain in use, often in combination. In this chapter, however, we focus on interactive video conferencing and asynchronous online learning delivered via course management software because these are the formats most commonly used today.

Interactive Video Conferencing

Distance education that relies on interactive video conferencing is synchronous—that is, the classes occur at a set time with the students and faculty present at their classroom locations. In the Unites States, most universities use room-based video conferencing, which connects two or more traditional classrooms in real time across a network. This setup requires that students travel to the video conferencing classroom. Each classroom is equipped with a camera to capture the faculty and/or students in that classroom, a monitor to broadcast this picture to the other classroom(s), and a sound system for transmitting voice communication between the rooms. In addition to this basic setup, classrooms often include a document projector and an Internet connection for transmitting images and slides across the network. The teacher is located in the originating or home classroom. The classroom(s) receiving the broadcast is referred to as the distance classroom(s).

In many ways, video conferencing is similar to the traditional classroom experience of both students and teachers—which is also its primary advantage. This approach requires less adjustment for both the teacher and the student compared to other distance education approaches. The main disadvantages include the set time of the class, the need to travel to the classroom, the cost of equipping the classrooms with the needed technology and sometimes the signal delay distortion.

In many cases, the course is transmitted to one or two other classrooms; however, the number of classrooms connected can vary greatly, with as many as 15 to 20 classrooms participating in a single session. This practice is referred to as multi-point video conferencing.

The functionality of the equipment in the classrooms can also vary greatly. For example, the camera may be focused only on the teacher and manually controlled by the teacher. Any movement requires the teacher to adjust the camera. In this setup, students in the distance classroom(s) see only the "talking head" or the images/slides. Remembering to switch the monitor between these two options is the responsibility of the teacher. Students in the home classroom see a group shot of the students in the other classroom. In a different setup, the camera focuses on sound. If the teacher is talking, the camera records the teacher. If the teacher moves, the camera follows him or her. If a student in either the home classroom or the distance classroom asks a question, the camera then focuses on the student.

In this environment, time on task and focus or attention are key factors for learning. Several factors in the classroom influence the time each student remains focused on the course content. Although many of these factors can be managed effectively, doing so requires a commitment on the part of students both as individuals and as a group.

Classroom Ambiance

The traditional classroom usually has a formal environment governed by protocols for behavior, such as raising your hand to talk or looking at the person who is talking. With video conferencing, students in the home classroom will experience much the same environment as students in a traditional classroom. There can be distractions from these expectations but they tend to be minor. For example, some faculty members have a tendency to talk to the distance class and forget to look at the students in the home room; others tend to forget the distance classroom. Some teachers have difficulty managing the technology and continuing to teach. With experience as well as feedback, these distractions tend to fade over time.

The ambiance in the distance classroom can be quite different. Usually a student worker, technician, or one of the students in the class is responsible for making sure the classroom is unlocked, for ensuring the equipment is turned on and working, for distributing handouts, and for performing other housekeeping tasks that are part of a smoothly running class. A distance education classroom can lack not just the physical presence of the faculty member, but also the psychological sense of presence that a faculty member communicates when he or she is physically present in the same room as the students. As a result, distance education classrooms have a tendency to become more informal and, in turn, more distracting. If the classroom sound system is muted, the faculty member may not be aware of background noise in the room such as side conversations between students or noise from food being consumed. This effect can be even greater if the faculty member has limited interaction with the distance education classroom.

Learning Engagement

In a traditional classroom, a teacher with strong lecturing skills can keep a classroom riveted on every word. Such a teacher paints a picture with words. As the students listen to the picture evolve, they are actively engaged with the topic being discussed. In contrast, watching a teacher on a monitor is very much like watching television. The student moves from active participant to passive observer; the talking head becomes a monotone and the mind begins to wander. To combat this effect, commercial television includes action. The action may be subtle, such as the changing camera shots with a news show, or there may be constantly changing screenshots, as is the case with many advertisements and fast-moving shows. Many times you will hear people comment, "That was a good show—it had a lot of action." Even with this emphasis on action, however, there is a tendency to engage in other activities while watching television. Note the number of people who read, eat, knit, or find other things to do while watching TV.

There are a number of things a teacher can do to increase the amount of interaction with students and focus the students on the topic; likewise, students can take steps to increase their individual interaction with the content. Each of the suggestions listed here will not work for every student. Review this list and select those that you believe will help you.

- Sit toward the front of the room, close to the monitor screen. This location will decrease the amount of visual distraction from others in the classroom.
- Take notes. Sometimes teachers may give students handouts in place of notes. These handouts may include the slides used to present the lecture or an overview of the lecture itself. Use these handouts to follow the lecture and write your notes on them, but do not let these types of handouts become a substitute for taking notes.
- If the teacher lectures directly from the textbook, be sure to read the chapter before class and then highlight the points the teacher is making during the class.

- Read the chapter before class and note key questions to ask the teacher.
- Turn off your cell phone and put it away so that you are not distracted with text messages.
- Avoid eating during the class, especially foods that tend to make you sleepy.
- Drink liquids that tend to keep you awake, such as coffee.
- If you are taking a late afternoon or evening class, and especially if you have been on the clinical unit before class, try to take a short nap followed by some exercise before class.
- Ask students to help by not holding side conversations or making distracting noises during the class.
- Create classroom activities that help focus others on the content. For example, before class, ask a group of friends to pick out the key points from today's class that will be on the next test. At the break, share these ideas.

Classroom Interaction

While transmission time has improved, there is a delay when data and voice are carried across the video conferencing network. This delay produces a trade-off between how much content can be covered and how much time can be spent on interaction. To maximize time and support the learning of all students in the class, students must use appropriate classroom etiquette:

- The monitor in the room where you are located will most often show the other classroom; the monitor in the other classroom will show your classroom. Because the people there are most likely looking at you, always assume you are on camera. Avoid inappropriate gestures, positions, or behavior.
- Most classroom microphones are fairly sensitive. Keep them mute unless you are speaking.
- In most video conferencing classrooms, the teacher will ask for questions at a specific point. Be sensitive to that reality and do not ask spontaneous questions throughout the class.
- Be sensitive to the time delay. Do not interrupt the teacher or other students.
- Keep your comments concise and your questions short. If you have a question that is of interest only to you, send it to the teacher in an email after class.
- When speaking look at the camera, speak in a normal tone and do not rush through your question or comment. Do not fidget or wear jewelry that creates noise.
- Assume the equipment is working. Do not ask if you are being heard.
- In larger and/or multipoint classes, give your name and location when you start to speak.
- Wear colors or, if you are in a uniform, wear a sweater or jacket with color.
- If technical problems affect reception in your classroom, let the teacher know.

Web-Based Course Management Programs

By removing the limitations of time and distance, Web-based course management programs have opened a whole new world of options for students of all ages and interests. In the early 1990s, browsers were new and had very limited availability, and the Internet was mainly accessed using text-based tools with no graphics. Thus the initial courses taught via this medium consisted of text-based lectures that were delivered by email to students. These initial courses demonstrated the potential of the Web-based format. One of the best-known examples is the course titled *Roadmap,* offered by Patrick Crispen beginning in 1994. The course consists of 27 classes spread over 6 weeks (Crispen, n.d.). An outline and access to the lectures can be seen at http://www.webreference.com/roadmap/.

Over the next few years, more than 500,000 people signed up for Roadmap and received their weekly email classes, learning how to use the Internet (Crispen, n.d.). Any one session of the course could have more than 10,000 students. The technical format for delivering the lecture was simple: an email message sent two or three times a week. The course and the content of each lecture were clearly presented and easy to follow. However, with 10,000 students in a class, participants did not ask questions or receive feedback. Put simply, students were on their own. While the software used to deliver Web-based distance education today provides much more functionality and even the automation of some feedback such as quizzes, this same principle still applies: The larger the student–teacher ratio, the less individual student support and feedback given.

A number of vendors now offer software applications for delivering a Web-based course. These applications provide an organizing structure for the following purposes:

- Presenting information including links to outside resources
- Encouraging interaction between students and with teachers
- Assessment of student involvement and learning

Table 11-2 lists a number of these vendors, along with links to their Web sites. The cost of these applications varies greatly, and as a result universities will sometimes change their standard application. This can cause real stress for both faculty and students. In addition, if you transfer or take a course at a different university, be prepared for the possibility that the new school will be using a different course management software (CMS).

The common functions of most of these applications are listed in **Table 11-3**. Course management software makes it possible for the educational experience to be asynchronous. That is, while the course may include some synchronous activities such as PC-based video conferencing, the great majority of learning will be asynchronous; this principle sets the culture for the course. In addition, with Web-based course management software, the structure of the course is no longer determined by the classroom setup, but rather by how individual professors

TABLE 11-2   WEB-BASED COURSE MANAGEMENT SOFTWARE VENDORS

Vendor or Package Name	URL	
A Tutor	http://www.atutor.ca/	Open source
Angel Learning	http://angellearning.com/	Commercial
Blackboard Inc	http://www.blackboard.com	Commercial
Claroline	http://www.claroline.net/	Open source
Desire2Learn Inc	http://www.desire2learn.com/	Commercial
Pearson eCollege	http://www.ecollege.com/index.learn	Commercial
ILIAS	http://www.ilias.de/	Open source
Moodle	http://moodle.org/about/	Open source
Open text: FirstClass	http://www.firstclass.com/	Open source
Scholar360	http://www.scholar360.com/	Commercial
Sakai Project	http://sakaiproject.org/portal	Open source
WebStudy	http://www.webstudy.com/	Commercial

organize the course content and learning experiences within the template of the software. In such an environment, key learning skills and habits can play a major role in ensuring your success.

Distance Education Learning Skills

To be successful in a distance education environment students must approach the educational experience with an appropriate attitude and effective distance education learning skills. This section provides an overview of these attitudes and skills.

Assume You Are in Charge of Your Learning

In a traditional classroom, many students expect the teacher to orient them to the expectations and requirements for the course. In distance education, the teacher will make this information available, but it is the students' responsibility to review and understand these materials. Appendix 11-1 provides an example of an online orientation and gives an overview of what you might expect to see in such an orientation. To meet this responsibility, start by looking over everything that is

TABLE 11-3 COMMON COURSE MANAGEMENT SOFTWARE FUNCTIONS

Content Delivery

- Internal Web pages
- Attached files such as lectures, presentation graphics, and spreadsheets
- External links
- Online assessment and testing
- Internal e-books

Communication Tools

- Discussion board
- Blog
- Internet email system
- Real-time chat
- Home pages and portfolios
- PC-based video conferencing

Group Work Tools

- Whiteboard
- Group work areas
- Document sharing

Productivity Tools

- Searching within the course
- Bookmarks
- Calendar
- Grade book and progress review

available in the course. Use **Table 11-4** as a guide for the types of information you should expect to find within your course.

Once you see how the professor has structured the course, go back and carefully read the materials that are posted. Many students find it helpful to print these materials and to highlight key points. Put any warning and due dates on your calendar. Be specific about the details of these requirements and prepare for problems. If an assignment is due at 5:00 P.M., do not wait until 4:55 P.M. to try to post the assignment. Waiting is one way to ensure your Internet service provider (ISP) will be unavailable. If an assignment is to be posted in a specific place in a certain way, make sure you understand how to do that. Sending the assignment at

TABLE 11-4   CONTENT AND STRUCTURE OF A DISTANCE EDUCATION COURSE

- A list of objectives, goals, or outcomes that describes what can be achieved from the course and how this will be useful
- Clearly outlined expectations for the projects and homework as well as an explanation of how each grade is achieved
- A variety of learning experiences guided through online information and resources
- Modules that organize topics into manageable units for learning
- Opportunity for interaction between the students and teacher
- A way to ask questions and receive answers
- Control, to some extent, of the learning environment so that the student can set the pace and progression through course modules
- Examples to facilitate understanding of material being studied
- The opportunity to practice using material and to apply material to problems or cases
- Feedback on practice and the use of the material
- Tools to help reflect on what is being learned and to guide setting the next steps in the learning process
- Resources in the form of hyperlinks, tables, charts, summaries, and references

the last minute via email to a busy teacher with many students in different classes is not a wise move.

Also, make sure you follow the file naming protocols required in the class. Professors use these protocols to manage several different assignments from different students and become frustrated when students do not follow their directions. Do not expect different professors to use the same organizing structures for their courses, the same rules related to assignments, or the same protocols for naming files. While these variations can be frustrating, they will help you become more flexible and more knowledgeable in the end.

Once you have reviewed the materials, make a list of your questions and post them for the class. You will want to review the materials first so you do not ask questions that the professor has already answered in the prepared materials. You want to post these questions in the class because most likely other students may have the same ones. In addition, you may get a quicker response because not only the professor but also other students may be able to answer your question(s).

Set Aside a Specific Time and Place for Learning

In a traditional class, you may read the content in the required readings, listen to the professor review this information, take notes on what the professor has said, and review your notes at least before the exam. A great deal of time is spent in reading, reviewing, and going to class. This consistent time on task usually leads to effective learning. In a distance education class, the repetitive process of reviewing materials must be done in a new environment. Reading, highlighting, and reviewing the assigned readings are important. Noting the relationship between the readings, posted lectures, and graphic presentations helps to reinforce the learning. Many times there are ungraded activities in a distance education course—but "ungraded" does not mean the activity is optional.

The learning process in a distance education class will not take any less time than the learning process in a traditional class. In fact, it may take more time. If a three-credit course requires 45 hours of class time and a student should spend an average of 2 to 3 hours studying for each hour of class, then a three-credit course requires at least 135 to 180 hours during the term. For a 15-week semester, that averages out to 9 to 12 hours *every* week. Many students will do well the first two to three weeks of the term, but then start to slack off. Once you miss a week or two of class, it can be very difficult to catch up in a traditional class—and even more so in a distance education course. Plan for that letdown after the first few weeks of class and push through that period.

Use Effective Communication Skills to Build Good Relationships with Others in the Class

In a distance education environment, communication depends heavily on the written word. First and lasting impressions are made based on how well you express yourself in writing. When you are posting comments and questions on a discussion board, excessive spelling and grammatical errors can give the impression that you are not a capable student. If this is a problem for you, prepare your remarks in a word processor and, after editing them, cut and paste the comments to the discussion board.

Consider alternative views when engaging in an online discussion. Always keep in mind that some of your ideas may actually be wrong. Even if you disagree, learn to understand what others are saying. If you disagree with someone, take your time and think about how best to express your ideas. Never respond when you are angry or upset. It is possible to disagree without being disagreeable. Try not to *react*, but rather to *respond*. One of the best ways to do so is to ask questions rather than to state your disagreement. If you feel a discussion is evolving into an argument, limit your comments and help move the discussion on to another subject.

When you post a comment, think about how others may interpret it. For example, "Many of the elderly have difficulty getting health information from the

Internet" sounds very different from "You cannot expect older people to be able to use the computer." If half of the students in the class are over 50 and you posted the second comment, you may get a negative reaction from your classmates.

Manage Your Stress

Taking a distance education class for the first time can be very stressful. Understanding (1) why it is stressful, (2) when the most stress can be expected, and (3) how relaxation activities can alleviate stress can be helpful in creating a successful learning experience.

The first few weeks of class are often highly stressful. During this period, you will be learning (1) the new content of the course, (2) how to learn in a distance education environment, (3) how to navigate the course management software used to deliver the course, and (4) new computer skills. Dealing with these four overlapping learning skill sets creates a fair amount of stress for most students. Many students, for example, express concern that they will miss an important assignment and fail the course. Because they are still learning how to communicate with their classmates, they often believe they are the only ones who are anxious. Some of this anxiety can be avoided by reviewing the university's technology requirements and participating in any online orientations provided by the university before starting the course. Most students get through this period by sharing their anxiety with other students, reviewing the materials they have been provided, and sharing their concerns with their professors.

The next anxiety-laden period occurs when the first major assignment or test is scheduled. If this is an assignment, review the directions and create a checklist of items that should be included. If a grading sheet is included with the assignment, make sure you address each point in the grading sheet. For example, if the professor has said you should document your sources, make sure you have included a set of references. If the first major graded activity is a test, practice taking online tests using the orientation materials provided by the university as well as self-administered tests available on the Internet. Table 11-1 provides some sources for practice tests. If the professor uses timed tests, use your own timer and do not depend on the course management software to alert you to the time or to stop the test if you go overtime.

The last stressful period in a course occurs during the last couple of weeks of class. Anxiety usually escalates if you have major assignments that you have not yet completed or if you are behind in the course. Planning ahead and leaving extra study time in your schedule during the last two weeks of class is the best way to manage this period. This advice works for on-campus courses as well!

Once you have made the adjustment to a Web-based distance education environment, you may discover you prefer this approach and the added flexibility it provides. As stated earlier in this chapter, it is assumed you will be continuing your education either to obtain an additional degree or just to remain competent in your field. Distance education is certainly one of the options you should consider for these endeavors. If possible, it is usually wise to take at least one (online) course before enrolling in a full-scale distance education program. Because this may not always be possible, know that motivated students who have never taken a distance education course often do very well in a distance education program.

Just as there is wide variation in the quality of traditional courses, so there is wide variation in the quality of courses or programs delivered by Web-based distance education. Selecting courses—let alone a complete program—can be an expensive process, so shop carefully.

Selecting a Distance Education Program

All distance education programs are not created equal. There are, of course, "diploma mills" that are not always easy to identify from a distance. In addition, excellent schools with well-earned reputations do not always carry that excellence forward when they turn a traditional educational program into a distance education program. That being said, distance education has introduced previously unavailable learning opportunities to students who want to continue their education. Once programs are discovered to be potential candidates to meet your needs, careful assessment of their quality is essential. The following questions provide an outline for that assessment.

Is the Program Accredited?

Accreditation is important from both the institutional perspective and the program perspective. Is the institution offering the program accredited, and is the educational program being offered also accredited?

In the United States, colleges and universities are accredited by one of several regional accrediting agencies. The Council for Higher Education Accreditation (CHEA) maintains a list of these agencies (which includes links to their Web sites) at http://www.chea.org/Directories/regional.asp. The appropriate regional agency is determined by the location of the university, not your location. For example, the University of Phoenix (http://www.phoenix.edu/), which has campuses in at least 40 states and an Internet presence in every state, is accredited by North Central Association of Colleges and Schools.

Specific educational programs in health care are accredited by specialty accrediting agencies. For example, nursing programs may be accredited by the National League for Nursing Accrediting Commission (NLNAC, http://www.nlnac.org) or by the Commission on Collegiate Nursing Education (CCNE, http://www.aacn .nche.edu/Accreditation/index.htm).

While it is important to determine if a program is accredited, it is also important to determine if that accreditation is meaningful. Accrediting agencies are private organizations and not subject to legal regulation. Thus, while a program may be accredited, the agency providing that recognition may be nothing more than a Web page. In other words, just as there are diploma mills selling degrees, so there are accrediting agencies selling accreditation.

Two resources can help you determine the quality of the accrediting agency listed by the educational program or institution you are considering. CHEA, a private organization, has developed a review process for ensuring the quality and effectiveness of accreditation agencies. The integrity of this list is well accepted by institutions of higher education. A list of accredited institutions, educational programs, and recognized accrediting agencies is provided on CHEA's Web site (http://www.chea.org/search/default.asp).

The U.S. Department of Education (USDE) also lists "regional and national accrediting agencies recognized by the U.S. Secretary of Education as reliable authorities concerning the quality of education or training offered by the institutions of higher education or higher education programs they accredit" (USDE, 2009). The USDE plays a key role in determining whether students attending an educational program are eligible for federal financial aid. A searchable database is provided by the USDE at http://ope.ed.gov/accreditation/.

Is Every Aspect of the Program Totally Online?

Many students assume that if a course or program is advertised as an online program, it is offered wholly by asynchronous Web-based distance education. However, that is not always the case. You may need to be on campus at some point in the program for orientation, video conferencing, or a clinical experience in a specific setting.

Be sure to ask if *all* of the courses and *all* of the course content are offered in an asynchronous Web-based format. Find out if you will need to be on campus at any point during the program. You may be required to come to campus for video conferences, testing, or a particular class. You may also discover that all students must come to campus for a specific activity such as orientation.

Always find out if there is a clinical component to the program and how it is completed. Many distance education programs will permit you to complete their clinical requirements in your local area. To do so, you may be expected to arrange a clinical experience that meets specific criteria. For example, a clinical course on physical assessment may require completing a set number of physical examinations under the supervision of a preceptor. Preceptors, too, must meet certain criteria. Finding a willing preceptor with the appropriate client access may be your responsibility. Facilitating communication between the preceptor and the faculty may be your responsibility as well.

If the program of interest includes requirements outside the department, ask if these courses are also offered online. For example, if the program of interest requires a statistics course offered by the math department, does the math department offer this course online? If not, what options does the university offer for meeting the requirement?

What Does the Program Cost?

Most universities will post the cost of tuition and fees on their Web sites, but it is not unusual for them to impose additional fees for courses and programs offered by distance education. To find the total cost, talk to personnel in the admissions office, financial aid office, and student accounts office. Ask about recurring costs, such as tuition, and about one-time costs, such as graduation fees. Ask if any fees are waived for distance education students. For example, if you are not on campus, are you still required to pay a recreation or health fee? Also, ask whether the costs are different for out-of-state students and if distance education students are considered to be out-of-state attendees. Universities may apply some very unique rules in this area. For example, until August 2008, part-time out-of-state distance education students at Slippery Rock University (http://www.sru.edu) paid 2% more than in-state students. In contrast, full-time distance education students paid the full out-of-state tuition—a difference of several hundred dollars.

Also consider indirect costs. For example, if you are required to be on campus for a week of orientation, what kind of housing costs might you expect? Will you have to pay shipping fees for books that are borrowed from the library? The financial aid office or other students who are already in the program may be helpful in estimating the indirect costs you might expect to pay.

Which Timelines Apply to the Program?

The best way to appreciate the timelines involved in a distance education program is to plan out the total program on a calendar. This plan should include the beginning and end dates of each course as well as any other requirements that are included in the program.

Begin this process by determining the number of courses and credits you will be required to complete. This varies between universities. For example, a nurse with an associate degree may discover that some universities accept the transfer of only 30 or 33 credits for their nursing courses. Other universities will transfer in the total number of credits completed at the community college, making no distinction between nursing and non-nursing courses.

Next, determine when the necessary courses are offered. Distance education programs do not always follow the traditional semester or trimester schedule. Sometimes courses can be started at any time and students can progress through the course or program at their own pace. Other universities offer specific courses during specific terms. For example, a course related to death and dying may be offered only in the spring term, and a public health course may be offered only in the fall term. In such a case, it is very important to plan your schedule for the total program based on when the required courses are offered.

As you develop your calendar, be realistic about the number of courses you can take at one time. Distance education courses often involve a greater time commitment than traditional courses. If you are working, going to school, and fulfilling other responsibilities, it is easy to become over-scheduled. Be especially careful if this is your first experience with distance education courses.

Are the Faculty Qualified?

When considering any type of educational program, you should always assess the qualifications of the faculty. In health care, this consideration includes both the academic preparation of the faculty and their clinical expertise. For example, the authors of this book have all taught computer literacy and health informatics courses. Each of the authors has more than 20 years of experience in teaching technology. Two of the authors have master's degrees in information science in addition to their master's degrees in nursing. Two of the authors were selected from more than 280 candidates to receive an HBOC Scholarship in Informatics; only eight candidates were selected for this honor each year the program existed.

In addition to these qualifications, the faculty teaching in a distance education program should be prepared to teach using this technology. Currently, there are no specific certifications or degrees given to a faculty member who teaches distance education courses. However, some questions can be asked to ascertain the university's quality in this area:

- Does the curriculum or course approval process in place at the university include any specific criteria for distance education courses?
- Does the university offer distance education preparation courses or workshops for faculty?
- Are faculty required to complete any type of preparation before teaching a distance education course?
- How long or how many courses have the faculty taught using distance education?
- Is there an administrative infrastructure to support faculty teaching with distance education technology? For example, is there a director of distance education or adequate instructional technology available to support faculty?

In addition to asking these questions, it is helpful to talk to current students. How do they evaluate the faculty and their distance education experience?

Are Distance Education Student Support Services Available?

Several student support services are part of a quality distance education program. First are library services. The American Library Association: American Association of College and Research Libraries (ALA: ACRL) has established standards for distance education library services (ALA:ACRL, 2008). **Table 11-5** includes several examples of university library Web sites listing their services for distance education

TABLE 11-5 EXAMPLES OF LIBRARY SERVICES FOR DISTANCE EDUCATION STUDENTS

Library	URL
Eastern Kentucky University	http://www.library.eku.edu/new/disted.php
NCSU Libraries	http://www.lib.ncsu.edu/distance/
Oregon Health and Science University Library	http://www.ohsu.edu/library/offcampus/distson.shtml
Southern Cross University	http://www.scu.edu.au/library/index.php/46/
University of Wisconsin: Cofrin Library	http://www.uwgb.edu/library/DE/index.asp

students. When looking at these sites, note the following points: (1) which resources are available in the library collection, (2) how distance education students get access to these resources, and (3) whether a librarian is available online to support student learning. Chapter 12 will help you evaluate the library collection available.

Other support services for distance education students should include the following:

- Online university and program orientation
- Technical orientation and support (What are the hours during which technical support is available?)
- Online registration, financial aid, student account services, and university ID card
- Academic advising and support
- Online student organizations and government
- Online book store access
- Career services assistance
- Writing assistance and/or workshops

One of the best ways to determine whether the university is "distance education friendly" is to assess the ease of finding information about online student support services on the university's Web site.

Is the Chemistry Right?

When selecting an educational program, certain intangibles may help you decide whether you will be comfortable and successful in the program. When a program is offered in the traditional format, you usually visit the school and talk to the people there. When selecting a distance education program, it is important to carefully assess these same elements from a distance. Talk to your previous or current faculty and ask their advice. Review the posted faculty biographical profiles and information. Telephone and/or email faculty members who teach in the program in which you are interested. How quickly and fully do they respond to your inquires? Find out if they understand your goals and your challenges. Keep in mind that they will be not only your future professors, but also your future role models. Problems in getting responses to your inquiries as a potential student are not a good sign. With distance education programs, faculty–student interaction is often a major factor in the success of students.

If you do not know any of the current students, ask for the names, phone numbers, and email addresses of some students who will share their experiences with you about the program. Use both telephone and email contacts to ask questions. Often you will get different kinds of information from these two modes of communication.

Summary

Successful distance education experiences occur when students are actively involved in their learning. This chapter identified the tools needed to be an active learner in a distance education course. It outlined a process and tools for assessing your distance education readiness. Criteria for selecting a best-fit distance education program were provided as well. The impact of distance education technology on the learning process was explained, and the chapter concludes by exploring required distance education learning skills.

References

American Library Association: American Association of College and Research Libraries. (2008). Standards for distance learning library services. Retrieved January 24, 2009, from http://www.ala.org/ala/mgrps/divs/acrl/standards/guidelinesdistancelearning.cfm.

Bates, T. (2007). What is distance education? *E-Learning and Distance Education Resources.* Retrieved February 14, 2009, from http://www.tonybates.ca/2008/07/07/what-is-distance-education.

Crispen, P. (n.d.). About Patrick Crispen. Retrieved January 20, 2009, from http://netsquirrel.com/crispen/about_crispen.html.

eLearners.com. (2009). Distance learning glossary. Retrieved January 24, 2009, from http://www.elearners.com/resources/glossary.asp.

Indiana University, Information Technology Service. (2003). Distance education student primer: Skills for being a successful online learner. Retrieved January 23, 2009, from http://ittraining.iu.edu/workshops/deguide/de_student_primer.pdf.

U.S. Department of Education (USDE). (2009). Accreditation in the United States. Retrieved January 23, 2009, from http://www.ed.gov/admins/finaid/accred/index.html.

APPENDIX 11.1 An Online Course Orientation Study Guide

■ **Introduction to Healthcare Informatics**
Class 1: Introduction to class

■ **Objectives**
At the completion of the class students will be able to:

1. List the basic computer skills used in this course.
2. Use Blackboard's course management software to learn about healthcare informatics.
3. Describe the course content, format, and evaluation procedures.
4. Define *healthcare informatics specialist.*
5. Identify students in this course.

The content in this first class follows the outline provided by the objectives. Read over the class objectives and expect to see content related to each objective throughout the study guide.

The first objective deals with basic computer skills. This first class in the course, *Introduction to Healthcare Informatics,* will not teach you basic computer skills used in this course. Rather, this class will acquaint you with the specific computer skills you will need to use in this course.

One of the documents that I am using in this class is a file called Technical Survey. Some of you may have received this document previously in the postal mail when you were admitted to the program. It is a survey we are using to plan our program orientation. What is important to us in this class is the content on the survey. The ideas about which questions should be asked came from three sources. First, we looked at the questions and help requests we were receiving from current students. Second, we asked the faculty which skills were needed in their individual classes. Third, we looked at surveys that were being used at other universities. From these three sources, we developed a list of computer skills used throughout the program. We, as a faculty, then used this list to develop the Technology Survey that is sent to all students on admission. Each term the student responses are used to update the online program orientation materials.

The Technology Survey is posted in the folder for class 1. Use this survey as a tool to assess your knowledge of needed computer skills. Keep in mind that very few students enter this program with all these skills. Throughout the program, when you run into the need for a specific skill, contact the student assistant for help. Also, let your teacher know that you are seeking help with a specific computer skill. While very few students enter this program with all these skills, most of them graduate with all these skills.

The second objective concerns using Blackboard. One of the files posted in the folder for class 1 is an orientation guide for Blackboard. Before you look at this file, I want to share a few comments with you. First, different people prefer to learn to use software in different ways. You may prefer to sign on and just explore the software; that is fine. Here is what you need to know:

- The URL is http://cde.sshe.edu:8082.
- Your user ID is the initial of your first name followed by your last name. For example, if your name is Mary Smith, your user ID is msmith. The program is case sensitive, so do not use capitals in the user ID.
- The password is the first name initial, middle name initial, last name initial followed by the last four digits in your Social Security number. There are no capital letters and no spaces. Mary Smith's password is mxs0000. When SRU does not know a student's middle initial, an x is assigned. If you try to sign in and have a problem, try substituting an x for your middle initial. You will not be able to see the password when you type it; instead, a row of stars will be substituted for the characters on the screen.

Once you enter this information, click OK and you will be taken to the front page of Blackboard. Select your course from here. A student user manual can be found under Tools. If you decide to follow this exploring approach, you still need to look over the Orientation to Blackboard file. There are some specific required activities in that document.

If you prefer a more guided approach, follow the step-by step directions in the Orientation to Blackboard file.

Whichever approach you use, there are two ways that you need to self-assess whether you have learned all the needed functions. I suggest you do both after you have finished reviewing the Blackboard software. First, look over the Blackboard orientation guide to see which functions were included in that guide. Second, look over the following list of needed skills. You will see some overlap between this list and the orientation guide, but between the two all needed skills and activities are identified.

Needed Blackboard Skills

1. Sign into the course.
2. Access the user's manual.
3. Navigate through each section of the course. Make a mental note about the types of information this professor puts in each section of the course.
4. Review the staff information, including on-campus and online office hours.
5. Access course information and course documents.
   a. Download the course materials for class 1.
   b. Open the downloaded course materials for class 1.
6. Access and exit a link in the External Links section of the course. Note that the external links open in a new window.
7. Send email from Blackboard.
8. Send a message within Blackboard.
9. Access the discussion board for class 1.
   a. Add a thread.
   b. Respond to another student's posting.
10. Complete your home page.
11. Edit your personal information, including checking your email address in Blackboard.
12. Take the sample quiz and access your quiz grades. **Unlike quizzes throughout the course,** the sample quiz can be retaken as many times as you like. The sample quiz points will not count in your final grade.

As you use Blackboard, you will also need to confirm that your computer is set up correctly for this course. You will find a link to computer testing area in the External Links for class 1. This may help you determine whether you need to install any additional plug-ins. Plug-ins are small, free programs that can be downloaded from the Internet and installed on your home computer. For this course, be sure Adobe Acrobat Reader is installed on your home computer. Links to plug-ins are provided in the External Links.

The third objective deals with orientation to this course. Some of this orientation will occur as a by-product of meeting objective 2. However, there are two activities that are specific to meeting this objective. **First, download and read the syllabus.** Second, post any questions you have on the Discussion Board for class 1. As described in the syllabus, posting on the Discussion Board counts for graded class discussion. This week, everyone is required to post two comments dealing with orientation. Your orientation posting can be a question, an answer to another student's question, or just a general comment on the course. Under Assignments, you will find guidelines related to posting on the Discussion Board.

The fourth objective deals with defining healthcare informatics. Notice on your syllabus that you are to read the preface in your textbook for this week's class. After you have read these pages, please share your thinking about this content on the Discussion Board for class 1 by posting two comments dealing with this orientation. You are also required to post a comment concerning the definition of healthcare informatics.

The fifth objective deals with learning who is in your class. You will be able to see their names as people post comments on the Discussion Board. If you go to Communications → Roster → List all, you will see the list of students in the class. Now click on anyone's name. Most likely, you found an empty student home page. Your last activity for this week's class is to complete your home page. The directions are found in the Student Manual. Remember—if you have a question or are not sure how to proceed, use the Discussion Board to get some help.

EXERCISE 1 Discovering Your Distance Education Readiness

- **Objectives**
  1. Use online self-assessments to identify your strengths and weaknesses as they relate to distance education.
  2. Develop strategies for managing your distance-education-related weaknesses.

- **Activity**
  1. Complete three of the self-assessment tests listed in Table 11-1.
  2. Using the results of these three tests, make a list of your strengths and weaknesses as a distance education learner.
  3. Using the distance education learning skills outlined in the chapter, create a list of strategies for maximizing your strengths and minimizing your weaknesses.

ASSIGNMENT 1 Evaluating Online Courses

- **Directions**
  1. Select an online course you are currently taking or use a search engine to search for online courses. You might try the terms "distance learning", "e-Learning", and "online courses."
  2. Table 11-4 lists the content you should expect to find in a online distance education course. Use this information as criteria for examining the online courses you selected to review. Note that you may not be able to access

all this information unless you enroll in the course, but there should be enough information in the marketing piece to give you a good idea of the course and its requirements.

3. Using Word, make a flyer listing each criterion. Beside or under each, identify how well the course you examined meets the criterion. Give enough information to lure someone to a good course or steer them clear of one that you think has not yet been well developed. Be sure that the course title and Web address appear on the flyer. Be creative with the design, and include graphics if you wish.

4. Submit the flyer to your instructor.

ASSIGNMENT 2 Finding Best-Fit Distance Education Programs

■ **Directions**

1. Use the content in this chapter to create a spreadsheet with criteria for evaluating distance education programs. The criteria that you develop should be listed in column A. Later in this assignment, you will list specific distance education programs in the header row across the top of the spreadsheet.

2. Share your spreadsheet with three other classmates and add any criteria that your spreadsheet is missing.

3. Do an Internet search and select five distance education programs that are of interest to you in furthering your education. These can be baccalaureate-, master's-, or doctorate-level programs. Do not select a certificate program.

4. Complete the spreadsheet with data gathered from the Web page for each program. Create a second worksheet (tab) with the same setup.

   a. On the first worksheet, use a rating scale from 1 to 5 to fill in the cells on the spreadsheet. The lowest rating of 1 is used when the criterion has not been met; 5 is the best rating possible. In row 7, create a formula for adding the points for each program.

   b. Use the cells on the second worksheet to record your comments and collect text-type data related to these criteria for each of the programs.

5. Note where there are gaps because the information is not available on the university or program Web site. If the information related to that criterion is not available, give the program a rating of 1. You can send an email inquiry to the admissions department with your questions that could not be answered from the Web page and change the rating based on the response you receive.

6. Using both the qualitative and quantitative data you have collected, select the program you believe is the best fit for you. Write a statement explaining why you selected this program. Be sure to refer to your criteria, including how they applied to this program.

Information: Access, Evaluation, and Use

Objectives

1. Define *information literacy.*
2. Demonstrate skills related to information literacy.
3. Define an information need, including concepts and terms that can be used to search for information.
4. Develop a variety of search strategies to locate and access information from published literature, "gray literature," and Internet resources.
5. Use a systematic approach to evaluate the quality of information obtained from a variety of sources.
6. Identify appropriate and inappropriate uses of information.
7. Explain general principles for documenting information resources.

Introduction

Staring in the late 1980s, a growing body of literature called for all health-care professionals to be "information literate." Examples of articles presenting this point of view are listed in **Table 12-1**.

Note the concepts reflected in these titles. Critical thinking, evidence-based practice, and lifelong learning all require information literacy. In 2001, the American Nurses Association (ANA) described information literacy as a required skill for all beginning nurses (Staggers et al., 2001). This call was repeated in 2008 in *Nursing Informatics: Standard and Scope of Practice Information* (ANA, 2008).

Information literacy is defined by the American Library Association (ALA, 2000) as the ability to recognize when information is needed as well

TABLE 12-1   CALLS FOR INFORMATION LITERACY

Author	Title of Article (Journal)	Year Published
L. M. Fox, J. M. Richter, and N. E. White	Pathways to Information Literacy (*Journal of Nursing Education*)	1989
S. M. Weaver	Information Literacy: Educating for Life Long Learning (*Nurse Educator Today*)	1992
J. Cheek and I. Doskatsch	Information Literacy: A Resource for Nurses as Life-Long Learners (*Nursing Education Today*)	1998
S. Kaplan-Jacobs, P. Rosenfeld, and J. Haber	Information Literacy as the Foundation for Evidence-Based Practice in Graduate Nursing Education: A Curriculum-Integrated Approach (*Journal of Professional Nursing*)	2003
T. Courey, J. Benson-Soros, K. Deemer, and R. A. Zeller	The Missing Link: Information Literacy and Evidence-Based Practice as a New Challenge for Nurse Educators (*Nursing Education Perspectives*)	2006
S. S. Baker, P. D. Boruff-Jones	Information literacy (*Radiologic Technology*)	2009

as the ability to locate, evaluate, and effectively use the needed information. The ALA has identified five information literacy standards for higher education. An information-literate person

- Determines the nature and scope of an information need.
- Effectively and efficiently accesses that information.
- Evaluates information and its sources critically and incorporates selected information into his or her knowledge base and value system.
- Uses information effectively for a specific purpose.
- Understands many of the economic, legal, and social issues surrounding the use of information and accesses and uses information ethically and legally.

These five standards, along with an emphasis on information related to health, provide the organizing structure for this chapter. The chapter begins with a discussion of how information can be effectively accessed. More specifically, it focuses on how to access information that has been stored in computer systems. The ability to access information makes it possible to find all types of information from a wide variety of sources. This information may, however, be accurate or inaccurate, objective or biased, current or outdated.

Inaccurate and misleading information does not come with a label indicating that there is a problem. In fact, many times the author will try to assure readers that the information appears to be very credible. The reader must determine the quality of the information.

Even good information can be misused. For example, the Internet includes many excellent sites with information about the importance of adequate vitamin intake during pregnancy. Referring a patient to one of these sites with no appreciation of the patient's ability to read and understand these data is a misuse of information.

Identifying an Information Need

Information needs come from a variety of sources. Common examples include a classroom assignment, a health problem in a family, or intellectual curiosity. In each case, the first step is to write a statement describing the question to be answered. Actually writing this statement down helps to clarify which specific information is needed. For example, if you were preparing to write a pamphlet on exercise for an elderly population, which information would you need? A statement of the information need might include these elements:

- Exercises that are valuable for elderly clients
- Exercises that should be avoided by most elderly clients
- Guidelines on writing for the general population, especially the elderly
- General health literacy levels of elderly clients
- Signs and symptoms that an elderly person is over- or under-exercising

Several other information needs can be identified as well. In addition, it is important to identify terms or phrases that can be used to find the information needed. How many different terms can be used for "elderly"? Each information need that is identified and the terms used to describe those needs will be useful in finding the required information.

Access

The process of accessing information begins by understanding how data are stored in the computer. Data are stored in an orderly and systematic structure called a database. As was explained in Chapter 8, a database is built of files that contain records. Each record refers to a specific entity and includes a set number of fields. Data related to the entity are stored in these fields. For example, if the entity is a journal article, the fields most likely include the author(s), article title, journal source, and an abstract of the article, along with several other fields that hold relevant data. The process of searching for data in a database involves matching specific attributes about the entity with the field where the piece of data is stored. For example, if a search request was looking for a book that was written by the author Joos, the database management system would search in the author field for the name Joos. Each time Joos was found in an author field, it would refer to a book written by Joos. However, if a record included Smith in the author field and Joos in the title field, this book would not meet the search criteria; this source would not be a book written *by* Joos, but rather a book *about* Joos.

A bibliographic database is a specific type of database designed to store information about articles, books, and other print materials. The fields in a bibliographic database include the title, author, abstract, date of publication, and other details about the item being indexed in the database. Increasingly, bibliographic databases also include full text of the article. **Table 12-2** lists bibliographic databases commonly used in health care.

The sources listed in Table 12-2 are only a few of the many important health-related bibliographic databases. Access to these databases may be provided by the group or organization that produced the database, or access to the database may be provided by an information vendor that has leased the database. Increasingly, information vendors are both producing the databases and providing access. **Table 12-3** lists examples of some information vendors in health care; most of these vendors produce their own databases as well as lease access to databases produced by other groups. **Table 12-4** provides examples of the databases offered by selected information vendors; the information in this table was collected from the Web sites of these vendors in January 2009. In a world of exploding information, there are constant changes in the content of databases that are offered by these vendors, so the information presented here may not be fully up-to-date.

Note the overlap in databases offered and the different descriptions for the same databases. Thus an individual journal may be indexed in several different databases. Vendors often combine databases along with other resources to create a discipline-specific package. One example is the Nursing Reference Center offered by EBSCO (http://www.ebscohost.com/thisTopic.php?marketID=1&topicID=860).

Although there are certainly a large number of databases and several vendors providing electronic access to healthcare information, including full-text access to many of the professional journals, there are some significant gaps in the online professional resources available. For example, vendors offer access to a number of online full-text medical books; however, the options for access to online books are limited for nursing and allied health. Examples of vendors that do offer such books appear in **Table 12-5**. Visiting the Web sites of these vendors demonstrates significant variation in the number and the currency of these e-books.

The company or organization that provides the access will determine the specific database management system and, in turn, the user interface employed for searching that database. Many users become confused about the difference between a bibliographic database and a bibliographical database management

TABLE 12-2   SELECTED BIBLIOGRAPHICAL AND FULL-TEXT DATABASES IN HEALTH CARE

Database	Description
AMED	The Allied and Complementary Medicine Database (AMED) includes journals in complementary medicine, palliative care, and several professions allied to medicine.
CINAHL	Provided by EBSCO, the Cumulative Index to Nursing and Allied Health Literature (CINAHL) database provides coverage of the literature related to nursing and allied health. More than 1600 journals are regularly indexed, along with publications from the American Nurses Association and the National League for Nursing. This database overlaps MEDLINE; however, there are several citations in CINAHL that are not included in MEDLINE.
ClinicalTrials.gov	ClinicalTrials.gov provides regularly updated information about federally and privately supported clinical research in human volunteers.
Cochrane Database of Systematic Reviews	This database produced by the Cochrane Library includes full-text articles reviewing the effects of health care. The reviews are highly structured and systematic, with evidence included or excluded to minimize bias.
EMBASE.com	This database includes worldwide literature on biomedical and pharmaceutical sciences.
LexisNexis	This resource is a full-text legal information service covering newspapers, magazines, wire services, federal and state court opinions, federal and state statutes, federal regulations, and SEC filings such as 10-K and 10-Q forms.
MD Consult	This full-text database provided by Elsevier Company includes medical texts, articles from clinical journals, peer-reviewed clinical practice guidelines with integrated MEDLINE searches, customizable patient education handouts, and a drug database of more than 30,000 medications.
MEDLINE	MEDLINE® (Medical Literature, Analysis, and Retrieval System Online), which is produced by the U.S. National Library of Medicine (NLM), is considered the primary bibliographic database of biomedical literature. It includes citations from more than 4600 journals, including those in the nursing, dentistry, veterinary medicine, pharmacy, allied health, and preclinical sciences fields. Increased coverage of life sciences such as aspects of biology, environmental science, marine biology, plant and animal science, and biophysics and chemistry began in 2000. By the end of 2001, most citations previously included in separate NLM specialty databases had also been added to MEDLINE.

(continues)

**TABLE 12-2   SELECTED BIBLIOGRAPHICAL AND FULL-TEXT DATABASES
IN HEALTH CARE** *(continued)*

Database	Description
MedlinePlus	Produced by the National Library of Medicine, this database of health information is designed for health professionals and consumers alike. It combines references from MEDLINE with extensive information from the National Institutes of Health and other sources on more than 650 diseases and conditions.
PsycINFO	Produced by the American Psychological Association, this database contains citations and summaries of journal articles, book chapters, books, dissertations, and technical reports in the field of psychology as well as the psychological aspects of related disciplines, such as medicine, psychiatry, and nursing.
SPORTDiscus	Produced by the Sport Information Resource Centre (SIRC), this database covers all aspects of sport, fitness, recreation, and related fields.

system. PubMed (http://www.ncbi.nlm.nih.gov/PubMed/) is an example of a bibliographical database management system. A World Wide Web retrieval service developed by the National Library of Medicine (NLM), PubMed provides access, free of charge, to materials indexed in MEDLINE. It also contains links to the full-text versions of articles at participating publishers' Web sites. Several other bibliographical database management systems can also be used to access

TABLE 12-3   ELECTRONIC INFORMATION VENDORS IN HEALTH CARE

Company Name	URL
EBSCO Informational Services	http://www.ebsco.com/home/
Elsevier	http://www.elsevier.com/
Gale Health Solutions	http://www.gale.cengage.com/Health/index.htm
OVID Technologies	http://www.ovid.com/site/index.jsp
ProQuest Company	http://www.proquest.com/
Stat!Ref	http://www.statref.com/
Thomson Reuters	http://www.thomsonreuters.com/

TABLE 12-4   EXAMPLES OF DATABASES OFFERED BY SELECTED INFORMATION VENDORS

Database Name	Focus and Content of the Database
Examples of Health-Related Databases Provided by ProQuest	
ProQuest Health and Medical Complete	Provides coverage of more than 1440 publications, with nearly1200 available in full text.
ProQuest: MEDLINE/ MEDLINE with Full Text	Includes the entire MEDLINE database with full text/full images for more than 200 MEDLINE-indexed titles.
ProQuest: Nursing and Allied Health Source	Provides abstracting and indexing for more than 780 titles, with more than 650 titles in full text, plus more than 12,000 full-text dissertations.
PsycINFO	Provides access to international literature in psychology and related disciplines.
Examples of Health-Related Databases Provided by Gale	
Health and Wellness Resource Center	Includes more than 700 health/medical journals with hundreds of pamphlets; 75% are full text. Also includes articles from 2200 general-interest publications.
Nurse Resource Center	Includes encyclopedia articles, journal citations, animations, medical illustrations, disease overviews, drug monographs, and sample care plans.
Examples of Health-Related Databases Provided by EBSCO	
CINAHL	Includes indexing for 2,928 journals, including more than 72 full-text journals.
Clinical Pharmacology	Provides drug monographs on all U.S. prescription drugs, over-the-counter drugs, and hard-to-find herbal and nutritional supplements.
Health Source Consumer Edition	Collection of consumer health information resources, including full text for more than 200 health reference books and encyclopedias dealing with topics such as aging, cancer, diabetes, drugs and alcohol, fitness, nutrition and dietetics, children's health, men's health, and women's health.
MEDLINE	Abstracts from more 4600 current biomedical journals.
PsycINFO	This database is the American Psychological Association's (APA) resource for abstracts of scholarly journal articles, book chapters, books, and dissertations. PsycINFO includes more than 2,200 periodicals and is the largest resource devoted to peer-reviewed literature in behavioral sciences and mental health.

TABLE 12-5	EXAMPLES OF VENDORS OFFERING e-BOOKS IN NURSING AND ALLIED HEALTH
Vendor Name	**URL**
NetLibrary	http://www.netlibrary.com/
Ovid Technologies (Lippincott/ Springhouse Nursing Collection)	http://www.ovid.com/site/catalog/ Collection/868.jsp
Rittenhouse Book Distributors: R2 Digital Library	http://www.r2library.com/public/ default.aspx
Stat!Ref	http://www.statref.com/

MEDLINE. Because vendors and information providers use different bibliographical database management systems and user interfaces, this book does not give specific commands for using them. Each bibliographical database management system will provide a help section, however. In addition, the library offering the database will offer assistance in using the databases in its collection.

General Principles for Searching

Two factors determine how much time and effort you need to exert when searching for information—your level of expertise with the topic and your knowledge of search strategies. An expert in a specific field will find it much easier to perform an efficient and focused search. For example, if you are an expert in maternity care and are looking for information about a specific complication of pregnancy, you could be expected to find the desired information very quickly because an expert knows the language and understands how knowledge is organized within the field.

If you are not an expert, then the process of searching for information is in many respects recursive. You usually begin by identifying a topic about which you want more information. For example, you may take a course on managed care and be assigned to write a report on a controversial issue related to managed care. As you begin the search for information on the topic of managed care, you will find related information that doesn't really apply to your assignment. At the same time, you may find that there is more information about this topic than you are able to use. In the process of selecting those materials that apply to your assignment and eliminating those materials that are not relevant, your search will become more focused. This initial exploration can be frustrating, but it is very important. It is during this initial stage that you become familiar with the terminology and the way in which the related information is organized. If your approach is to look for a few related articles or Internet sites and then stop your search there, you will miss a significant portion of information about both the topic and the organization of information in that field.

Indexing, Standard Languages, and Keywords

A record within a database will include several fields. The database management system that interfaces with the database will offer you the opportunity to search on these fields. Database management programs are usually designed for both experienced and inexperienced users. The experienced user will understand both the concept and the procedure for searching on specific fields. For example, many literature database management systems are designed so that you can search for a specific author. In these systems, you enter a command such as "au-Nelson" or "a-Nelson". The search results from these systems would include all materials in that database that were written by an author with the last name of Nelson.

At the same time, these same literature database management systems are accessible to users who are less familiar with these concepts. With these systems, any term that is entered in the search field will be compared to several fields. For example, one would enter the term "Nelson"; if this term occurred in the title, author, or even abstract field, it would be included in the search results. When the database management system offers the opportunity to search on a specific field, the fields and commands found in **Table 12-6** may be applicable.

The two fields that are most frequently confused are keywords and subject. Both of these fields identify the topic discussed in the reference being accessed. However, keywords and subject terms are developed very differently. Using the

TABLE 12-6   FIELDS THAT ARE COMMONLY SEARCHABLE IN BIBLIOGRAPHICAL DATABASES

Abbreviation	Field
Au or A	Author
Ti or T	Title
Yr	Year Published
Pb	Publisher
K	Keyword
Su	Subject

same term as a keyword and then as a subject term will often produce overlapping, yet different search results. Keywords are terms that may have been selected by the author, the publisher, or the developer of the literature database management system to identify the topic of the article. Some literature database management systems are designed so that any word appearing in the title, author field, and/or abstract will function as a keyword. However, keyword terms are not standardized in any way. For example, an article about cirrhosis may be indexed using the keywords "liver," "hepatic disease," or "cirrhosis." The same article in different literature database management systems may have different keywords associated with it.

Subject terms, by comparison, are standardized. Individuals who are experts in understanding indexing and taxonomy concepts develop these terms in a systematic process. Standard sets of subject terms are often referred to as a controlled vocabulary. An example of such a controlled vocabulary is MeSH (Medical Subject Headings), which is used in indexing MEDLINE. Thus there are people who read each article found in the database and then select the specific indexing terms from the controlled vocabulary.

If you use a subject term as part of your search, you can expect to find all of the materials that relate to that term as identified by the index or taxonomy expert. In contrast, because keywords are not standardized, searching on a keyword may lead to incomplete results. For example, you may use "cancer" as a search term and miss all of the articles related to cancer that were indexed using the keyword "neoplasm." If you explore the interface of the different database management systems, you will usually find helpful tools for identifying the subject terms.

It is also important when planning a search strategy to understand that different databases may be indexed with different subject terms. For example, CINAHL (Table 12-2) has its own controlled vocabulary that is different from MeSH. As a consequence, the same article may be indexed under different terms in CINAHL and in MEDLINE.

By understanding how keywords and subject terms differ, it becomes possible to maximize the advantages of both indexing approaches when developing a search strategy. By using terms and concepts that were developed in clarifying the information need, you can select a specific database or group of databases. For example, if the information need is related to the concept of nursing diagnosis, CINAHL would be a better choice of database than PsycINFO.

Because most library information systems permit the user to search several databases at the same time, the next step is to use the library information system to indicate which databases to include in the search. The identified terms are entered into the library information system as keywords. The resulting hits from the search are reviewed to find those references that fit best with the information need. These best-fit citations are then examined to determine the subject terms that were used to index these references. If you are searching across several databases at the same time, keep in mind that different databases may be indexing the same concept using different terms. Also, more than one subject term will be used for each article. For example, an article describing the types of injuries that occur when children are abused will be indexed on subject terms related to trauma, children, and abuse. Select the subject term that fits best with the identified information need. A new search using the subject term will result in a more comprehensive list of hits, although that list of hits may include too many or too few references.

Boolean Search Strategies

Several approaches can be used to expand or exclude references from search results. These approaches are built on the concept of Boolean search strategies. Chapter 8 introduced these concepts, which are explained in more detail here.

AND

By searching on two topics and placing the word **AND** between the two topics, you will be able to find materials that deal with both topics. For example, if you are searching for information dealing with computers and nursing diagnosis, your search might look like this: **computers AND "nursing diagnosis."** In many systems, placing the plus symbol (+) in front of both terms works the same way as using the Boolean AND between the terms. The option "Find or use all terms" also functions the same as using AND between the terms. Each of the citations that is listed in the search results will be about both computers and nursing diagnosis. The Boolean AND is used to narrow the search results to a more focused group of hits.

You may have noticed the quotes around the phrase "nursing diagnosis" in the previous search. Using quotes usually results in the terms being treated as a single phrase rather than as two separate terms. If "nursing diagnosis" is seen as two separate terms, any article that indexed with the term "nursing" and the term "diagnosis" would be included in the search results. When quotes are used to identify the phrase, the two terms must appear next to each other in the source to be included in the search results.

OR

Sometimes a concept can be represented by several different, yet closely related terms. Many of these terms would have been identified when analyzing the information need. For example, the concept "abuse" is related to the terms "intimate partner abuse (IPA)," "family abuse," and "family violence." If the Boolean term **OR** is used between each of these terms in a search, the

	citations in the search result will include references indexed on any of these terms. OR is used to expand a search. Many search engines offer the option "any of the terms," which will provide the same results as using OR between terms.
Truncation	Sometimes your topic may have several words with the same base—for example, "nurse," "nursing," and "nurses." In such a case, using truncation may be more efficient than using the Boolean OR. With truncation, you type the beginning of the term and then use a symbol to indicate that you are searching for any citation that includes a term beginning with these letters. The specific symbol will depend on the specific database management system in use. Symbols commonly used for this purpose include the asterisk (nurs*), question mark (nurs?), and dollar sign (nurs$). Remember that when you use truncation. your search results will include every term that begins with the beginning letters. For example, which other terms begin with the letters "nurs" in addition to the terms "nurse," "nurses," and "nursing"?
NOT	The Boolean term **NOT** is used to eliminate references. For example, you may be interested in information about assistive heart devices but do not want citations dealing with pacemakers. In this case your search would be "**assistive heart devices**" **NOT pacemakers**.
NEAR	The term **NEAR** is used when the terms should be located within the next few words. For example, you may be looking for information on teaching people about computers. In this case, **teaching NEAR computers** might be a useful search phrase.

Figure 12-1 demonstrates the Boolean concepts of AND, OR, and NOT. Several other operators can also be used to expand or limit a search. These strategies are usually explained in the help section of the library information system or the Internet search site.

Search Sites and Engines

The Internet contains a vast amount of information. However, there are important differences between the information found on the Internet and the information resources found in an academic library even if accessed over the Internet. **Table 12-7** compares the key differences.

Search sites are places on the Internet where you go to find information. Search engines are software used to find and index information. Several hundred search sites and engines are available on the Internet. **Table 12-8** provides examples of URLs for general and specific types of search sites. Although each has a different

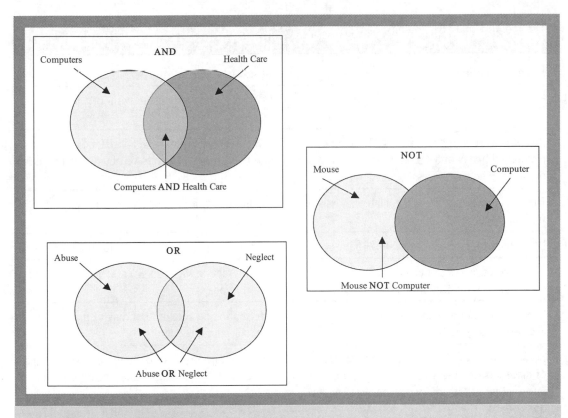

Figure 12-1 Understanding Boolean Search Strategies

interface or appearance, all of them share certain features. Understanding how to use search sites begins by understanding relevant terms.

Directory	A directory is a hierarchical grouping of topics and related Web links organized by subject and related concepts. Directories are created by people who searched the Web and then grouped the links by subject. Not all search sites include directories.
Gray Literature	Gray literature includes works that are not formally reviewed and have not appeared in standard, recognized publications. Because it is not widely distributed, gray literature is difficult to locate or is not available for study. Examples of gray literature include some government documents, conference proceedings, online journals, and other valuable resources (CrosRef.org, n.d.).
Hits	Hits are a list of links that are returned as search results when a search engine is used.

TABLE 12-7   KEY DIFFERENCES BETWEEN LIBRARY AND INTERNET RESOURCES

Library Resources	Resources on the Internet
Resources go through a review process.	Many resources are posted without a review process.
Resources are purchased by the library and distributed free or at a discount to those individuals or groups who have access to that library.	A wide variety of financial approaches are used and these may not always be obvious to the user.
There is a professional staff available to assist in finding resources.	The Internet does not usually provide personal assistance.
Library resources are indexed and organized.	There is no organizational plan for the Internet.
Library resources are selected to ensure a comprehensive collection related to key topics.	The Internet provides an eclectic hodgepodge of information.
Information found in a library can usually be accessed at a later date.	Information on the Internet may or may not be available at a later date.
Because the review process and the preparation of materials for library use takes time, the information in the library may not be completely up-to-date.	Newer information can be found on the Internet; however, it may or may not be accurate.
Most information in the library is dated so that the user can tell how old or new the information is.	Information on the Internet may or may not be dated. If it is dated, the date may reflect the date the page was updated, rather than the date the content was updated.

Meta-directory	A meta-directory (sometimes called a directory of directories or directories of directories) is a directory of links to other directories. An excellent health-related example of a meta-directory can be seen at http://www.sldirectory.com/searchf/medicine.html#top.
Meta-search Engines	Meta-search engines are not really search engines, but rather search sites that the user's query and search the Web with several different search engines at one time. These sites permit one-stop searching and, therefore, are gaining in popularity. Examples are included in Table 12-8.
Query	A query is the combination of terms that the user enters into a search engine so as to conduct a search.

TABLE 12-8   EXAMPLES OF SEARCH SITES BY TYPE OF SEARCH SITE

General Search Sites	Health-Specific Search Sites
Google: http://www.google.com	MedHunt: http://www.hon.ch/MedHunt/
Yahoo: http://www.yahoo.com	MedNets: http://www.mednets.com/
Ask: http://www.ask.com	PubMed: http://www.ncbi.nlm.nih.gov/entrez/query.fcgi
Teoma: http://www.lycos.com/	Entrez: http://www.ncbi.nlm.nih.gov/gquery/gquery.fcgi
Microsoft: http://www.live.com	MEDBOT: http://www-med.stanford.edu/medworld/medbot/info.html
Meta-search Sites	**Academic Search Sites**
Dogpile: http://www.dogpile.com/	Academicinfo: http://www.academicinfo.net/
Webcrawler: http://www.webcrawler.com/	Google Scholar: http://scholar.google.com/
Clusty: http://clusty.com/	Infomine: http://infomine.ucr.edu/

Ranking   Ranking is a process of indicating how relevant a hit may be. Many times a search sites will organize the search results based on their rankings. However, the methods used by search engines to rank sites vary. For example, the number of times a site is linked from other sites can be used to determine ranking. Some search sites sell ranking placement; thus ranks need to be viewed with caution. On January 15, 2009, a search for **nursing AND computers** on Google (www.google.com) returned 11,900,000 hits. In contrast, the same search conducted on August 31, 2004, returned 1,990,000 hits. If you spent 24 hours a day and 10 seconds looking at each site, it would take you more than 3.5 years to skim over all these hits. Because most people can take the time to look at only one to three screens, the process used to select the hits that appear on these first screens can be very important. Examples of how different search sites rank hits can be seen at http://www.lib.berkeley.edu/TeachingLib/Guides/Internet/SearchEngines.html.

Robot   Robots (also called spiders or crawlers) are used to create a database of links that are accessed when you conduct a search. These special computer programs can search the Web, locate links, and then index the links to create a database. Indexing

	is usually carried out by using the words in the URL and title of the HTML file and counting the frequency of words used at the Internet site. Some robots search the full text of a source; others review only a portion of the site. If there is no link to a site, these robots can't find and index it.
Search Engine	A search engine is the software that is used to search a database. On the Internet search engines use robots to search for and index Web sites. Sometimes this term is also used to mean a search site.
Search Site	A search site is a server or a collection of servers dedicated to indexing Web pages, storing the results, and returning lists of links that match particular queries. The indexes are normally generated using spiders. Sometimes the terms "search site" and "search engine" are used to mean the same thing, but they are really two different concepts.
Stop Word	A stop word is a word that is ignored in a query because the word is so commonly used that it makes no contribution to relevancy. Examples include *and, get, the,* and *you.*

Using a search engine begins by accessing the search engine site on the Internet. There are several ways to find sites. For example, most academic libraries provide links to several sites. Some examples of sites with search engines include these:

- http://www.noodletools.com/index.php
- http://www.searchenginecolossus.com
- http://www.internettutorials.net/engines.asp

Select any of the search sites from your university library or one of the options above. On the home page of the search site, you will find a field or box where search terms are entered to create a query. Before you try your query, it is often helpful to access the help section of the Web site (it is sometimes referred to as "search tips"). Because each search site is different, you will find some variations and unique features on each one. Think of a car as an analogy: Each model is different, but all models share many common functions. The process for searching is very similar to the process you used when doing library searches.

In many cases, your first searches will result in a large list of irrelevant hits. One of the reasons for this result is that many search engines automatically assume OR is intended between any of the words in the query. Thus, if you are looking for information about University of Virginia, on many search sites you will get results that include "university" and "Virginia"; only some of these sources will contain both terms and relate to your desired subject. The power searches, search tips, or help included with the search site can assist you to narrow your search. Boolean search strategies will also help you focus your search. Many search engines use a plus sign (+) in front of the term for AND and a minus sign (–) in front of the term for NOT. A blank space between terms can be considered as either an AND or an OR, depending on the search engine.

Evaluation of Information

Although finding information that is specific to your topic can be a challenge, finding quality information can be even more of a challenge. It is your responsibility to ensure that you use only high-quality information. The attributes of quality information provide a basis for developing criteria to evaluate information.

Information Attributes

Information attributes apply to all information from any source. These attributes are used to develop criteria for evaluating the quality of information.

Timely

Information that is timely is true at this point in time. In other words, it is as current now as when it was written. For example, in 1992, the Agency for Health Care Policy and Research (AHCPR) released clinical practice guidelines on urinary incontinence. At that time, approximately 20 clinical practice guidelines had been published by this division of the U.S. government. You may be able to find a copy of them in your library. As of January 15, 2009, four of these clinical guidelines were still posted; only one of the four had been updated. These guidelines can be found at http://www.ncbi.nlm.nih.gov/books/bv.fcgi?call=bv .View. ShowSection&rid=hstat2.part.4408. As noted on this Web page, the government agency has been renamed the Agency for Healthcare Research and Quality (AHRQ).

The concept of timely can be relative. For example, if you were writing a paper on the history of Florence Nightingale or the medical treatment of soldiers during World War II, something dated 10 years ago might still be correct and therefore still timely. However, if the topic was the current treatment modalities for breast cancer, an article written 10 years ago would no longer be timely. When you access information on the Internet or in a library, always check the date of the information at the site of the information. A word of caution applies when you do so: Always make sure that the date reflects the date the content was updated, not the date the Web page was published.

Accurate

Information is accurate when it does not contain errors or misleading information that could lead you to an incorrect conclusion. For example, using the search phrase "HIV does not cause AIDS" will result in several hits for sites that dispute a relationship between acquired immune deficiency syndrome and the human immunodeficiency virus. These sites contain inaccurate information.

Verifiable

Verifiable information can be checked at more than one source; that is, there is consensus among experts and consistency in how the data are reported. Verifiable information is usually supported by quantifiable data. An example of verifiable information is data related to the current nursing shortage. In this case, you might check government statistics, predictions from your professional organization, and health foundations such as the Pew Foundation to find verifiable information about this trend. While they may present slightly different numbers or predictions, each of these sites will confirm the existence of a nursing shortage.

Accessible

Accessibility refers to how easy it is to obtain the information. For a number of years, MEDLINE was not generally available to the public. In the first six months that access to MEDLINE was offered free on the Internet, one-third of all searches were conducted by the general public as opposed to professional healthcare providers. With the addition of MedlinePlus (http://medlineplus.gov/), this resource has become accessible to a widely diversified audience.

Information is considered accessible if you can enter a search term looking for information, and the desired information is found in your search results. Four factors have a major influence on accessibility.

The first factor relates to the terms or language used to store the information. If you are using a bibliographical database, which words are in the title or in the abstract? How was the document indexed? If the information is located on the Internet, access depends on which words are used on the Web page and the approach to indexing used by the Internet search engine. For example, does the Internet search engine search the whole document or just the first paragraph?

A second factor that determines accessibility is the number of references that refer to the original document. In a bibliographical database, references appear in the footnotes to an entry. Sometimes it is possible to click a footnote and be linked directly to the article. On the Internet, access is also determined by links. If several Web pages link to a document, you are more likely to find them either by browsing or by using a search engine.

The third factor that determines accessibility is your ability to focus the search. Initial searches often find either too much or too little information. One of the most effective approaches is to find one document that includes information you find useful and then use the information from this document to find additional material.

A fourth factor that will determine accessibility is the functions added to the search engine software. For example, EBSCO has added reference linking, which in turn offers three ways to link a particular article to other related resources. First, if a reference cited in the references list of the original article is in the EBSCO database, a direct link from the cited reference to the actual reference is provided. Second, clicking on a reference link at the top of the screen will create a list of references that were cited in the original article. Finally, clicking the name of an author will create a list of other materials published by that same author.

Freedom from Bias

Biased information has been altered or modified in an attempt to influence the reader. Sometimes the bias is blatant and easy to identify. To confirm this point, do an Internet search using the term "abortion" or "gun control"; both topics generate strong opposing opinions. Look at several sites to determine if information is accurate and free from bias. Bias is easier to identify when you disagree with the opinion being expressed or when the information is clearly inaccurate. Sometimes, however, the information is accurate and the bias is subtle. For example, information provided by a drug company about one of its pharmaceutical products will most likely include information about side effects—but it may appear in small print near the end of the document. In contrast, the indications for which the drug is used may appear in larger print at the beginning of the document and be reinforced with a graphic. Each time the drug is referred to in the document, the trade name will be used as opposed to the generic name. These formatting choices are intended to influence you to consider the indications for the drug before its side effects and to think of the trade name before remembering the generic name.

Comprehensive

Comprehensive information is complete. Because there is always more that can be said about any topic, it can be difficult to determine if the information is comprehensive. Information is not comprehensive if missing details mislead the reader. For example, suppose there are two hospitals in your local community where coronary artery bypass surgery is done, and one hospital has a higher postoperative death rate than the other. This information could lead you to conclude that one hospital provides better care than the other does. However, if the first hospital is a community hospital that takes only low-risk patients and the second hospital is a major medical center that cares for high-risk patients, the death rate data may not give a comprehensive picture of the quality of care at either hospital.

Precise

Information is comprehensive if all the details are provided. The information lacks precision, however, if the details are not specific. For example, a map on the Internet may include the specific street where a clinic is located, yet fail to provide the street number for the clinic. Precision occurs when the details provided meet the specific information needs of the reader.

Appropriate

Appropriateness refers to how well the information answers your questions. Is the information on target? For example, you may be looking for information on preparing clinic nurses for a new information system. You may be able to find a great deal of information about the new system, but nothing that helps you to prepare the new users for engaging with it. The information that is found is precise, timely, and accurate, and meets all the other criteria of quality information, but it does not focus on the specific information needed; that is, it does not answer the specific question that was asked.

Clear

Information lacks clarity if the same information can be interpreted in more than one way. For example, consider the following disclaimer: "There are several sites on the Internet that provide health information. Some sites provide quality information, while others do not. This is one of these sites." The reader is left to decide if this site provides good- or poor-quality information.

Criteria for Evaluating the Quality of Online Information

Knowing information attributes can help you evaluate the information you find online. Using those attributes, you can evaluate the source of the information, determine its accuracy and currency, and identify how easy it was to access and use the information online.

Source

When accessing and using information on the Internet, try to start with a reliable source. Reliable sources are usually verifiable and accurate. The source of the information on the Internet refers to both the author of the information and the location where the information is found on the Internet. Many times these two factors overlap. For example, you may find information about the role of weight in diabetes on an Internet site maintained by the American Diabetic Association or you might find the information on the personal sites of individuals well known for their research on diabetes and weight. Many times personal sites use a ~ symbol (called a tilde) in the URL to direct you to a personal directory.

When evaluating the author as a source, it is helpful to identify the author's name, title or position, degrees or education, and professional affiliation. Remember that this information may be included as part of the information on the Web pages, yet not be accurate. The author could state that he or she is the chairperson of the department of a major university and in reality be a 10-year-old child learning to design a Web page. It is up to you, as the user of the information, to validate the source.

The URL is your major clue for the location of the information. Let's look at the following URL: http://www3.widener.edu/Academics/Libraries/ Wolfgram_Memorial_Library/Evaluate_Web_Pages/659/.

The use of the *http* protocol indicates this site is located on the World Wide Web. *www3* is the specific name of the server where the information is located. *widener* is the name of the institution where the server is located. *edu* indicates that this is an educational site. *Academics/Libraries/Wolfgram_Memorial_Library/Evaluate_Web_Pages/659/* is the directory path on the server where the Web page is located.

If you look around this Web site, you will see and hear a great deal of excellent information reinforcing the content in this chapter. The Wolfgram Memorial Library information literacy resource applies to all types of online information. By comparison, the Western Connecticut State Libraries site provides an excellent example of how these principles can be applied in nursing and in the support of evidence-based practice (http://library.wcsu.edu/web/assistance/research/nursing/tutorial/).

Currency

Current information has been updated as new information has evolved. With the ongoing knowledge explosion, keeping current is a major challenge in health care. In January 2009, the U.S. Department of Health and Human Services published the results of a research study dealing with relevant consumer Web sites with guidelines for treating acute otitis media, or ear infection. The study reported that 32 months after the latest guidelines were released, only 32% of the relevant Web sites had been updated (Holland & Fagnano, 2008).

There are three dates that can be important to consider when evaluating a Web site. The first is the original date when the information was generated. For example, if the site quotes clinical guidelines, when were those guidelines produced? Second is the last date on which the content or information was updated. This is not the same as the last time the page was modified, which is the third date to consider. Design features on the page may be modified and a new date put on the page; however, the information may not have been updated at the same time.

Another clue that the information is current is the reliability of the links. There are two ways to evaluate the links. First, do they function? Links on the Internet change constantly. If a site is not being well maintained, the links will become outdated and no longer function. Second, does this site link to current information? On a well-maintained site, links that no longer connect to quality information are removed. If historical data are maintained, they should be identified as such. Note the following example posted at http://www.health.gov/scipich/:

> On April 28th, 1999, the Science Panel on Interactive Communication and Health (SciPICH), an independent body convened by the U.S. Department of Health and Human Services (HHS), released its final report, *Wired for Health and Well-Being: The Emergence of Interactive Health Communication.*
>
> The Panel is no longer active, and this site is maintained for historical purposes only.

Ease of Navigation

Quality information is usually organized in a logical format. Logical technical approaches are then used to guide the user through the information. The navigation aids employed may be as simple as a table of contents that provides an overview of the information in the document or as complex as the use of multiple frames. Sometimes a site map is used to provide an overview of the information at the site. Color and graphics can also be used to help (or hinder) the navigation of a site. A site may be comprehensive, but if the site is not well organized and the navigational aids do not function well, you may never find the quality information located on the site.

Because a search engine may send you anywhere in the site, effective navigational aids are important. They provide a clear overall picture of the Web site as a whole as well as an at-the-moment location. A menu, a site map, arrows, and buttons should all flow together to provide direction. Standard terms such as "Home" and "About" are easier to understand than terms that are unique to a specific Web site.

Objective Information

Objective information is free of bias. Of course, the Internet is an excellent place for the expression of opinions as well as advertisement of ideas, products, and positions. Biases on the Internet are acceptable if they are clearly stated. For example, http://www.democrats.org/index.html is the URL for the Democratic Party; http://www.rnc.org/ is the URL for the Republican Party. You would naturally expect to find very different opinions on these sites.

Errors

Several of the criteria already listed will help you determine if an online resource is error free, but other clues may also be helpful in this regard. First, watch for errors in spelling and grammar. If a site is sloppy with these kinds of details, it may also be sloppy with the accuracy of the information provided. Second, be cautious if the information is found on only one site and no other information verifying it exists at other sites. For example, an Internet site might describe a malaria epidemic in Alaska. Malaria is caused by a parasite that is transmitted from person to person by the bite of an infected *Anopheles* mosquito. These mosquitoes can be found in almost all countries in the tropics and subtropics. Given these facts about the cause of malaria, do you think that it is likely a malaria epidemic could occur in Alaska?

Health-Related Information on the Internet

Not all health information is created equal, and not everything out there is correct. When knowledgeable people have "surfed" the Web, they have found dangerously misleading or incomplete health information that looks quite legitimate on the surface. The medium itself contributes to the problem. A good designer can make any Web page look slick and professional. While poor design can indicate poor information, good design does not guarantee good information. Information on a Web site may be no more reliable or credible than something heard at a party or on a talk show. While much of the health information on the Internet was posted to help people, not all of it will be good for everyone.

Additional Criteria for Health-Related Information

The criteria discussed earlier in this chapter deal with any information found on the Internet. They also apply to healthcare information, though they are not *specific* to healthcare information. Some unique criteria do apply when the information is health related, however.

Intended Audience

Does the site clearly state who the intended audience is, including the skills and knowledge needed to interpret the information provided by the site? This information is often included in an area titled "Mission" or "About us." Many sites will identify information as being appropriate for the general public or for health-care professionals.

Confidentiality of Personal Information

Many healthcare sites collect personal healthcare data. For example, many sites include self-assessment areas. A quality site will clearly state which data are being collected and how those data will be used. Remember that anyone can publish anything on the Web, however—including a statement of privacy that is incomplete or inaccurate. Be sure you know the site and the sponsors of that site before you provide personal information to an Internet site.

Source of the Content/References

An Internet site that provides health information needs to be able to document the source of that information and the relationship of that source to the information. The name of the organization or institution responsible for the content should be clear. The author's name, credentials, and personal or financial connections that could be a source of real or potential bias should be clearly indicated on the page. In addition, the Web page should provide an easily located way to contact the author of the page. As a user of that information, you need to evaluate the source of the information and determine whether the sources listed are, in fact, real. The references list itself may include references that do not exist.

Sensitivity to the Health Literacy of the Intended Audience

As defined in *Healthy People 2010*, "Health literacy is the degree to which individuals have the capacity to obtain, process, and understand basic health information and services needed to make appropriate health decisions" (U.S. Department of Health and Human Services, 2000). Basic to health literacy is the ability to read and comprehend information. Several tools can be used to evaluate the reading level of materials posted on the Internet. The word processing application presented in this book includes one such tool. You can learn more about this tool by using the help function with Word and searching on *readability statistics*. Comprehension is a more difficult question: It depends on the healthcare background of readers and their ability to understand and effectively use the information being presented. Because the Internet can be accessed by anyone, it is important for any healthcare-oriented site to address this issue. It is also helpful if the intended audience is specifically identified.

Recognition by Other Authorities

An excellent site with quality information will be recognized by other sites. If there are no links to a site and no references to it, you should be concerned. For example, the Consumer and Patient Health Information Section (CAPHIS) of the Medical Library Association maintains a list of the top 100 sites related to health care; this list is located at http://caphis.mlanet.org/consumer/index.html.

Sites Containing Healthcare Information Criteria

The quality of healthcare information on the Internet is of great concern to many healthcare providers. A number of sites located on the Internet provide guides for evaluating healthcare information.

Rollins School of Public Health at Emory University has developed a form that can be used to evaluate health-related sites on the Internet. The form (located at http://www.sph.emory.edu/WELLNESS/instrument.html) is designed to help health educators and clinicians evaluate the appropriateness of Web sites for the health education of their clientele.

Other organizations accredit or recognize sites that meet specific criteria. One of the most well known is Health On the Net Foundation (HON, http://www .hon.ch/home.html), a nonprofit organization located in Geneva, Switzerland. Among its many activities, HON has developed a code of conduct for providers of healthcare information. The code is not intended to rate the quality or the information provided by a Web site; rather, it defines a set of rules designed to make sure the reader always knows the source and the purpose of the data being read. You will note that Emory University's entry includes a reference to this code of conduct on its evaluation form.

The Utilization Review Accreditation Commission (URAC, http://www.urac .org/) is another independent, nonprofit organization offering accreditation, certification, and other quality improvement activities for companies providing health services and information on the Internet. Its benchmarking activities cover health plans, preferred provider organizations, medical management systems, health technology services, health call centers, specialty care, workers' compensation, Web sites, and HIPAA privacy and security compliance, among other areas.

Using Information

The final step in information literacy is making effective use of information. In this book, the discussion of effective use is limited to documenting information from the Internet.

Documenting Internet Sources

All information accessed on the Internet should be documented just as one would document information from any other source. Failure to document is plagiarism: Plagiarism is the act of stealing another person's ideas or work and presenting it as your own. The Internet has made it easier to plagiarize another's work and has created additional issues regarding attribution of sources. As a result, students do not always realize they are stealing. For example, it is easy to forget that the copyright laws also protect information posted on the Internet. These laws can even apply to email messages posted to an online discussion group. Because documentation of Internet-based information has become an increasing concern, several Web sites have been developed to help deal with this issue. One example can be seen at http://www.nwmissouri.edu/library/SERVICES/PREVENT.HTM.

Citing Internet Information

Just as it is easy to post information on the Internet, so it is also easy to remove that information. As a consequence, the citation for information obtained from the Internet should include some additional data, such as the date on which the information was developed. This information should be provided by the Internet site; if it is not, the citation should indicate that the information source is not dated. Also, because data are frequently removed from the Internet, the citation should indicate the date on which the information was accessed. Several Internet sites give specific directions for formatting an Internet citation and including these dates.

The American Psychological Association (APA) is one of the most commonly used formats for citing healthcare information. The APA maintains a Web site that includes information on how to use the APA format to cite Internet resources; it is located at http://www.apastyle.org. Many university libraries and writing centers provide additional help with APA style; see http://owl.english.purdue.edu/owl/resource/560/01/ as one such example.

In addition to the APA format, there are other accepted citation formats. Several of these are demonstrated on a site maintained by the General Library at the University of Texas at Austin. This site is located at http://www.lib.utexas.edu/refsites/style_manuals.html.

Like the University of Texas at Austin, many libraries include this type of information on their Web sites. Often they will include a list of links to guidelines for citing Internet resources. Two sites that demonstrate this approach include http://www.nova.edu/library/eleclib/eref.html#cite and http://library.lafayette.edu/help/citing/webpages; the second site includes a list of components that should be included in any Internet citation.

Summary

This chapter explored the concept of information literacy and outlined strategies needed to identify an information need, find information, evaluate the quality of information, and cite information from the Internet. Quality health care requires good information. As a healthcare provider, it is your responsibility to search for the latest high-quality information and make appropriate use of that information in providing care to your patients. It is also your responsibility to educate patients about safe and effective approaches for becoming informed consumers of health-related information.

References

American Library Association. (2000). Information literacy competency standards for higher education. Retrieved August 28, 2004, from http://www.ala.org/ala/acrl/acrl-standards/standards.pdf.

American Nurses Association. (2008). *Nursing informatics: Scope and standards of practice.* Silver Spring, MD: Nursesbooks.org.

CrossRef.Org. (n.d.). CrossRef glossary. Retrieved January 31, 2009, from http://www.crossref.org/02publishers/glossary.html.

Holland, M. L., & Fagnano, B. A. (2008). Appropriate antibiotic use for acute otitis media: What consumers find using Web searches. *Clinical Pediatrics, 47*(5), 452–546.

Staggers, N., Gassert, C., Kwai, J. L., Milholland, K., Nelson, R., Senemeier, J., Stuck, D., & Welton, J. (2001). *Scope and standards of nursing informatics practice.* Washington, DC: American Nurses Publishing.

U.S. Department of Health and Human Services. (2000). *Healthy People 2010.* Washington, DC: U.S. Government Printing Office.

EXERCISE 1 Using a Search Site

■ **Objectives**

1. Use the help section of an Internet search site.
2. Conduct an Internet search using Boolean search strategies.
3. Identify a directory, search directory, meta-directory, and meta-search site.

■ **Activity**

1. Access a search site.
   a. **Type** the following URL in your browser **Location** or **Address** text box: **http://www.yahoo.com**. You are now on the home page of Yahoo.
   b. On this page, locate the following four areas: (1) Help, (2) Advanced Search, (3) the area where you enter your query, and (4) the list of subjects within the directory.
2. Use a directory.
   a. **Click** the subject area that deals with **Health**. The next page will be a subdirectory.
   b. **Click** one of the topics from the subdirectory. Look at the URL of the page to see if there is a path statement that will tell you how deep you are in the directory. The path may look something like this: http://health.yahoo.com/health/centers/women/index.html.
3. Use a home navigational aid.
   a. **Click** the **Home** link to return to the Yahoo home page.
   b. **Find** the **Help** section. Does all the help relate to searching Yahoo?
   c. Did you learn anything new on this page?
4. Use the advanced search capability.

    a. **Click** the **Back** button on your browser to return to the Yahoo home page.

    b. Find the **Advanced Search** area again.

    c. Look around in this section and note the various ways that you can focus a search.

    d. **Click** the **Back** button to return to the Yahoo home page.

5. Find and become oriented to new search engines.

    a. Use Yahoo to find at least two other **search engines** on the Internet.

    b. Use the same approach demonstrated with Yahoo to orient yourself to the new search sites.

6. Conduct a search.

    a. Go to the **search engine** you prefer.

    b. Design a query to search for **search engine or site tutorials**.

7. Compare online tutorials.

    a. **Select** a **tutorial** from the hits on your search and one of the following URLs:

    http://academics.sru.edu/library/tutorials/internet/intro.htm

    http://www.monash.com/spidap.html

    http://www.pandia.com/goalgetter/

    http://liblearn.osu.edu/tutor/

    b. **Complete** the two tutorials.

    c. Which of the two did you find most informative? Why?

    d. As you are looking for a site with tutorials for search sites or engines, be sure to at least take a quick look at this site: **http://www.lib.berkeley .edu/TeachingLib/Guides/Internet/FindInfo.html**.

8. Use meta-search sites classifications.

Meta-search sites can be classified in many ways. Examples include classification by topic searched (medicine, law, art), by the way in which sites are found and indexed (robots and people), and by number of search engines used simultaneously to conduct the search. Several sites on the Web provide lists of links to several search engines. These sites classify the search sites in a variety of ways.

    a. Locate at least three Web sites that include 15 or more search sites.

    b. Locate Web sites where the search sites are grouped under certain headings.

    c. Create a table that includes columns for (1) the sites, (2) the classification, and (3) an example of a search sites in that classification.

    d. Search sites may be classified in more than one way, so your groupings or classifications may overlap. Here are some sites to get you started. Do not include these sites or sites listed in Table 12-8 in the five sites that you located for this exercise.

    http://en.wikipedia.org/wiki/List_of_search_engines

    http://www.pandia.com/powersearch/

EXERCISE 2 Evaluating Information on the Internet

■ **Objectives**

1. Using the criteria described in this chapter, develop a tool that can be used to evaluate the quality of information on the Internet.
2. Evaluate the effectiveness of the tool for a user who has limited health literacy.

■ **Activity**

1. Evaluate information sites.
   Review three sites from the following list:
   http://www.virtualsalt.com/evalu8it.htm
   http://www.ala.org/ala/alsc/greatwebsites/greatwebsitesforkids/
       greatwebsites.htm
   http://www.ahrq.gov/data/infoqual.htm
   http://www.uic.edu/depts/lib/lhsu/resources/guides/web-evaluation.shtml
2. Develop a tool that can be used to evaluate related information on a Web site.
   a. Using information from the selected sites and this chapter, design a tool for evaluating Web pages.
   b. Select two wellness-related Internet sites that provide information for the general public. One site should have high-quality information; the other site should have inaccurate information.
   c. Ask a high school student or college freshman, who would be expected to have a limited healthcare background, to review the sites using your form.
3. Answer the following questions.
   a. Did the student collect information for all sections of your form?
   b. When information was missing, did the student note this fact? For example, if the date the page was last updated was missing, did he or she note this omission?
   c. Did the student validate the data or information that was collected? For example, if the author of the information at the Internet site indicated that he or she was a college professor, did the student check the directory of the college to see if the person was listed?
   d. Was the student able to differentiate the quality of the information at the two sites?
   e. If the student was correct, which factors influenced the student in making this decision? In other words, how was he or she able to recognize the quality of the information?
   f. If he or she was incorrect, which factors misled the student? Remember the student may be correct about one page and not the other.

g. From this experience, how would you revise your form? What would you stress if you were teaching patients to evaluate information on the Web?

ASSIGNMENT 1 Evaluating Healthcare Information on the Internet

■ **Directions**

1. Begin this assignment by designing two forms for evaluating health-related information at an Internet site. Design one form that can be used by a healthcare provider. The second form should be designed for use by the general public. The forms should be no longer than two pages and should include directions for use.

2. Pilot-test both forms with at least five users. Exercise 2 should be helpful to you in planning your pilot.

3. Write a paper about this project that includes the following information: Explain the rationale for the design and content of each form. Describe how you selected your users and what happened when you pilot-tested the forms with them. Outline your findings or the results of your pilot test. Redesign the forms based on your pilot and include the revised forms as an appendix to your paper. Don't forget to cite references using the appropriate format.

4. After the paper is completed, design a poster presentation based on the paper. You may find PowerPoint helpful for this part of the assignment. Present the poster presentation to your classmates.

5. Turn in both the paper and the poster presentation.

ASSIGNMENT 2 Understanding Boolean Search Strategies

■ **Directions**

1. In each of the three diagrams shown in Figure 12-1, the light gray area represents the hits you can expect with Boolean search strategies.
   a. Use the following three search strategies with a general Internet search site:
      i. (Nurses AND Computer)
      ii. (Nurses OR Computers)
      iii. (Nurses NOT Computers)
   b. Write a brief statement explaining how and why the results from these three search strategies are different.

2. Use the same three search strategies to search a health-related database in your school library. Explain how these results are different from your Internet search.

Privacy, Confidentiality, Security, and Integrity of Electronic Data

Objectives

1. Discuss the concepts of privacy, confidentiality, security, and integrity as they apply to the management of electronic data.
2. Recognize common threats to privacy, confidentiality, security, and integrity of data stored in electronic systems.
3. Apply effective procedures for protecting data, software, and hardware.
4. Follow Health Insurance Portability and Accountability Act (HIPAA) principles for protecting healthcare information.
5. Discuss healthcare security issues related to the Internet and the role of healthcare providers in protecting patient data.

Introduction

This chapter identifies threats to privacy and confidentiality as well as integrity and security of information. *Privacy* refers to a person's desire to limit the disclosure of personal information. *Confidentiality* deals with the healthcare provider's responsibility to limit access to information so that it is shared in a controlled manner for the benefit of the patient. *Security* refers to the measures that organizations implement to protect information and systems. *Integrity* refers to the accuracy and comprehensiveness of data.

The code of ethics for healthcare professionals consistently demonstrates that ensuring the confidentiality and privacy of patients, clients, and consumers information, is a major responsibility of healthcare providers. Meeting that responsibility is impossible if the healthcare provider does not understand how to follow current regulations and apply effective procedures for protecting electronic data. This chapter clarifies the regulations for protecting healthcare information. In addition, healthcare providers are responsible for ensuring the security and integrity of patient data; this chapter describes procedures for protecting data, software, and hardware.

Using Computer Systems for Storing Data

With rare exceptions, all healthcare institutions manage and store data in automated systems. These data, which relate to clients, employees, and the institution, are interrelated and interdependent. A threat to any data element in these automated systems can be a threat to the clients, the employees, and the institution. More importantly, the legal and ethical implications related to storing personal data are of primary concern.

Concerns with confidentiality and security are not limited to healthcare information systems. Many personal PCs now store a significant amount of confidential data. Data stolen from these personal systems can be a major source of problems. Identity theft occurs when someone uses another person's personally identifying information, such as a Social Security number, to commit fraud or other crimes (Federal Trade Commission a, n.d.).

A specific type of identity theft—a medical identify theft—is of special concern for healthcare providers. Medical identity theft occurs when someone uses another person's personal information without that individual's knowledge or consent to obtain or receive payment for medical care. Victims of medical identity theft may discover that their medical records are inaccurate. This inaccuracy is not only medically dangerous for the victim, but can also affect his or her ability to obtain insurance coverage or benefits (Federal Trade Commission b, n.d.).

Concerns with data integrity and security are not limited to healthcare or personal data, of course. Most of the files that have been created on a computer represent hours of work that can be very difficult to replicate. For example, if a student has spent several hours completing a term paper that is destroyed by a computer virus, it may be difficult to convince the instructor that a virus "ate the paper."

Four major concerns arise in conjunction with electronically stored data, be it data stored on a healthcare information system, on an Internet server, or on a personal computer:

- Providing for privacy and confidentiality of data
- Ensuring the integrity of the data
- Protecting the hardware and software that are used to manage and store these data
- Recognizing and prosecuting criminal abuse of computer data and equipment

Privacy and Confidentiality

To protect privacy and confidentiality, issues relevant to data storage and use must be addressed. Problems of ensuring privacy and confidentiality of data include data protection issues and data integrity issues. Data protection issues include accessing of data for unauthorized use and unnecessary storage of data. Data integrity issues include incomplete or inaccurate storage of data and intentional or accidental manipulation of data.

Personal Privacy and Confidentiality

With the advent of computers, numerous companies, institutions, and government agencies maintain databases containing personal data. For example, personal information related to education is stored in university computers, including data related to learning disabilities and financial need. Information related to personal driving records is stored by the Department of Motor Vehicles; Social Security benefits information is stored by the Social Security Administration; and mail-order companies store personal information such as phone numbers, addresses, and items that have been ordered as well as credit card numbers. Insurance companies maintain extensive information on their customers' personal health care. Knowing which data are stored is an important first step in protecting individual privacy.

When individuals complete warranty or registration forms that ask for their names, addresses, and other information, these data may be sold to other companies. Simply using the Internet generates information about the individuals—where they go on the Net, who they interact with via chat rooms and online discussion group, and which products they buy. Several organizations have evolved to respond to these issues; **Table 13-1** lists several of the better-known organizations. Notice that all of these groups were established in the early 1990s, just as the Internet was becoming available to the general public. While each of these groups has taken a different approach to protecting online privacy, all include as one of their approaches education of the general public. For example, the Center for Democracy and Technology (CDT) offers a detailed online privacy guide designed specifically for consumers ("CDT'S Guide to Online Privacy," 2009).

Currently many organizations share personal data from their databases. By sharing information across these databases, it becomes possible to create a personal profile of an individual that is more extensive than the individual might imagine. An example of the data being shared can be seen in the small-print leaflets concerning privacy that are mailed with credit bills or bank statements. Another excellent example in health care is provided by the MIB Group, Inc. (MIB). MIB is an association of more than 500 U.S. and Canadian life insurance companies. By sharing information, these companies work together to ensure

TABLE 13-1   ORGANIZATIONS PROTECTING ONLINE PRIVACY

Name	URL	Description
Center for Democracy and Technology (CDT)	http://www.cdt.org/	CDT, founded in 1994, works to promote democratic values and constitutional liberties in the digital age by building consensus among parties interested in the future of the Internet and other new communications media.
Electronic Frontier Foundation (EFF)	http://www.eff.org/	EFF, founded in 1990, focuses on defending free speech, privacy, innovation, and consumer digital rights. EFF's primary approach is in the courts, bringing and defending lawsuits "even when that means taking on the U.S. government or large corporations."
Electronic Privacy Information Center (EPIC)	http://epic.org/	EPIC is a public interest research center established in 1994 to focus public attention on emerging civil liberties issues and to protect privacy, the First Amendment, and constitutional values.
Privacy International (PI)	http://www.privacyinternational.org/	PI is a human rights group formed in 1990 as a watchdog on surveillance and privacy invasions by governments and corporations.
Privacy Rights Clearinghouse (PRC)	http://www.privacyrights.org/	PRC is a nonprofit, consumer information and advocacy organization established in 1992.

the accuracy of health information supplied on a person's insurance application ("MIB: About Us," 2009). Because many people do not know they have a record with MIB, few checks and balances exist to ensure the accuracy of this information. For example, an individual may be refused life insurance and never know that the reason he or she was not insured was the presence of inaccurate information in the MIB file.

Patient Privacy and Confidentiality

Because many people believe that information they share with their healthcare providers is held in confidence, they may assume a level of protection that does not exist. Once that information is documented in a medical record, however, the actual confidentiality of that information is determined by who has access to those data. Healthcare information is shared not only with physicians, nurses, and other healthcare providers, but also with insurance companies and government agencies such as Medicare or Medicaid. Legal access to these records is obtained when individuals agree to let others see them, usually by signing consent forms or blanket waivers when receiving health care.

With the increasing use of technology, medical information is stored in a variety of computer databases, both in local institutions and in other places serving a number of healthcare institutions. In passing PL 104-191, the Health Insurance Portability and Accountability Act of 1996 (HIPAA), Congress included provisions for a standard unique health identifier for each individual, employer, health plan, and healthcare provider in the healthcare system. To date, a process for issuing standard unique health identifiers for individuals has not been developed or accepted.

HIPAA applies to medical records maintained by healthcare providers, health plans, and health clearinghouses only if the facility maintains and transmits records in *electronic* form. A great deal of health-related information exists *outside* of healthcare facilities and the files of health plans and, therefore, is beyond the reach of HIPAA. While the law also includes penalties for infringement of the integrity and confidentiality of data, privacy advocates remain concerned about secondary uses of medical information by employers or others with unauthorized access (Private Rights Clearinghouse, 2008).

Under both the HIPAA and the Patriot Act, there are certain circumstances when police are permitted access to medical records without a warrant (Burke & Weill, 2005). Although HIPAA requires that you be informed about how your records may be used without your consent, it does not require that you be informed when your records are actually shared. In addition, the Patriot Act includes provisions that do not allow you to be told if your medical records are shared under the provisions of this act (Roach, Hoban, Broccolo, Roth, & Blanchard, 2006).

Safety and Security

Protecting the safety and security of patient data involves identifying the threats to computer systems and initiating procedures to protect the integrity of the data and system. The two main types of threats are those to the integrity of data and to the confidentiality of the data. These threats can result from accidental or intentional human actions or natural disasters. Destruction of data, hardware, and software by natural disasters include damage by water, fire, or chemicals; electrical power outages; disk failures; and exposure to magnetic fields.

The types of human actions that result in these threats can be divided into five areas ("For the Record: Protecting Electronic Health Information," 1997).

Innocent Mistakes

Innocent mistakes are errors made by people who have legal access to the system and who, in the process of using the system, accidentally disclose data or damage the integrity of data. Examples can be as simple as a physician recording data in the wrong medical record or a lab sending a fax to the wrong phone number. In school, it may take the form of a teacher entering the wrong grade on the student's academic record. Several incidences of accidental disclosure of medical data have been documented by M. Eric Johnson in a paper titled "Data Hemorrhages in a Health Care Sector." Examples cited of accidentally posting medical data to the Internet include the Wuesthoff Medical Center in Florida, which posted information on more than 500 patients; the Tampa-based WellCare Health Plans, which posted information on 71,000 Georgia residents; and the University of Pittsburgh Medical Center, which posted names and medical images of nearly 80 individuals (Johnson, 2009).

Inappropriate Access by Insiders for Curiosity Reasons

Sometimes people with legal access to the system make an intentional decision to abuse their access privileges. Browsing is a problem with many electronic record systems—and health records are not immune to this problem. In this type of access, the person looks at medical records for the expressed purpose of satisfying his or her own curiosity; the access to the medical record provides no benefit to the patient. The auditing functions in many healthcare information systems, however, make it easy to identify these browsers and discipline those individuals. In educational institutions, an information technology professional may occasionally browse his or her son's or daughter's academic record in clear violation of Family Educational Rights and Privacy Act (FERPA) regulations. A current example of this type of access was demonstrated by the inappropriate access of Nadya Suleman's medical records after she gave birth to octuplets. In May 2009 California health regulators fined Kaiser Permanente's Bellflower Hospital $250,000 for this violation (Ornstein, 2009).

Inappropriate Access by Insiders for Spite or for Profit

In 2002, Al Roker, the weatherman on NBC's *Today Show,* had gastric bypass surgery to treat obesity. He told neither his mother nor his colleagues at the TV station. He was admitted using a different name. Roker describes his experience with privacy of medical data on a Web site he maintains:

> The *National Enquirer* had a hospital employee violate my privacy and break several laws in providing them with my surgical and hospital information. Good for them. I'm sure they're proud (Roker, 2004).

The story in the *National Enquirer* included Roker's preoperative weight, the time of surgery, and several other personal data items. In 2008, Farrah Fawcett, under treatment for cancer, experienced the same type of a violation while a patient at UCLA. In April 2008, the *Los Angeles Times* reported that a UCLA employee accessed her records more often than her own doctors. This employee pleaded guilty to federal felony charges of selling the information to the *National Enquirer* (Ornstein, 2009). These are just two of the many examples of documented inappropriate access by insiders for profit. Healthcare professionals play an important role in protecting patients from this type of exploitation.

Unauthorized Intruders Who Gain Access to Patient Data

Many hospitals rely on physical security, software, and user education to protect the information stored inside a computer against unauthorized intruders. For example, the computers may be located where it is difficult for others to access or use them. Passwords and firewalls are also used to control access. In addition, the computers automatically log off all users after a few minutes of inactivity.

Vengeful Employees and Outsiders

Examples of data incursions by vengeful individuals include vindictive patients or intruders who mount attacks to access unauthorized information or damage systems and disrupt operations. For this reason, most hospitals terminate employees' computer access before informing them they are being let go and physically escort the terminated employees off the premises.

Computer Crime

Computer crimes include a wide range of illegal activities, from computer intrusion into a computer system (i.e., hacking) to child pornography or exploitation. Some of these crimes require a certain level of technical skill, but many are as simple as sending an email with false or misleading information. Such crimes may be perpetrated by an individual; others are carried out by large organized crime groups and even governments. Victims range from vulnerable individuals or organizations to corporations and government institutions that are vital to the infrastructure of the country. In creating the Office of Cybersecurity and announcing the position of Cybersecurity Coordinator to deal with the risk posed by these dangers President Obama stated:

> In short, America's economic prosperity in the 21st century will depend on cybersecurity.

And this is also a matter of public safety and national security. We count on computer networks to deliver our oil and gas, our power and our water. We rely on them for public transportation and air traffic control. Yet we know that cyber intruders have probed our electrical grid and that in other countries cyber attacks have plunged entire cities into darkness. (Obama, 2009)

Several government agencies are involved in investigating these types of crimes and the new office is charged with improving the coordination of these agencies. **Table 13-2** lists several of these agencies, their URLs, and their missions. As computer crimes have evolved, so have the language and terms used to discuss these crimes. **Table 13-3** defines a number of these terms as well as a few data protection terms.

Prosecution of Computer Crime

It is difficult to detect and prosecute many computer crimes. Many times the person initiating the criminal act is not located in this country and may not be subject to U.S. laws. A key resource for understanding computer crime and related issues is maintained by the U.S. Department of Justice; its Web site includes a section especially designed for children (http://www.cybercrime.gov/rules/kidinternet.htm). Although the terms in Table 13-3 are more readily identified with computer crime in areas other than health care, all types of crime can and do occur within healthcare computer systems.

Some computer crimes are detected but not reported. When data are stolen, the information is not always seen as valuable; thus those responsible for its theft may not be prosecuted. Many times, an institution will be more concerned with the poor publicity that can result from disclosure of this event.

Although methods for tracking entry into computer systems are becoming increasingly sophisticated, discovery of computer crime may be difficult. Laws are catching up, but still lag behind computer technology and associated crimes. In some situations, there are questions about who "owns" data. Many of the early laws that were developed in this area, therefore, were designed to protect individuals from having data about them stored in a computer without their knowledge.

Selected Laws Related to Computing

Freedom of Information Act of 1970: This law allows citizens to have access to data gathered by federal agencies.

Federal Privacy Act of 1974: This law stipulates that there can be no secret personal files; individuals must be allowed to know what is stored in files about them and how it is used. This act applies to government agencies and contractors dealing with government agencies but not the private sector.

U.S. Copyright Law of 1976: This law stipulates that it is a federal offense to reproduce copyrighted materials, including computer software, without authorization.

TABLE 13-2   GOVERNMENT AGENCIES FOCUSED ON PREVENTING AND PROSECUTING COMPUTER CRIMES

Agency	URL	Mission
Computer Crime and Intellectual Property Section, United States Department of Justice (CCIPS)	http://www.cybercrime.gov/	The CCIPS is responsible for implementing the Department of Justice's national strategies in combating computer and intellectual property crimes worldwide, including electronic penetrations, data thefts, and cyberattacks on critical information systems.
Internet Crime Complaint Center (IC3)	http://www.ic3.gov/default.aspx	IC3 is a partnership between the Federal Bureau of Investigation (FBI), the National White Collar Crime Center (NW3C), and the Bureau of Justice Assistance (BJA). IC3's mission is to serve as a vehicle to receive, develop, and refer criminal complaints regarding the rapidly expanding arena of cybercrime.
National White Collar Crime Center (NW3C)	http://www.nw3c.org/	NW3C is a congressionally funded, nonprofit corporation whose mission is to provide training, investigative support, and research to agencies and entities involved in the prevention, investigation, and prosecution of economic and high-tech crime.
United States Secret Service, Electronic Crimes Task Forces and Working Groups	http://www.ustreas.gov/usss/ectf.shtml	The common purpose of these groups is the prevention, detection, mitigation, and aggressive investigation of attacks on U.S. financial and critical infrastructures through the use of schemes involving new technology.
United States Postal Service (USPS)	http://postalinspectors.uspis.gov/	Many computer crimes involve both the mail and the Internet. The USPS investigates crimes dealing with mail fraud.

TABLE 13-3 TERMS RELATED TO COMPUTER CRIME AND DATA PROTECTION

Term	Definition
Cracker	A hacker who illegally breaks into computer systems and creates mischief.
Cybercrime	The use of the Internet or other communication technology to commit a crime of any type.
Data diddling	Modifying valid data in a computer file.
Denial of service	Any action or series of actions that prevents any part of an information system from functioning—for example, using several computers attached to the Internet to access a Web site so that the site is overwhelmed and not available.
Encryption	A method of coding sensitive data to protect those data when they are sent over the Internet.
Firewall	A piece of hardware or a software program used to protect computers from unauthorized access via the Internet.
Hacker	Originally referred to a compulsive computer programmer; now it has a more negative meaning and is often confused with "cracker."
Identity theft	A crime in which someone uses another person's private information to assume his or her identity.
Keyboard loggers	Either hardware or software installed on a computer to log the keystrokes of an individual. A keyboard logger can be used to monitor computer activities such as time spent on the Internet or to collect personal information such as passwords.
Logic bomb	A piece of program code buried within another program, designed to perform some malicious act in response to a trigger. For example, the trigger can involve entering a data or name.
Opt out	A number of measures designed to prevent users from receiving unwanted products or services. For example, if you signed up for a free journal on the Internet, you may want to opt out of receiving emails and product announcements from companies that advertise in this journal. In many cases, the default is that you opt in.
Phishing	Pronounced "fishing"; the creation of a replica of a legitimate Web page to hook users and trick them into submitting personal or financial information or passwords.
Sabotage	The purposeful destruction of hardware, software, and data.

(continues)

TABLE 13-3 TERMS RELATED TO COMPUTER CRIME AND DATA PROTECTION *(continued)*	
Term	**Definition**
Salami method	A method of data stealing that involves taking little bits at a time.
Software piracy	Unauthorized copying of copyrighted software.
Spamming	The act of sending unsolicited electronic messages in bulk. The most common form of spam is that delivered in email as a form of commercial advertising.
Theft of services	The unauthorized use of services such as those provided by a computer system.
Time bomb	Instructions in a program that perform certain functions on a specific date or time, such as printing a message or destroying data.
Trapdoors	Methods installed by programmers that allow unauthorized access into programs.
Trojan horse	Instructions in a program that add illegitimate functions; for example, the Trojan horse program may print out information every time information on a certain patient is entered.
Virus	A program that, once introduced into a system, replicates itself and causes a variety of mischievous outcomes. Viruses are usually introduced from infected external storage devices, email attachments, or downloaded files.
Worm	A destructive program that can fill various memory locations of a computer system with information, clogging the system so that other operations are compromised.

Electronic Communication Privacy Act of 1986: This law specifies that it is a crime to own any electronic, mechanical, or other device used primarily for the purpose of surreptitious interception of wire, oral, or electronic communication. This law does not apply to communication within an organization such as email between employees.

Computer Security Act of 1987: This law mandated that the National Institute of Standards and Technology (NIST) and U.S. Office of Personnel Management (OPM) create guidance on computer security awareness and training based on functional organizational roles. In response, the NIST created the Computer Security Resource Center (http://csrc.nist.gov/index.html).

U.S. Copyright Law of 1995, Amendment: This amendment protects the transmission of digital performance over the Internet, making it a crime to transmit something for which you do not have proper authorization.

National Information Infrastructure Protection Act of 1996: This law established penalties for interstate theft of information.

U.S. Copyright Law of 1997 (No Electronic Theft Act): This addition to the copyright act creates criminal penalties for copyright infringement even if the offender does not benefit financially.

Digital Millennium Copyright Act of 1998: This legislation placed the United States in conformance with international treaties that prevail in other countries around the world. It provided changes in three areas: protection of copyrighted digital works, extensions of copyright protection by 20 years, and the addition of criminal penalties and fines for attempting to circumvent copyright protections. In addition, it provides for copy protection for the creative organization and structure of a database, but not the underlying general facts in the database; requires that "Webcasters" pay licensing fees to record companies; and limits Internet service providers' (ISPs') copyright infringement liability for simply transmitting information over the Internet.

Children's Online Protection Act of 2000: This law requires Web sites targeting children younger than age 14 to obtain parental consent before gathering information on children.

USA Patriot Act of 2001: This act gives federal officials greater authority to track and intercept communications for law enforcement and foreign intelligence. With this act, law enforcement agencies now require fewer checks to collect electronic data.

Homeland Security Act of 2002: This act established the Department of Homeland Security as an executive department of the United States. It also expanded and centralized the data gathering allowed under the Patriot Act.

Cyber Security Enhancement Act (CSEA) of 2002: This act was passed along with the Homeland Security Act and reduced privacy by allowing an ISP to voluntarily hand over personal information from its customers to a government agency. Previous to this act a warrant was required (SANS, 2004).

Controlling the Assault of Non-solicited Pornography and Marketing Act of 2003 (CAN-SPAM Act): This act establishes a framework of administrative, civil, and criminal tools to help U.S. consumers, businesses, and families combat unsolicited commercial email or spam.

Computer Fraud and Abuse Act (CFAA) of 1984, Amended in 2008: This law specifies that it is a crime to access a federal computer without authorization and to alter, destroy, or damage information or prevent authorized access. The 2008 amendment clarified a number of the provisions in the original section 1030 and criminalized additional computer-related acts. For example, a provision was added that penalizes the theft of property via computer that occurs as a part of a scheme to defraud. Another provision penalizes those who intentionally alter, damage, or destroy data belonging to others; this part of the act covers such activities as the distribution of malicious code and denial-of-service attacks. Finally, Congress included in the CFAA a provision criminalizing trafficking in passwords and similar items (CCIPS, 2007).

Identity Theft Enforcement and Restitution Act of 2008: This act lowers the bar for what is considered punishable identity theft crimes, thereby making it easier for prosecutors to bring charges against cybercriminals. It also makes it easier for identity theft victims to be compensated, even for costs that are indirectly associated with the harm incurred from the theft.

Protection of Computer Data and Systems

The privacy and confidentiality of data as well as the safety and security of the entire system can be protected by procedures initiated by the healthcare agency. Steps taken by individual healthcare providers are also important in maintaining data security. Agency responsibilities include protecting data from unauthorized use, destruction, or disclosure, and controlling data input and output. Individuals are also accountable for managing data responsibly.

To protect data from unauthorized use, destruction, or disclosure, agencies should take the following steps:

1. Develop ongoing educational programs to ensure that users understand their responsibilities.
2. Restrict access to data by requiring passwords, personal identification numbers, and/or callback procedures.
3. Develop encoding procedures for sensitive data.
4. Use transaction records to document access and routinely audit these records.
5. Develop biometric methods such as electronic signatures, fingerprints, iris scans, or retina prints to identify users.
6. Protect systems from natural disasters; locate them in areas safe from water and other potential physical damage.
7. Develop backup procedures and redundant systems so that data are not lost accidentally. In many cases data stored on an individual PC's hard drive is not backed up when the network file servers or other hospital servers are backed up; instead, the individual is responsible for developing a system to back up these data.
8. Develop and enforce policies for breaches of security.
9. Store only needed data.
10. Dispose of unneeded printouts by shredding.
11. Develop alerts that identify potentially inaccurate data such as a weight of 1200 lb or a blood pressure of 80/130 mm Hg.

To manage data responsibly, individuals should follow these guidelines:

1. Avoid distractions and other factors that may result in data entry errors.
2. Refuse to share a password or sign in with another person's password.
3. Attend implementation/orientation classes and clearly understand institutional policies and procedures.
4. Keep the monitor screen and data out of view of other persons.
5. Develop passwords that include numbers and letters and are not easy to identify.
6. Keep your own password and means of access to data secure.
7. Report unusual computer activity and potential breaches of security.
8. Encourage patients to understand their rights to privacy and confidentiality.
9. Keep harmful materials such as food, drink, and smoke away from computers.

Tools for Protecting Your PC

Most healthcare agencies store information on large computers and have policies for protecting these data. However, PCs and laptops are spread throughout the institution and are much more difficult to monitor. With the increased connectivity that prevails today, many of these PCs are connected to a LAN, thereby creating an intranet. In addition, many of these computers are connected to the Internet. Although this type of increased connectivity makes it easier to monitor PCs, it also increases their risk of exposure, whether in the form of inappropriate access or in the form of worms and viruses. Now that the Internet is used to access information, including health information, it is important to know how to safeguard that information on the PC. The tools discussed next may be used to protect a PC.

Antivirus Software

Computer viruses are malicious software programs that replicate themselves as they spread from one computer to another. They carry a payload that can destroy files, damage hardware, and/or launch an attack on other computers. Often the user is not aware that his or her computer has been infected with a virus until the damage is done. Antivirus software scans the computer, email, and downloaded files to identify and disable virus software. Several companies produce and sell this type of software. Students should check whether free versions are available from their university or ISP before purchasing any of these programs.

The majority of new computers are now sold with antivirus software already installed. There is wide variation on how long this software is current and able to be updated on a regular basis. Sometimes the coverage is a trial version that remains valid for only a few weeks or months. New viruses, however, are being developed and spread every day. Therefore, when installing new antivirus software, make sure that you configure this software to obtain regular updates and perform scheduled scans of your computer. Updates require that your computer be able to access the Internet and download new files from the vendor for your antivirus software. Most antivirus software will alert you when your subscription for updating is running out and new software must be obtained. An increasing number of antivirus software vendors are bundling anti-spyware software with the antivirus software.

Anti-spyware Software

By definition, a spyware program is a type of computer software designed to install itself on your computer and then send personal data back to a central service without your permission or knowledge. The information is secretly obtained by logging keystrokes, recording Web browsing history, and scanning documents on the computer's hard disk. **Table 13-4** lists the symptoms indicating that a virus infection might be affecting a computer.

Adware is a specific type of spyware designed to collect data for targeted advertisements directed to your computer. As this type of software is becoming more powerful, there is increasing concern about the amount and type of personal data collected by many well-known companies without the knowledge of Internet users. For example, Google, in describing a new program announced in their official blog, wrote, "We think we can make online advertising even more relevant and useful by using additional information about the websites people

TABLE 13-4   SYMPTOMS OF A VIRUS AND/OR SPYWARE
• Computer performance is slow
• Recurring pop-up ads appear
• Your home page changes and resets back to the same home page after this change is corrected
• Anti-spyware or antivirus software is turned off
• New or different browser icons appear
• The Windows system freezes or crashes
• Emails are returned that you never sent
• The hard drive light is constantly lit
• The Windows Control Panel Add or Remove Programs feature shows the presence of a new program
• Frequent alerts from your firewall signal an unknown program or process trying to access the Internet

visit." Given the large number of people who search the Internet for health information, collecting these kinds of data raises important issues.

Cookies are small pieces of data that a Web site puts on your computer. They usually consist of a string of characters that identifies you to the site—something like an account number. Cookies can be useful and make the Internet more efficient. In most cases, cookies do not send personal information back to a central server, but third-party cookies may be used to track Web sites that you visit and report those visits to other third-party Web sites such as those described above. Anti-spyware software identifies and deletes spyware.

Firewall

A firewall is a piece of hardware or a software program created to secure the interactions between an organization's inside network of computers and the external computer environment. It achieves this goal by blocking access to the networked computer from the Internet and by blocking programs on the computer from accessing the Internet. By blocking access to your computer, a firewall can prevent a hacker or malicious software from gaining access to your computer. It can also prevent these types of problems from persisting on your computer and spreading to others.

Both the Windows Vista and Windows XP operating systems include a built-in firewall that should be turned on at all times. If you are accessing a network, such as a wireless network in your home, be sure that the network is also protected by its own firewall. To access the firewall in Windows, go to **Start**, **Control Panel**, and **Security**. Windows Vista will also let you select specific programs that can access your computer or access the Internet from your computer. For example, automatic updates that are part of your antivirus and anti-spyware software, as well as Windows access, require free passage through the firewall.

Web Browser Security Settings

Because your browser is your connection to the Internet, it is important that you configure your browser to ensure your computer's protection. This protection can include a phishing filter, a pop-up blocker, notification that a Web site is trying to download files or software onto your computer, and notification if a program's digital signature is current and correct when you are trying to download a program or files. Your browser can also provide you with a 128-bit secure connection for activities such as interaction with online medical sites. With this protection, when you visit a Web site whose URL starts with "https," a small padlock symbol appears in the browser window. This symbol indicates that the Web site is secured using a digital certificate issued by one of the few trusted Certification Authorities (CAs).

Because each browser has its own procedure for configuration, you must look around on the browser to find the appropriate settings; use the browser's help section to ensure that you have provided your computer with the highest level of protection possible. Note that some sites that you might access, such as your school's email or course management software for online courses, may require certain settings be turned on. For example, Blackboard—a type of course management software for delivering online and Web-enhanced courses—requires that cookies and JavaScripts be enabled for that Web site.

Password Protection

You can control who has access to all of the files on your computer by password-protecting the computer itself. In addition, individual files can be password protected. However, be sure to use good password design to ensure your password is not easily guessed and one that you can remember. Files protected by passwords are lost if you can't remember the password. They can NOT be reset by IT like your network password. **Table 13-5** provides guidelines on creating strong passwords.

If you are using a home wireless network like those provided by many broadband services, make sure the network is password protected. If it is not password protected, anyone with a wireless card can access the connection when in range.

TABLE 13-5   DO'S AND DON'TS FOR CREATING STRONG PASSWORDS

- Use at least eight (or more) characters.
- Combine letters and symbols.
- Use both lowercase and uppercase letters.
- Select characters from the whole keyboard.
- Use a blank password only if your computer is physically secure.
- Do not use the same password for several different accounts.
- Do not rely on Web sites emailing you your "lost or forgotten" password on a regular basis.
- Write the password down and store it in a safe place.
- Change the password regularly.
- Do not use your password on public computers.
- Avoid using your name, Social Security number, birth date, or other data that can be associated with you in your password. This includes names spelled backward.
- Avoid dictionary words or common communication abbreviations such as LOL or ICU.
- Do not repeat characters.
- Create a complete sentence and use the first letter from each word with numbers in the middle.

User Guidelines for Protecting Your PC

While some of the same guidelines related to safety and security of larger computers are important for the PC, additional guidelines apply when you seek to protect the PC system and its data. Often individuals are concerned about the privacy of information on their computers and about the information that may be accessed on their PCs when they use the Internet. The following is a summary of action steps to protect the data on your PC.

Protecting Your Email
- Configure your virus checker to scan all email and downloaded files as they come in.
- Install a virus checker to routinely scan your computer's hard drive(s).
- Do not open email or attachments if you do not know the sender.
- If you use a filter to screen your mail, remember to empty the mailbox where the junk mail is being sent.
- Scan all email attachments before opening them. Do *not* set your mailer to automatically open attachments.
- Use whatever methods your email system provides to protect your mail from snooping, tampering, and forgery.

Downloading Files
- Download data only from reputable systems that are regularly checked for viruses.
- Develop a habit of scanning suspect files, downloaded files from unknown sites, and data storage devices given to you by others before opening the files.

Using the Internet
- Install and routinely update a firewall.
- Do not stay connected to the Internet for long periods when access to the Internet is not being used.
- If others have access to the computer, install a password so that the password is required to sign on to the Internet.
- Don't tape passwords on the wall or hide them under your keyboard.
- Use only reputable online backup services.

Protecting Your Computer Hardware and Software
- Use an approved surge protector. Remember—a power strip may or may not provide surge protection.
- Load only sealed software from a reputable vendor.

Protecting Your Data
- Regularly perform system backups and rotate the storage media used for the backup procedure.
- If data are lost due to a virus, scan the backups before installing them to ensure you are not reinstalling the virus.
- Do not store backups in the same area as the computer.

- Store sensitive data on a secure external hard drive, and store the hard drive in a locked area.
- Name sensitive files cryptically.
- Hide important files by using utilities and other devices.
- Shred paper output before disposing of it.
- Label storage media such as CDs and DVDs so that you have easy access to the contents of a disc.
- Eliminate old or unnecessary backup files.

Protecting Your Personal Identity

- Examine the implications of where your email address is listed and the use of other information you provide to your online service provider and other Internet resources you use.
- Never give out personal information on a chat room or an online discussion group.
- Check **NO**. Many online companies give you the option to have your email address be used for sending future information. Check **No** if you do not want that service and want to ensure that your email address is not passed on to others.
- Use the secure server when you are given that option. A secure server provides additional protection when you are sending private information such as a credit card number via the Internet.
- Keep one credit card for Internet use only. Some credit card companies will issue a second card with a different number for just this purpose.
- Look for the padlock icon. When you are sending data to a private Internet site, such as your bank, look for the padlock icon on the screen. This icon signifies your data are encrypted and you are on a secure site. Alternatively, look for the http to be https for a secure server.
- Know the policies related to using email. If you transfer messages from your ISP to your own computer, you will have more privacy protection than if you leave those messages on the provider's server.
- Recognize that to make some Web sites work, you will need a cookie on your computer. A cookie—a small file sent to your hard drive when you interact with certain Web sites—contains information about what you did on that Web site and, in some instances, communicates personal preferences when on the site. Cookies do not scan your hard drive and are read only by the site or site group that originally sent the file. These may be deleted either manually or automatically by some spyware programs.

Providing Patient Care via Computer

While most healthcare providers are well aware of the computer as a tool for documenting care and managing the healthcare record, that application is only the beginning of how computers are used to deliver care and communicate with patients, clients, and consumers. Three key areas of health care now dealing with major security issues in electronic communication include (1) the electronic transmission of personal health information (PHI), (2) the use of the Web as a health information and emotional support resource, and (3) the use of email between healthcare providers and clients.

Federal Regulations and Guidelines for the Exchange of Personal Health Information

In their early days, healthcare information systems consisted of individual computer systems designed for specific functions. Over time, however, healthcare providers began networking these islands of information. The early networks were simple. For example, one of the early interfaces involved connecting the lab to the clinical units so that lab results could be quickly transmitted back to the clinical unit.

Today, the United States is building a National Health Information Infrastructure (NHII). NHII is a comprehensive network of interoperable network systems transmitting clinical, public health, and personal health information, with the goal of improving decision making by making health information available when and where it is needed (U.S. Department of Health and Human Services, n.d.). Needless to say, a major concern is the security of the personal health data within the NHII.

The Health Insurance Portability and Accountability Act of 1996 (HIPAA), which has as its goal the simplification of the administrative processes used to transmit electronic health information, represents a major step forward in building the needed security standards, policies, and procedures. This law established standards for transmitting health data, including standards for transmitting PHI. These standards were the first federal regulations to address privacy and security of PHI. In December 2008, the U.S. Department of Health and Human Services' Office of the National Coordinator for Health Information Technology released *The Nationwide Privacy and Security Framework for Electronic Exchange of Individually Identifiable Health Information*:

> The principles below establish a single, consistent approach to address the privacy and security challenges related to electronic health information exchange through a network for all persons, regardless of the legal framework that may apply to a particular organization. The goal of this effort is to establish a policy framework for electronic health information exchange that can help guide the Nation's adoption of health information technologies and help improve the availability of health information and health care quality. The principles have been designed to establish the roles of individuals and the responsibilities of those who hold and exchange electronic individually identifiable health information through a network (Office of the National Coordinator for Health Information Technology, 2008, p. 1).

On the same day this document was released, the Office of Civil Rights published the new HIPAA Privacy Rule guidance documents consistent with *The Nationwide*

Privacy and Security Framework for Electronic Exchange of Individually Identifiable Health Information (Privacy and Security Framework). These new guidance documents discuss how the Privacy Rule can facilitate the electronic exchange of health information (U.S. Department of Health and Welfare, Office of Civil Rights, 2008). The principles underlying both of these documents are listed in **Table 13-6**.

The Web as a Health Information and Emotional Support Resource

Web sites are fast becoming a major—if not *the* major—source of health information for the general public. Discussion boards and online discussion groups on the Internet are also emerging as a major source of emotional support for those facing difficult health issues. The use of Web sites as communication tools and related security issues are discussed in Chapter 10.

Email and Security Issues

While many physicians and other healthcare providers have been hesitant to use email communication with patients, increasing numbers of patients are requesting this form of communication. Patients are especially interested in scheduling appointments, renewing prescriptions, and getting the answers to health questions via this medium. Healthcare providers are often reluctant to engage in such communication because of concerns related to security issues, malpractice, and the possibility they will not be able to manage the increased workload.

Nevertheless, increasing numbers of healthcare providers are now using this resource to communicate with patients. Two factors have encouraged this change. First, HIPAA requires that email be encrypted. Second, Danny Sands, a primary care physician, and others have become champions for patient–physician email communication; as a result of their work, the American Medical Association and the American Medical Informatics Association have developed email guidelines. These and other guidelines can be accessed at http://134.174.100.34/. Safe use of email communication, however, requires educating both the healthcare provider and the healthcare receiver.

Summary

Storing data and exchanging data via the computer raises several privacy, security, and confidentiality concerns. This chapter focused on issues related to confidentiality and privacy of data, as well as methods to ensure the integrity of data, software, and hardware. Securing computers and the data they store poses a challenge both for large healthcare information systems and for individuals using PCs. The development of the Internet has created a whole new level of opportunity—and a source of concern. Protecting the privacy of patients and the integrity of their health-related data depends on carefully drafted laws and on educating both the provider and the consumer of health care.

TABLE 13-6   PRINCIPLES OF *THE NATIONWIDE PRIVACY AND SECURITY FRAMEWORK FOR ELECTRONIC EXCHANGE OF INDIVIDUALLY IDENTIFIABLE HEALTH INFORMATION*

Principle	Description
Individual access	Individuals should be provided with a simple and timely means to access and obtain their individually identifiable health information in a readable form and format.
Correction	Individuals should be provided with a timely means to dispute the accuracy or integrity of their individually identifiable health information, and to have erroneous information corrected or to have a dispute documented if their requests are denied.
Openness and transparency	There should be openness and transparency about policies, procedures, and technologies that directly affect individuals and/or their individually identifiable health information.
Individual choice	Individuals should be provided with a reasonable opportunity and capability to make informed decisions about the collection, use, and disclosure of their individually identifiable health information.
Collection, use, and disclosure limitation	Individually identifiable health information should be collected, used, and/or disclosed only to the extent necessary to accomplish a specified purpose(s) and never to discriminate inappropriately.
Data quality and integrity	Persons and entities should take reasonable steps to ensure that individually identifiable health information is complete, accurate, and up-to-date to the extent necessary for the person's or entity's intended purposes and that the information has not been altered or destroyed in an unauthorized manner.
Safeguards	Individually identifiable health information should be protected with reasonable administrative, technical, and physical safeguards to ensure its confidentiality, integrity, and availability and to prevent unauthorized or inappropriate access, use, or disclosure.
Accountability	These principles should be implemented, and adherence assured, through appropriate monitoring and other means and methods should be in place to report and mitigate nonadherence and breaches.

Source: The information in this table was developed from information taken from the following Web page: http://healthit.hhs.gov/portal/server.pt?open=512&objID=1173&parentname=CommunityPage&parentid= 34&mode=2&in_hi_userid=10732&cached=true.

References

Burke, L., & Weill, B. (2005). *Information technology for the health professions.* Upper Saddle River, NJ: Prentice Hall.

Center for Democracy and Technology (CDT). (2009). CDT's guide to online privacy: Getting started: Top ten ways to protect privacy. Retrieved January 2, 2009, from http://www.cdt.org/privacy/guide/.

Computer Crime and Intellectual Property Section (CCIPS), United States Department of Justice. (2007). Prosecuting computer crimes. Retrieved January 3, 2009, from http://www.usdoj.gov/criminal/cybercrime/ccmanual/index.html. (This manual is maintained online and can be downloaded as a PDF file. The online version of the manual includes sections that have been added since the copyright date of 2007, including the section referenced here.)

Federal Trade Commission a. (n.d.). Fighting back against identify theft: About identify theft. Retrieved January 2, 2009, from http://www.ftc.gov/bcp/edu/microsites/idtheft/consumers/about-identity-theft.html.

Federal Trade Commission b. (n.d.). Fighting back against identify theft: Resolving specific identify theft problems. Retrieved January 2, 2009, from http://www.ftc.gov/bcp/edu/microsites/idtheft/consumers/resolving-specific-id-theft-problems.html.

For the record: Protecting electronic health information. (1997). Retrieved September 24, 2004, from http://www.nap.edu/openbook/0309056977/html/54.html.

Google. (2009). Making ads more interesting. Retrieved May 31, 2009, from http://googleblog.blogspot.com/2009/03/making-ads-more-interesting.html.

Johnson, E. M. (2009). Data hemorrhages in the health-care sector. Paper presented at Financial Cryptography and Data Security '09 the Thirteenth International Conference of International Financial Cryptography Association. February 23–26, 2009. Retrieved May 31, 2009, from http://fc09.ifca.ai/papers/54_Data_Hemorrhages.pdf.

MIB: About us. (2009). Retrieved January 2, 2009, from http://www.mib.com/html/about_mib_inc.html.

Obama, B. (2009). Remarks by the President on securing our nation's cyber infrastructure. Retrieved May 31, 2009, from http://www.whitehouse.gov/the_press_office/Remarks-by-the-President-on-Securing-Our-Nations-Cyber-Infrastructure/.

Ornstein, C. (2009). Kaiser hospital fined $250,000 for privacy breach in octuplet case. *Los Angeles Times*, May 15, 2009. Retrieved May 31, 2009, from http://www.latimes.com/news/local/la-me-privacy15-2009may15,0,2916906.story.

The Privacy Manager. (2003). Medical records put on flyer. Retrieved January 2, 2009, from http://groups.google.com.ua/group/comp.society.privacy/browse_thread/thread/06b60505cc04bbf2.

Private Rights Clearinghouse. (2008). Fact sheet 8: Medical records privacy. Retrieved January 2, 2009, from http://www.privacyrights.org/fs/fs8-med.htm.

Roach, J. R., Hoban, R. G., Broccolo, B. M., Roth, A. B., & Blanchard, T. P. (2006). *Medical records and the law* (4th ed.). Sudbury, MA: Jones and Bartlett.

Roker, A. (2004). Al's journal. Retrieved January 2, 2009, from http://www.alroker.com/journal_archive_display.cfm?journal_id=5527.

SANS Institute. (2004). Federal computer crime laws. SANS Institute, InfoSec Reading Room. Retrieved May 31, 2009, from http://www.sans.org/reading_room/whitepapers/legal/federal_computer_crime_laws_1446?show=1446.php&cat=legal.

U.S. Department of Health and Human Services. (n.d.). FAQs about NHII. Retrieved January 3, 2009, from http://aspe.hhs.gov/sp/NHII/FAQ.html.

U.S. Department of Health and Human Services, Office of the National Coordinator for Health Information Technology. (2008). Nationwide privacy and security framework for electronic exchange of individually identifiable health information. Retrieved January 2, 2009, from http://www.hhs.gov/healthit/privacy/framework.html.

U.S. Department of Health and Human Welfare, Office of Civil Rights. (2008). The HIPAA privacy rule and health information technology (HIT). Retrieved January 2, 2009, from http://www.hhs.gov/ocr/hipaa/hit/.

EXERCISE 1 Applying Ethical Concepts in Using Computers

■ **Objectives**

1. Apply ethical concepts in making decisions about the use of computers in commonly encountered situations.
2. Clarify your personal attitude about the ethical use of computer hardware and software.

■ **Activity**

As a professional in health care, you will be expected to make ethical decisions about the appropriate use of computers. Start this exercise by first reviewing the codes of ethics posted on the following sites. As you review these documents, pay special attention to the sections on privacy and confidentiality. If you do not understand the concept of ethics, use this definition obtained from Merriam-Webster Online dictionary: "the discipline dealing with what is good and bad and with moral duty and obligation" (Ethic, 2009). It is a set of standards that tells us how we should behave.

Professional Association	URL for the Code of Ethics
American Medical Association (AMA)	http://www.ama-assn.org/ama/pub/physician-resources/medical-ethics/code-medical-ethics.shtml
American Medical Informatics Association	http://www.amia.org/inside/code#
American Nurses Association	http://nursingworld.org/ethics/code/protected_nwcoe813.htm
Association for Computing Machinery (ACM)	http://www.acm.org/about/code-of-ethics
International Medical Informatics Association (IMIA)	http://ethics.iit.edu/codes/coe/int.medical.informatics.assoc.html

Professional Association	URL for the Code of Ethics
National Association of Social Workers (NASW)	http://www.socialworkers.org/pubs/code/code.asp
American Occupational Therapy Association	http://www.aota.org/Practitioners/Ethics/Docs.aspx
American Health Information Management Association	http://library.ahima.org/xpedio/groups/public/documents/ahima/bok1_024277.hcsp?dDocName=bok1_024277

Beside each situation below, place a check by the term that best reflects your opinion of the behavior of the individual. Provide your reasoning for each of your answers.

1. Kevin, a student who is enrolled in a computer class for which a lab fee is charged, gives his password to Beth, another student who is not enrolled in the class. The password allows access to the school computer. The unauthorized student uses three hours of computer time in a time-sharing environment.

   Kevin (enrolled in class):
   Ethical___ Unethical___ Computer crime___
   Beth (not enrolled in class):
   Ethical___ Unethical___ Computer crime___

2. A physical therapist gives his password to a friend who is a graduate student in PT so that she can review a patient record and extract the data needed for a clinical paper. The graduate student has access to the paper record when he is in the clinical unit.

   Physical therapist:
   Ethical___ Unethical___ Computer crime___
   Graduate student:
   Ethical___ Unethical___ Computer crime___

3. A copy of a commercial word-processing package distributed as part of class materials is given to a friend who will be taking the course next term.

   Ethical___ Unethical___ Computer crime___

4. Using a computer terminal, a healthcare worker breaks a security code and reviews confidential patient data. No use is made of the information. "I was just curious" is the response when caught.

   Ethical___ Unethical___ Computer crime___

5. Brian is creating a Web page and finds a terrific background on another page. He copies the background to use on his page.

   Ethical____ Unethical____ Computer crime____

6. Several healthcare providers are collaborating on an important research study. The Hospital Board of Review has been slow to give permission for data collection via computerized patient records. The research team members, who are experienced with computer systems, decide to go ahead and begin data collection while waiting to hear from the Review Board.

   Ethical____ Unethical____ Computer crime____

7. Terry lurks on an online discussion group that provides a thought-provoking discussion about AIDS. The student takes some of the ideas from the online discussion group and incorporates them into a paper he is writing, but does not include the source so as to ensure the privacy of people on the list.

   Ethical____ Unethical____ Computer crime____

8. Judy downloads a file that is labeled shareware, useable for 45 days; if further use is desired, payment is requested. Judy really likes the program and continues to use it after the trial period without sending any payment.

   Ethical____ Unethical____ Computer crime____

9. Dr. Bob is teaching a computer course. The university purchased a site license for 25 copies of the software he is distributing to students. However, 25 students are registered for the course. Dr. Bob makes a copy of the software for himself and distributes one copy to each student.

   Ethical____ Unethical____ Computer crime____

10. James is completing his senior year as a nursing student in a BSN program. A patient he has cared for a few weeks ago obtained his email address from the online university directory and has sent him an email. In the email the patient discussed new and potentially serious symptoms. James forwards the email to the charge nurse on the unit where the patient was treated and to the senior resident involved in the patient's care.

    Ethical____ Unethical____ Computer crime____

Reference:
Ethic. (2009). In *Merriam-Webster Online Dictionary*. Retrieved June 10, 2009, from http://www.merriam-webster.com/dictionary/ethic.

EXERCISE 2 Discovering Personal Information on the Internet

■ Objectives
   1. Gain an appreciation of the personal information available on the Web.
   2. Understand the options you have and do not have in protecting your private information.

■ Activity
   1. Use an Internet search engine to search for your professor's name on the Internet. Now search for the names of the authors of this book. Then search for your name. Note what information you found in each case and what you were able to learn about these people and yourself. Did you find any sites that offered information for a price?
   2. Go to **www.google.com** and put in your home phone number or your parents' home phone number with the area code in the following form: 1233451790. Click on the map. Were you able to locate your home?
   3. Go to **Google Earth** and download the software needed to use this service. Did you see the following option: *Help make this software better by sending anonymous usage statistics and crash reports to Google.* What do you think would be the advantages and disadvantages of checking this box? Were you able to find your home? Was there a familiar car in the driveway or on the road in front of your home?
   4. Search at **www.zabasearch.com** using your name, your parents' names, and your professor's name. Were you able to find information on each of these people? Do you know if the information is accurate?
   5. Using your word processor, write a brief paper explaining what you learned from this exercise and your reaction to this information. Save this file as **Chap13-Ex1-YourLastname**. If you are using a discussion board, respond to the discussion thread on this exercise.

EXERCISE 3 Copyright and Privacy Issues

■ Objectives
   1. Describe copyright restrictions and the fair use doctrine.
   2. Identify methods for adhering to copyright law when writing a research paper.
   3. Identify some potential security problems when surfing the Web.

■ Activity
   1. Copyright.
      a. Access the following Web sites: **http://www.lib.utsystem.edu/copy right/** and **http://www.copyright.gov/circs/circ01.pdf**. Complete the tutorial on the first site and review the second site.

    b. Answer the following questions, typing the answers in Word:

      1. What is a copyright?

      2. What is fair use?

      3. What is the public domain?

      4. What are the guidelines for including information in a research paper to be in compliance with the copyright law?

      5. How do you cite a Web site in a reference list? How do you cite an email message?

    c. Call the file **Chap13-Ex3-YourLastname**. Submit it as directed by your professor.

2. Privacy.

    a. Use several different Internet search sites to search for your name and the name of one of your professors.

      ■ List each fact you were able to learn about yourself from this search.

      ■ Write a description of your professor using only the information you were able to find on the Internet. If you were unable to find any information about your professor, do the exercise using one of the authors of this book.

    b. Discuss your reaction to the information you found about yourself and your professor (or the author). Consider whether any of the information you found would be helpful or would hinder you if you were applying for a position in health care.

    c. Add this information to the file from part 1, creating a second document called **Privacy**.

EXERCISE 4 Preventing Computer Crime

■ **Objectives**

1. Apply information about computer crimes to prevent these crimes in commonly encountered situations.
2. Understand current laws as they apply to computer crimes.

■ **Situation**

During the school year, you are living in a dorm and share a computer with your roommate. The rest of the time, you live at home and share a computer with your family. In both cases, you are concerned that you as well as the other persons involved are at risk of being the victim of a computer crime.

■ **Activity**

1. Review the materials that are available from the sites listed in Table 13-1 and Table 13-2.

2. Search for Web sites that provide information about protecting your computer, data, and software, such as **http://www.microsoft.com/athome/security/computer/default.mspx?wt.svl=Left_nav**.

3. Write a set of guidelines that can be used in each situation described in the scenario.

4. Describe how you would encourage others to use these guidelines.

5. Save this document as **Chap13-Ex4-YourLastname**. Submit it as directed by the professor.

ASSIGNMENT 1 Using Internet Materials

■ **Directions**

1. You are a part of a student group that has been assigned the task of developing some guidelines for using materials on the Internet in such a way as to prevent copyright infringements.

2. Go to some of the following addresses, or find your own sites, to help you develop your guidelines:

   http://www.templetons.com/brad/copymyths.htm

   http://www.bitlaw.com/copyright/fair_use.html

   http://palimpsest.stanford.edu/bytopic/intprop/#faq

   http://www.lib.byu.edu/departs/copyright/tutorial/intro/page1.htm

   http://www.plagiarism.org/

3. Use a Word brochure template and create a three-panel, two-sided brochure that lists those guidelines. Use a variety of fonts, bold, italics, underlining, graphics, and other formatting features so that the brochure has an eye-catching format. See **Figure 13-1** for an example template. Be creative.

4. Save the file as **Chap13-Assign1-YourLastName**. Submit your brochure as directed by your professor.

ASSIGNMENT 2 Computer Use Guidelines

■ **Situation**

You are expecting an influx of newly hired personnel who will use the laptops now available in your healthcare agency. You want to encourage their use, yet protect the agency from misuse of this equipment. There is a variety of software available on CD-ROMs as well as on the hard drives of the computers. You expect the new personnel will use this equipment to prepare patient summaries, develop quality assurance reports, document supply inventories, and record patient visits.

Your charge is twofold: (1) prepare a handout of guidelines and (2) prepare a short PowerPoint-based orientation to the laptops including these guidelines. This presentation will be shown during the employees' orientation.

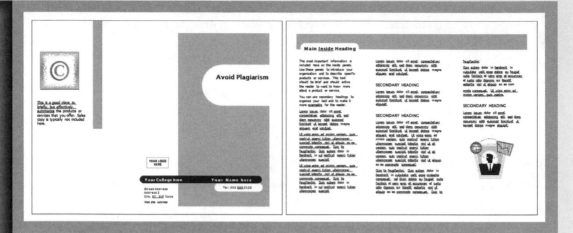

Figure 13-1 Sample Brochure Template

■ **Directions**

1. Use Word to prepare a separate list of issues and guidelines that you can give to the new users. Your guidelines should help increase awareness of how they can use the laptops in ways that will protect patient privacy and confidentiality and that will promote the safety and security of the computer data and equipment. Make sure to format the guidelines appropriately, including any graphics that might reinforce them.

2. Save this file as **Chap13-Assign2-Lastname.docx**. Submit your list of safety and security issues and your guidelines to your instructor.

3. Because you know that some of the newly hired people are already oriented to multimedia, create a short PowerPoint presentation that will be shown during their employee orientation. This presentation will also be loaded on the laptops to provide a quick reference for them. Make sure to follow the guidelines for quality presentations. Set the program to run automatically.

4. Save this presentation as **Chap13-Assign2-Lastname.docx**.

ASSIGNMENT 3 Issue Critique

■ **Directions**

1. Select one of the following statements to critique:

   a. "There is nothing wrong with breaking security if you accomplish something useful and leave things the way you found them."

   b. "The healthcare agency owns the data in its computers and, therefore, is free to do whatever it chooses with those data."

    c. "In the long run, when simple rules are followed, computer records are more secure than hard copy records."

    d. "There is nothing wrong with breaking security if the only records you are looking at are your own."

2. Use Word to prepare a one- to two-page paper identifying points that support or refute the statement you select. End the paper by stating your position and your reasons for that position.

3. Save the file as **Chap13-Assign3-YourLastname**. Submit your paper.

> NOTE: If this course has an online component, this assignment may be part of a discussion forum requirement, where you will support or refute the statement selected and respond to classmates' posts.

ASSIGNMENT 4 Email Guidelines

■ **Situation**

In the school that your children attend, the school nurse has reported that both students and teachers are sending her email using both the school intranet and the Internet. You have been asked to help the nurse write a set of email guidelines for the teachers and the students.

■ **Directions**

1. Use Word and create these guidelines. Run a readability index on the document to be sure that the reading level is appropriate for the students.

2. Save the file as **Chap13-Assign4-YourLastname**. Submit the guidelines.

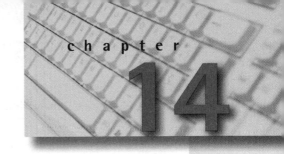

Healthcare Informatics and Information Systems

Objectives

1. Define healthcare informatics using the concepts of data, information, knowledge, and wisdom.
2. Describe automated healthcare delivery systems.
3. Discuss types of healthcare data and explain how the integration of these data influences the effectiveness of healthcare information systems.
4. Identify selected types and levels of computer-related personnel.
5. Differentiate between computer literacy, information literacy, computer-assisted instruction, and healthcare informatics.

In 2002, more than 150 experts from health professions education, regulation, policy, advocacy, quality, and industry attended a Health Professions Education Summit. Their goal was to assist the Institute of Medicine (IOM) Committee on Health Profession Education Summit to develop strategies to ensure that educational systems for health professionals were consistent with the principles of the twenty-first-century health system. Based on this summit, key position papers, and other resources, the IOM issued a seminal report titled *Health Professions Education: A Bridge to Quality* (Greiner & Knebel, 2003).

The report stated that doctors, nurses, pharmacists, and other health professionals are not adequately prepared to provide the highest-quality and safest medical care possible. To meet this challenge, the report called upon educators as well as accreditation, licensing, and certification organizations to ensure that students and working professionals develop and maintain proficiency in five core areas: patient-centered care, interdisciplinary teams, evidence-based practice, quality improvement, and informatics.

The IOM publication established the need for healthcare professionals to be computer, information, and informatics literate and called upon the health professions to make this a reality. Several of the health professional organizations have taken up this call. For example, the Joint Task Force of the American Health Information Management Association (AHIMA) and the American Medical Informatics Association (AMIA) focused on the education of healthcare workforce as shown in the follow example:

> There are several important cross-cutting issues, including the wide variety of health professionals—from physicians and nurses to therapists and admissions staff—who are or will be using Electronic Health Records (EHRs) as part of their day-to-day activities. This, in turn, has an impact on the broad range of training needed, from basic computer literacy to more sophisticated computer applications and health (AHIMA & AMIA, 2008, p. 5).

In nursing, this call was answered by the American Nurses Association (ANA), the National League for Nursing (NLN), and the American Association of Colleges of Nursing (AACN). The ANA's report *Nursing Informatics: Scope and Standards of Nursing Informatics Practice* (2008) identified informatics competencies that are required of all nurses. "These competencies are categorized in three overall areas: computer literacy, information literacy, and professional development/leadership" (ANA, 2008, p. 36).

In 2008, both the NLN and the AACN documented the need for computer, information, and informatics literacy within nursing. The AACN stated in the revised *Essentials of Baccalaureate Education for Professional Nursing Practice* that "Computer and information literacy are crucial to the future of nursing" (2008, p. 17). The NLN went one step further, pointing out the need for nursing faculty and administration to be prepared to provide the needed education. The NLN's recommendations for faculty and administration preparation are outlined in the position paper entitled *Preparing the Next Generation of Nurses to Practice in a Technology-Rich Environment: An Informatics Agenda.*

This book is designed to support healthcare professionals in mastering the computer and information literacy skills needed for safe and effective healthcare delivery. This chapter introduces the healthcare provider to the discipline of healthcare informatics and automated systems commonly used in health care.

Defining Healthcare Informatics and Related Terms

Healthcare informatics is defined as "the study of how healthcare data, information, knowledge, and wisdom are collected, stored, processed, communicated, and used to support the process of healthcare delivery to clients, providers, administrators, and organizations involved in healthcare delivery" (Englebardt & Nelson, 2002, p. xx). It is concerned with the application of information and computer science concepts and theories to the delivery of health care. Healthcare informatics is an interdisciplinary science developed from the integration of information science, computer science, cognitive science, and the healthcare sciences.

Information science focuses on the study of information generation, transmission, and use. The study of information as a science is usually considered to have originated with Shannon and Weaver's (1949) theory of information. Their work focused on the communication of information. Shannon and Weaver's communication model demonstrates the transmission of a message from a sender to a receiver and is the standard used in teaching communication concepts to healthcare providers. Since their work was published, the study of information theory has been approached from several different conceptual frameworks. The primary information model used to explain healthcare informatics was established by Blum (1986). Blum, in giving a historical overview of computers in health care, found the model useful in grouping medical applications according to the objects they processed. He identified three groups of applications: data processing, information processing, and knowledge processing.

Using Blum's model, Graves and Corcoran (1989), in their classic article, "The Study of Nursing Informatics," proposed that nursing informatics includes nursing data, information, and knowledge. Later that same year, Nelson and Joos (1989) proposed the addition of wisdom to this continuum.

Understanding the definition of healthcare informatics requires an understanding of several key terms—*data, information, knowledge,* and *wisdom*—as well as an appreciation of the interrelationships between these concepts. In 2008, the ANA *Nursing Informatics: Scope and Standards of Practice* included wisdom in defining the meta-structures of nursing informatics. The terms and their interrelationships are illustrated in **Figure 14-1**.

Data

Data are raw facts. They exist without meaning or interpretation. Data are the attributes that healthcare professionals collect, organize, and name. The individual elements in a history and physical or a nursing assessment are data elements. For example, the observation that a patient's hair is red, that his weight is 150 pounds, or that his blood sugar is 200 are attributes or raw facts that can be interpreted in many different ways. By itself, each piece of these data is meaningless. The red hair may be the result of illness, a hair color product, or just the natural color. The weight may be too high, too low, or the ideal weight for this individual. Depending on the circumstances, this blood sugar could be normal, indicate that the patient is improving, or indicate that the patient is becoming sicker. The process of populating the fields in a database, as described in Chapter 8, involves entering these types of data elements into the database.

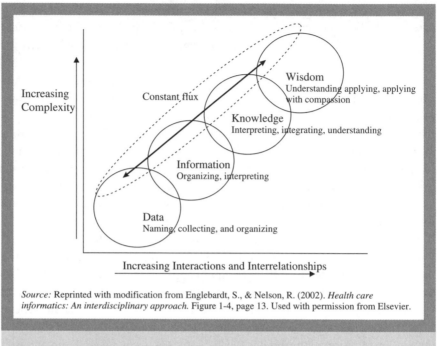

Source: Reprinted with modification from Englebardt, S., & Nelson, R. (2002). *Health care informatics: An interdisciplinary approach.* Figure 1-4, page 13. Used with permission from Elsevier.

Figure 14-1 Data-to-Wisdom Continuum

Information

Information is a collection of data that has been processed to produce meaning. Techniques that are used to process data include classifying, sorting, organizing, summarizing, graphing, and calculating. A number of tools are used to process data, including paper and pencil, short-term memory, and computers. Many of the exercises in this book demonstrate how computers can be used to present, classify, sort, organize, summarize, graph, and calculate data to produce meaningful information. These processes prepare data so that they can be interpreted. The actual interpretation of the data is a cognitive process whereby data are given meaning and become information. Several factors, including education, attitudes, emotions, and goals, influence how these data are interpreted. As a result, each individual gives a unique interpretation to the same collection of data. The various interpretations can be similar, or they can be surprisingly different; however, they are never the same.

For example, suppose a person with newly diagnosed type 2 diabetes has a blood sugar of 350. The client, the physician, and the nurse each place a different significance on this data element; each provides a different interpretation. In other words, this data element is meaningful, but the meaning is different for each individual involved. The physician may interpret this data element as a need for more insulin, the nurse may interpret it as a need for additional patient education, and the client may assume that this blood sugar level is a temporary result attributable to the cake that was eaten the evening before the blood was drawn.

An information system is a system that processes data, organizing the various elements into meaningful units of information. This definition of an information system does not require that the system be automated. However, in healthcare informatics, the focus is on automated information systems that are used in the delivery of care. Many different types of automated healthcare information systems exist, several of which are described later in this chapter.

The key point to remember is that information from these systems may be interpreted and used differently by different healthcare providers. For example, a chart that tracks the increased independence of a client after a cerebral vascular accident presents vital nursing information. This same chart, when interpreted by the physical therapist, provides key rehabilitation information. Although members of both of these disciplines use the same information to make important decisions about the patient's plan of care, the chart has a different significance for the nurse and for the physical therapist. This is why the development of effective interdisciplinary documentation systems that are basic to the electronic health record requires the involvement of each of the healthcare disciplines as well as clients.

It is also important to realize that the same data can produce different types of information. For example, a hospital information system processes order entry data to produce billing information. These same data may be processed by a clinical information system to develop a clinical pathway. Each of these information systems is using the same data, but the information produced is quite different in each case.

Knowledge

While information is built from data, knowledge is built from information and data. Knowledge is a collection of interrelated pieces of information and data. In this aggregation, the interrelationships are as important as the individual items of information. An organized collection of interrelated information about a specific topic is usually referred to as a knowledge base. For example, the statement "This student has a good knowledge base in anatomy" would not sound correct if the word "base" was removed from the statement.

The information in a knowledge base is organized or structured so that interrelationships can be identified. For instance, the table of contents in any textbook provides an outline of a knowledge base. An effective lecture explains how various facts or pieces of information interrelate. By understanding the information and the interrelationships, the learner can understand the concepts and theories that are inherent in the specific knowledge base being explained.

Once the learner develops a knowledge base, the learner uses this knowledge to interpret new data or even reinterpret old data, thereby producing new information. An individual's knowledge base plays a major role in determining how data and information are used in the process of decision making. For example, a diabetic client with an extensive knowledge base about diabetes could be expected to make different decisions than a person with a limited knowledge base in this area.

A professional with an extensive knowledge base is usually referred to as a specialist or expert. In this discussion, a knowledge base is more than just a large collection of information: It also includes the interrelationships between the pieces of information that produce the knowledge base. An expert has built mental processes that provide quick access to a wide array of interrelationships. As a result, the expert has access to a new level of knowledge. An expert looks at a patient and sees the patient and his or her problems as a whole; in other words, the expert has a gestalt view. In contrast, a novice looks at the same patient and sees only pieces of the information. A novice does not have the quick mental access to all of the interrelationships that the expert has and cannot always see the entire picture of what is happening with a patient. Whereas an expert can look at a client and understand immediately just how sick or anxious that client is, a novice may see the same patient and collect the same data, yet not reach the same conclusion.

This difference is one reason why the teaching–learning process in a clinical setting can be such a challenge. The teacher, who has an expert background, will process the same data and information differently from the student. The student will have no idea how the teacher was able to reach a diagnosis, and the teacher may not understand why the student could not see the "obvious."

The same gap can often be seen between healthcare providers and clients. The client's ability to understand and use health information in making healthcare decisions is referred to as health literacy. "Health literacy is defined as the degree to which individuals have the capacity to obtain, process, and understand basic information and services needed to make appropriate decisions regarding their health" (IOM, 2004, p. 2).

A knowledge base can be stored and shared using a variety of media, including oral communication, textbooks, and online databases. As a person gains information, it is added to his or her internal knowledge base. It is this internal knowledge base that one first uses to interpret information and to make decisions. An individual will not go beyond this internal knowledge base unless that person determines that there is an information or knowledge gap. It is very difficult for even an expert to identify what is not known, especially in an area such as health care, where the amount of new knowledge and information is exploding. As a result, there is a keen interest in developing the information literacy skills of healthcare professionals as well as automated decision support systems that can identify information gaps and tap into external knowledge bases.

Automated decision support systems are systems that process information, identifying and demonstrating pertinent interrelationships. These systems may be as simple as the bar chart in **Figure 14-2**, which identifies overtime hours in a healthcare institution, or as complex as a fully automated staffing system. Complexity in this situation refers to how much of the knowledge base is stored in the automated system and to the automated rules used to process the data. With a decision support system, the individual's knowledge base interprets the bar chart. Different nurse managers looking at this same bar chart can and do reach different conclusions about staffing on these units.

Although decision support systems can help in the decision-making process, they do not make decisions. For example, an automated scheduling system can be used to generate a work schedule for staff in a clinical setting. The automated system will likely contain an extensive online knowledge base. The system will "know" several facts about the staff as well as the institution's staffing rules. However, the scheduling system will not decide who will work when. Instead, the professional in charge is responsible for approving the schedule.

Decision support systems are an aid to the decision maker. They provide the decision maker with a more complete picture of the interrelations between the information being considered. Ultimately, though, it is the decision maker who

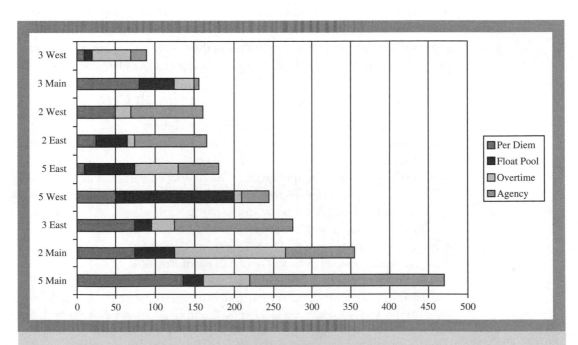

Figure 14-2 Hours of Overtime and Supplemental Staff Used by Clinical Units

interprets the information and decides what action to take. For example, a clinical support system may generate a list of assessment items for a patient with a head injury. This list can be very helpful in ensuring that the healthcare provider does not forget to check a specific assessment item. However, the healthcare provider is still responsible for ensuring that the patient receives a comprehensive and appropriate assessment including areas that are not on the checklist but are nevertheless important because of the patient's overall health status. This is the key difference between a decision support system and an expert system: The healthcare provider makes the decision, not the automated system.

Wisdom

In health care, ethical decision making that ensures cost-effective quality care requires more than an empirical knowledge base. Knowing when and how to use this knowledge is referred to as wisdom. Knowledge makes it possible for a caregiver to explain the stages of death and dying; wisdom makes it possible for the caregiver to use theories related to death and dying to help a terminal patient express anger and frustration. The development of wisdom requires not only empirical knowledge, but also ethical, personal, and aesthetic knowledge.

Currently, there is no way to automate wisdom, although certain aspects of this concept are being built into automated systems. Expert systems are knowledge-based systems that include built-in procedures for determining when and how to use that knowledge. In the future, the development of decision support systems for experts will require a better understanding of the concept of wisdom and the ways in which wisdom influences the decision-making process of expert practitioners.

Automated Information Systems in Health Care

Computer technology has now been infused into almost every aspect of healthcare delivery. Automation in health care began in the late 1960s and early 1970s with systems that were designed to meet specific needs within health care. In most institutions, financial applications were developed first—for example, payroll, billing, and general ledger programs. They were followed by institution-wide applications to manage admission, discharge, and transfer (ADT) processes as well as applications to support the various clinical departments such as laboratory, radiology, or pharmacy. These departmental systems were usually stand-alone systems and were referred to as islands of information.

The first attempts at communication between these stand-alone applications consisted of order entry/results reporting systems. These systems, which were built on the ADT system, were located on the clinical units and communicated with the departmental systems. A unit clerk or nurse selected a patient from the ADT system and entered new orders. These orders were then communicated to the appropriate department. Once the orders were completed, the results were communicated back to the clinical units. In these early systems, a unit clerk or staff nurse was responsible for entering orders that physicians had handwritten on a paper chart.

Today these original order entry systems serve as the basis for computerized provider order entry (CPOE) systems that enable clinicians (e.g., physicians, nurses, therapists, pharmacists) to enter orders for tests, medications, services, or other clinical processes directly into the healthcare information system. To ensure increased accuracy and implementation of evidence-based healthcare delivery, these systems are often supplemented with decision support systems (Agency for Healthcare Research and Quality, 2008).

As the functions performed by the different types of healthcare information systems have expanded, and as the need to integrate the data managed by stand-alone systems has become obvious, larger integrated systems with new and expanded functions have emerged. These new and innovative systems often exist alongside older legacy systems. As a result, modern-day healthcare information systems range from small stand-alone systems (i.e., a scheduling system used to make appointments in a private office) to fully integrated healthcare information systems (i.e., electronic health records maintained by large integrated health delivery systems).

Here, the discussion of automated systems used in health care is divided into three sections. First is an overview of selected types of automated applications used in health care. It is followed by a discussion of the types of data that are processed in automated healthcare information systems—including a discussion of levels of integration. Finally, the systems are discussed in terms of healthcare computing roles.

Automated Applications Used in Healthcare Delivery

This section reviews the types of applications commonly used in healthcare delivery. It is becoming increasingly difficult to classify these diverse applications into specific categories. As vendors have increased the scope of functions offered within their products, their niches have increasingly overlapped. In addition, several information systems companies have been purchased or merged. As a result, many of their products have been integrated or merged. For the purposes of our discussion, automated information systems used in health care will be grouped into five types: healthcare information systems (also known as backbone systems), clinical information systems, administrative information systems, consumer information systems, and personnel management systems.

Healthcare Information Systems

While healthcare automation is increasingly more decentralized—a scheme made possible by network connections between systems—healthcare information systems (HISs) continue to form the backbone of that network within healthcare institutions. Healthcare information systems were originally developed for hospitals. Today, however, they may be located in nursing homes, rehabilitation centers, clinics, private offices, or any other healthcare institution. There are four primary functions for HISs.

First, HISs are often the backbone or primary system used to integrate or interface with the various applications throughout the organization. They communicate information between the point of care or clinical units and the various departments within the institution. This functionality can include sending patient orders to hospital departments and reporting results back to patient health records, as well as requesting supplies and equipment for clinical units or offices. As part of the communication function, HISs may also support the institution's intranet.

Second, HISs manage the ADT process. In doing so, they track the location of all patients while maintaining their demographic data.

Third, these systems almost always interface with the financial systems that are used to track the charges and billing process for the institution.

Fourth, they are used to produce a number of administrative reports that support the daily operations of the institution as well as long-term planning. For example, HISs may be used to print out a list of patients' dietary orders, which in turn can be used to distribute meal trays or track institutional food costs.

Clinical Information Systems

Clinical information systems are used to process patient data and support patient care. Examples of functions in clinical information systems include collecting patient assessment and health status data, developing plans of care, managing order entry processes and results reporting, tracking treatments including medication administration records, developing work lists, and producing reports such as patient problem lists.

Clinical department systems support the daily work of clinical departments as well as populate the appropriate sections of the electronic health record (EHR) through results reporting. The most commonly automated clinical departments include laboratory, radiology, cardiology, and pharmacy. Clinical departmental systems accept patient orders; report results; schedule patients, equipment, and rooms; print labels and work lists; and maintain inventories. The primary benefits of these types of systems include improved efficiency of the department and communication with the clinical units or points of care.

Documentation systems collect assessment and patient status data from a variety of healthcare providers and are increasingly used as interdisciplinary communication tools. The primary uses for these systems include documentation of patient data and the development of plans of care as well as related work lists. These systems can be interfaced to automated monitoring devices, thereby capturing vital signs and other data that are entered directly into the clinical record. Their primary benefit includes improvements in the quality of the documentation through the use of prompts, thereby increasing access to comprehensive client data.

In many healthcare institutions, the clinical information system, documentation system, and healthcare information system are now being integrated to create an EHR. EHR systems grew out of the concept of a computer-based patient record. The EHR is a complete collection of an individual's health-related data. Increasingly, these data are being shared across the total institution, including clinics and private physicians' offices.

The data are collected and managed by an EHR system much as a database management system manages a database. Data from an individual's EHR can be stored in a clinical data repository, which can be conceptualized as a warehouse or large database where all data elements from all the different systems could be stored. This scheme makes it possible to integrate the data and to obtain a different level of information. For example, by integrating the clinical data with the financial data, it becomes possible to evaluate the cost of each problem on the patient problem list. For these systems to be truly effective, a data dictionary that defines each element is required. An example of an EHR as it appears on a computer screen of a provider is depicted in **Figure 14-3** and **Figure 14.4**.

Although the development of the EHR has been evolving for several years, the development of these systems was stimulated in 2003 when U.S. Department of Health and Human Services Secretary Tommy G. Thompson announced a government initiative to build a national electronic healthcare system that would allow patients and their doctors to access their complete medical records anytime and anywhere they are needed (U.S. Department of Health and Human Services, 2003). In 2008, the agenda of the newly elected President Barack Obama provided strong support for the continued development of healthcare information systems, including EHRs.

The Obama Biden will:

> **Lower Health Care Costs by Investing in Electronic Information Technology Systems:** Use health information technology to lower the cost of health care. Invest $10 billion a year over the next five years to move the U.S. health care system to broad adoption of standards-based electronic health information systems, including electronic health records (http://change.gov/agenda/technology_agenda/, 2008).

Administrative Information Systems

Administrative information systems automate the management of data used in the daily operations of the institution as well as data used for strategic and long-range planning. They can be institution-wide systems, such as financial systems, or they can be specific to certain functions, such as acuity or patient classification systems used for staffing.

Classification systems use patient data to classify patients based on the amount and type of care required. For example, a patient with new second- and third-degree burns over 60% of the body may require 6 hours of professional nursing

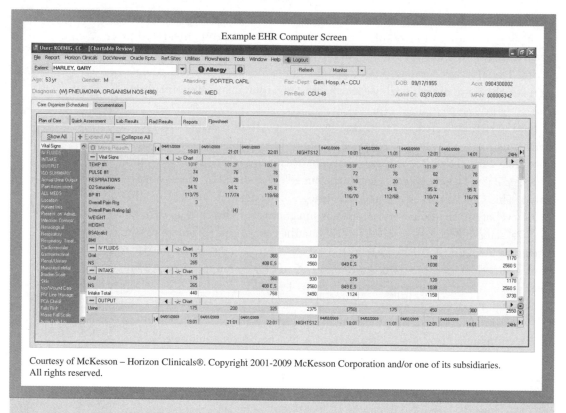

Courtesy of McKesson – Horizon Clinicals®. Copyright 2001-2009 McKesson Corporation and/or one of its subsidiaries. All rights reserved.

Figure 14-3 Example EHR Computer Screen

time during every 8-hour shift. In contrast, a patient who is three days postoperative from open-heart surgery may require 2 hours of professional nursing time per 8-hour shift. The data from classification systems can be used to decide the amount and type of staff assigned to a clinical unit.

Quality assurance systems attempt to measure and report on cost-effective quality care, resulting in a high level of patient satisfaction. Examples of data that are processed in quality assurance systems include patient outcomes or variance reports, performance indicators for providers, infection reports, incident reports, patient satisfaction results, and costing data. These data can be reported for individuals or in aggregate format.

Material management systems are used to manage the supplies and other inventory of an institution. The goal of these systems is to ensure that the right supplies are at the right site with a minimum of overhead costs. These systems can include an online catalog that can be searched, an automatic interface to budget systems, automatic reordering of supplies, and alerts that can be issued when there is a significant increase or decrease in inventory orders or costs.

Example Ambulatory Care Computer Screen

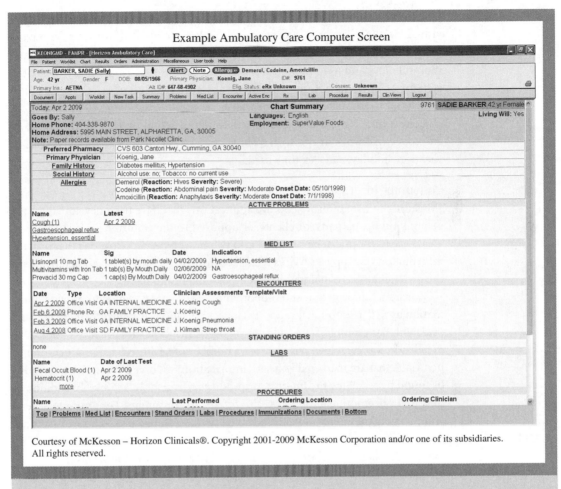

Figure 14-4 Example Ambulatory Care Computer Screen

Financial systems include a combination of information systems that are used to manage and report the financial aspects of the institution. These include systems that track income-related data, such as those related to billing and contract monitoring; systems used to develop and monitor capital and operating budgets; and systems that track costs to the institution such as payroll and cost accounting. Financial systems usually interface with the ADT and personnel systems. For example, the payroll system typically interfaces with the time-and-attendance or scheduling system to track who has worked and during which hours they worked.

Personnel Systems

Personnel systems include a combination of systems that are used to track the characteristics of employees and/or the use of these employees within the institution.

Human resources management or personnel records systems maintain individual employee records. For example, healthcare institutions must know the home address, salary, job title and description, professional license number and renewal date, and a number of other details about each employee. Automated systems make it much easier to maintain accurate data and to search for information about individual employees as well as groups of employees.

Scheduling systems are used to schedule the actual dates and times that an employee will work or not work. These systems can keep a historical record of vacation, holiday, and sick time used.

Consumer Information Systems

Consumer information systems are applications that have been developed for the general public, patients, or clients, as opposed to the traditional care providers. These applications can be classified into two basic types: applications that provide information or support services related to health care and applications that assist the general public in maintaining their personal health data.

Consumer information and support applications are designed to provide information as well as emotional support. These applications vary greatly in quality and oversight. For example, state and federal government agencies provide a number of excellent resources. However, there are a number of health-related products of limited value that are marketed as health information resources. Examples can readily be found by searching the Internet for products useful in weight loss. In addition to information, emotional support is also offered to consumers. For example, several voluntary organizations provide moderated virtual groups where cancer patients can provide information and support for each other, such as the Cancer Survivors Network maintained by the American Cancer Society (http://csn.cancer.org/).

Personal health records (PHR) are applications designed for patients to maintain copies of their own healthcare information. The need for EHR and especially records that can be accessed by patients at the point of need was clearly demonstrated in the aftermath of Hurricane Katrina. One month after the storm, most of the 1 million people displaced by the storm had no medical records, making it dangerous and difficult for healthcare providers working in disaster medical centers and community hospitals to care for these patients (Mann, 2005). The very few patients who were able to provide their own healthcare records were at a significant advantage. PHR applications are being developed by traditional healthcare institutions, insurance companies, employers, and outside vendors such as Google and Microsoft.

Applications established by healthcare institutions can interface with the institution's EHR, thereby ensuring a more comprehensive PHR. A well-designed example of this approach is demonstrated by the Cleveland Clinic (http://my.clevelandclinic.org/eclevelandclinic/mychart/default.aspx). Using MyChart, patients at this facility can see test results and a list of their medications, view reminders and health information, make appointments, request renewals of medications, and engage in many other health-related activities.

Patient-owned PHR applications have also been developed by a number of vendors. Some of these applications store these data on patients' computers; others offer backup services or store these data on the vendor's server. Because the data in these applications are entered by the patients themselves, these PHR are not protected by HIPAA regulations. This issue raises questions about how individual data as well as aggregated patient data may be accessed and used for marketing and other purposes. Examples of larger vendors working in this arena include Microsoft (http://www.healthvault.com/), Google (www.google.com/health), and WebMD (http://www.webmd.com/phr). While these types of PHRs are not currently regulated by HIPAA this is an area of concern as demonstrated by the February 25, 2009, minutes of the Department of Health and Human Services National Committee on Vital and Health Statistics Subcommittee on Privacy, Confidentiality and Security, posted at http://www.ncvhs.hhs.gov/090225t1.htm, and may clearly be regulated in the future.

Setting-Specific Systems

These systems may include any of the functions already discussed (e.g., clinical, financial, and personnel information management); however, the functions are customized for the specific setting. Examples of setting-specific systems include home health systems, physician office systems, outpatient or ambulatory care clinics, nurse center clinics, and emergency room systems.

Types of Automated Data Used in Healthcare Information Systems

To fully understand the impact of automated systems on health care, it is imperative to consider the types of data that are processed. For the purposes of discussion, these data are classified into five major types. Four of these have previously been identified (Nelson, 2004). However, it is important to realize that any one piece of data by itself is without meaning and can, in fact, fall into all of these classifications, albeit in a slightly different way in each case.

Clinical or Client Data

These data include all data that are related to an individual client. A comprehensive collection of the client data is stored in the EHR. An example of this type of data would be a patient's blood pressure or a list of the patient's problems.

Financial Data

These types of data include all of the fiscal data related to the operation of the healthcare institution. Examples include the patient's bill or the budget for an individual unit.

Human Resources Data

These data include all data related to employees as well as individuals who have a contractual relationship with the institution such as physicians, nurses, students, or volunteers.

Material Resources Data

These data refer to all of the tangible resources used in the operation of the healthcare institution—everything from supplies that are purchased externally to supplies that are created internally.

Intellectual Data

These data comprise the factual data that are stored in the various discipline- or subject-specific databases. Examples include a database with information about medications or a database with published articles and research results.

Levels of Data Sharing

The various types of data described previously are processed using healthcare applications. The effectiveness of these applications in supporting quality, cost-effective health care is influenced by the level of data sharing made possible by the overall logic and physical design of the total healthcare information system.

Stand-alone systems do not share data or information with any other computer system. These systems tend to be developed when departments do not trust the institution's systems or when institutional systems do not process data in the format needed by the department. For example, a department may have frequent changes in its work schedule that are difficult to process in the institutional systems. A PC-based scheduling system developed in that department would be a stand-alone system. If the schedule for an employee is changed in the department's system, that change will not be reflected in any other institutional system; for example, the personnel and payroll systems would still show the original schedule. Stand-alone systems result in data redundancy in the system and database discrepancies—and those discrepancies can become a source of conflict between departments and personnel.

Interfaced systems maintain their own database while sharing data across a network. For example, a laboratory system may be interfaced with a HIS; in such a case, the patient orders from the HIS are passed directly to the laboratory system, and the laboratory results are passed directly back to the HIS. When several department systems are interfaced, the results have been referred to as spaghetti. Because most of these interfaced systems are purchased from different vendors and the computer systems are constantly being updated, maintaining the interface-related code becomes a constant battle, and patient data can get lost in this complexity.

Integrated systems share a common database. The clinical data repository or warehouse system discussed earlier is such a system. All of the data related to a client, employee, or financial system are stored in one repository. Although this is a simple concept, the process of building a repository is very complex.

Most healthcare institutions operate with a combination of stand-alone, interfaced, and integrated systems. Data are shared at four different levels.

Level 1 data sharing involves integration of a specific institution service or function. For example, an executive information system may pull census, personnel, and financial data together to present an overall picture of the institution's operational status. A product-line system may integrate patient data from several different systems to track how patients in that product line move through the organization.

Level 2 involves sharing data for an individual healthcare institution. Sometimes all patient data are shared in this way; at other times, the sharing involves all institutional data including financial, personnel, and tangible resources.

Level 3 involves the sharing of data across all institutions within the larger organization, a type of system referred to as an enterprise-wide system. This level of sharing has become increasingly important with the development of integrated healthcare delivery systems. The best example of this level of integration is the application used by the Veterans Health Administration. The integrated system of software applications that support patient care at Veterans Health Administration healthcare facilities is called VistA. A key component of VistA is the Computerized Patient Record System (CPRS); CPRS is a longitudinal health record that follows the patient through all VA treatment settings. This application has been installed at all VA Medical Centers since 1997. A keystone to the future of this system is the ongoing development of the Health Data Repository (HDR). The HDR will be a national databank for standardized, patient-specific clinical data on all patients in the VA system (Department of Veterans Affairs, 2008).

Level 4 involves sharing data outside of the institutions owned by the enterprise. These applications serve as regional or community health information networks. Connecting regional or community networks together creates a national network or "network of networks." Such an effort has been undertaken by the U.S. federal government, for example:

> The Nationwide Health Information Network (NHIN) is being developed to provide a secure, nationwide, interoperable health information infrastructure that will connect providers, consumers, and others involved in supporting health and healthcare. This critical part of the national health IT agenda will enable health information to follow the consumer, be available for clinical decision making, and support appropriate use of healthcare information beyond direct patient care so as to improve health (U.S. Department of Health and Human Services, n.d.).

With this level of integration, a patient's record could be accessed from any healthcare institution. For example, if a person living in Pennsylvania was in a car accident in Florida, his or her healthcare record could be accessed from the emergency room in Florida.

In its early stages, healthcare computing relied on stand-alone systems. Today, these systems are becoming increasingly integrated. This sharing of data across disciplines within health care is one of the factors increasing the overall move toward integration of services. As this trend continues, healthcare information systems are becoming more generic. For example, they are becoming patient-focused systems rather than medical or nursing systems. Although this trend is improving the comprehensiveness of the data, one approach to managing patient data will not meet the information needs for all disciplines. How to develop an integrated, patient-focused healthcare information system that meets the information needs of different disciplines is an important applied research question in healthcare computing.

Healthcare Computing Personnel

There are several levels and types of personnel who work in healthcare computing. Some personnel have their primary background in computer and information science, whereas others have their primary background in health care. A few are prepared in healthcare informatics. The educational preparation of people in healthcare computing varies from on-the-job training to postdoctoral preparation.

Chief Information Officer or Director of Information Services

The chief information officer is administratively responsible for the operation of the information services department. Depending on the organization, this individual may be part of the executive team responsible for strategic and long-range institutional planning as well as the day-to-day operation of the department.

Systems Analysts

Systems analysts work with users to define their information needs and design systems to meet those needs. Their education is usually in information or computer science with knowledge of health care acquired from on-the-job experience.

Programmers

Programmers design, code, and test new software programs as well as maintain and enhance current applications. These individuals usually receive their educational preparation in computer science or as on-the-job training.

Systems or Network Administrators

Systems administrators are responsible for planning and maintaining multiuser computer systems on a local area network. These individuals may have an associate or baccalaureate degree in computer or information science. They are often certified in the use of the software application used to manage the network.

Microcomputer Specialists

Microcomputer specialists support personal computer users throughout the institution. They may install new software, troubleshoot or repair personal computers, answer user questions, and train users on new software.

Computer Operators

There are several types of computer operators. The title "computer operator" usually refers to an individual who actually runs a mainframe or minicomputer; these individuals usually have minimal interaction with healthcare providers. Microcomputer (PC) operators, by comparison, work closely with users. They troubleshoot, upgrade, and repair computers as well as install software. Network managers provide this same type of service for local area networks.

Informatics Specialists

Informatics specialists are healthcare professionals who have completed additional education related to the field of informatics. These individuals have a degree in their healthcare profession and have become experts in the use of computers in health care. Examples include specialists in medical informatics, dental informatics, veterinary informatics, and nursing informatics. These specialists integrate their respective health science specialty with cognitive science, computer science, and information science to manage and communicate data, information, knowledge, and wisdom in the delivery of healthcare services.

Summary

Literacy is the ability to read, write, and use numbers skillfully enough to meet the demands of society. Computer literacy is the ability to use a computer skillfully enough to meet the demands of society. Like literacy, the scope and depth of computer literacy needed by any one person can vary extensively. One person can be very literate with word processing, but unable to use any other program. Another person may have a general knowledge of several different programs. In today's automated world, all people need to have at least a basic understanding of computers. Healthcare professionals, like all other educated people, need a basic level of computer literacy.

Information literacy refers to the ability to access, evaluate, and use information. With the advent of computers, information literacy requires the ability to access databases, especially literature databases and the largest database of all—the Internet. Once information has been accessed, the information-literate individual needs the ability to evaluate the information effectively and to recognize inaccurate and incomplete information. This task is especially difficult if the reader has a limited knowledge base related to the information being accessed. Finally, information literacy requires the ability to use the information.

Healthcare informatics is a field specific to health care. It uses tools from information science, computer science, cognitive science, and the healthcare sciences to help manage healthcare institutions and deliver quality health care.

This book provides the reader with a foundation in computer and information literacy. It concludes by introducing the reader to the discipline of healthcare informatics.

References

Agency for Healthcare Research and Quality. (2008). Computerized provider order entry. Retrieved December 22, 2008, from http://healthit.ahrq.gov/portal/server.pt?open=514&objID=5554&mode=2&holderDisplayURL=http://prodportallb.ahrq.gov:7087/publishedcontent/publish/communities/k_o/knowledge_library/key_topics/health_briefing_02062006010308/computerized_provider_order_entry.html.

American Association of Colleges of Nursing. (2008, October). The essentials of baccalaureate education for professional nursing practice. Retrieved December 2008 from http://www.aacn.nche.edu/Education/pdf/BaccEssentials08.pdf.

American Health Information Management Association (AHIMA) & American Medical Informatics Association (AMIA). (2008). Joint Work Force Task Force: Health information management and informatics core competencies for individuals working with electronic health records. Retrieved December 21, 2008, from www.amia.org/files/shared/Workforce_2008.pdf.

American Nurses Association. (2008). *Scope and standards of nursing informatics practice.* Silver Spring, MD: NurseBooks.org.

Blum, B. I. (1986). *Clinical information systems.* New York: Springer-Verlag.

Department of Veterans Affairs, Office of Enterprise Development. (2008). VistA-Health eVetMonograph: 2008–2009. Retrieved December 23, 2008, from http://www.va.gov/vista_monograph/docs/2008VistAHealtheVet_Monograph.pdf.

Englebardt, E., & Nelson, R. (2002). *Health care informatics: An interdisciplinary approach.* St. Louis: Mosby.

Graves, J., & Corcoran, S. (1989). The study of nursing informatics. *Image: Journal of Nursing Scholarship, 21*(4), 227–231.

Greiner, A., & Knebel, E. (Eds.). (2003). *Institute of Medicine: Committee on the Health Professions Education Summit. Health professions education: A bridge to quality.* Washington, DC: National Academies Press. http://www.nap.edu.

Institute of Medicine, Committee on Health Literacy. (2004). Health literacy: A prescription to end confusion. Retrieved May 31, 2009, from http://www.nap.edu/catalog.php?record_id=10883.

Mann, D. (2005). Katrina shows need for electronic health records. *WebMD Health News.* Retrieved December 23, 2008, from http://www.medscape.com/viewarticle/513215.

National League for Nursing. (2008). Position paper: Preparing the next generation of nurses to practice in a technology-rich environment: An informatics agenda. Retrieved December 21, 2008, from http://www.nln.org/aboutnln/PositionStatements/informatics_052808.pdf.

Nelson, R. (2004). Incorporating new technology: Nursing informatics. In L. Caputi & L. Engelmann (Eds.), *Teaching nursing: The art and the science* (pp. 555–588). Glen Ellyn, IL: College of Dupage Press.

Nelson, R., & Joos, I. (1989, Fall). On language in nursing: From data to wisdom. *PLN Visions,* 6.

Shannon, C. E., & Weaver, W. (1949). *The mathematical theory of communication.* Urbana: University of Illinois Press.

U.S. Department of Health and Human Services. (n.d.). Nationwide Health Information Network (NHIN): Background. Retrieved December 23, 2008, from http://www.hhs.gov/healthit/healthnetwork/background/.

U.S. Department of Health and Human Services. (2003). News release: HHS launches new efforts to promote paperless health care system. http://www.hhs.gov/news/press/2003pres/20030701.html.

EXERCISE 1 Literacy, Computer-Assisted Instruction,
and Healthcare Informatics

■ Objectives
1. Differentiate between computer literacy, information literacy, computer-assisted instruction, and healthcare informatics.
2. Identify available software programs, both generic and those specific to health care.
3. Describe uses of each type of software.

■ Activity
1. Use your word processing skills to create tables to answer the questions in parts 3, 4, and 5 of this activity; answer question 6 at the end of the document. Place your name in a header on the right side of the document.
2. Make a list of software programs that are available to you as a student in your current curriculum. Include the programs and databases in your library for accessing reference materials, software you were required to purchase as a student, and any software offered at a discounted price by your school or university. This compilation will serve as the master list for this exercise.
3. Identify the applications on your list that are not specific to health care. For example, a word processing program can be used in any field, not just health care. Classify the identified programs by their primary purpose. For example, Microsoft Word would be classified as a word processing program. Write a brief statement explaining how each type of software would be useful for a healthcare student or employee.

LIST OF SOFTWARE PROGRAMS

Program Name	Health Care	Purpose	Useful
	___Yes ___No		
	___Yes ___No		
	___Yes ___No		

HEALTH-RELATED DATABASES

Database	Literature Referenced	Background Needed

COMPUTER PROGRAMS TO TEACH HEALTH CONTENT

Program	Literacy Level

4. Make a list of the health-related databases in your library and briefly explain which type of literature is referenced in these databases. For example, how does the literature indexed in MEDLINE differ from that indexed in CINAHL? Give a brief description of the background or knowledge base the reader should have to evaluate the quality of information included in the references in each database.

5. Identify applications or computer programs that are used to teach health-related content in your curriculum. Select five of these programs, and describe the level of computer literacy necessary to use each program.

6. Identify one program that can be used to explain the concepts inherent in healthcare informatics. Explain how you would use this program to explain healthcare informatics concepts.

7. Save this file as **Chap14-Ex1-LastName**. Submit it electronically or as a printout to your instructor.

EXERCISE 2 Data, Information, Knowledge, and Wisdom

■ **Objective**

1. Develop personal definitions of healthcare data, information, knowledge, and wisdom.

■ **Activity**

Work in small groups (three to five people) to develop an answer for each of the following questions. These questions may also be used in a discussion forum in a course management program for online courses.

1. When patients complete a health assessment form, have they provided you with data or with information? Explain your answer.
2. Does knowing a patient's diagnosis provide you with information or knowledge? Will your answer differ if you are referring to a medical or a nursing diagnosis?
3. What is your definition of healthcare knowledge? How does healthcare and medical knowledge differ from nursing knowledge and from pharmacy knowledge? How are they the same?
4. Can wisdom be taught? Explain your answer.
5. Give a personal example of a time when an instructor or teacher demonstrated wisdom as opposed to knowledge.

ASSIGNMENT 1 Healthcare Informatics: Job Descriptions

■ **Directions**

The healthcare setting where you are employed has decided to purchase and implement an EHR system. Because computer and healthcare informatics content was included in your basic education program, you have been added to the implementation team with the title of Informatics Specialist. Your first assignment is to write your job description. You have been referred to the following reference and Web sites:

- American Nurses Association. (2008). *Scope and standards of nursing informatics practice.* Silver Spring, MD: NurseBooks.org.
- http://www.amia.org/ni-wg/ni-wg-roles
- http://jobsearch.monster.com/?inter_js=no
- http://www.amia.org/inside/initiatives/workforce.asp

1. Using a search site, search for a **job description template**.
2. **Download** the template and use it to create the following items:
    - A brief description of the job
    - A list of required and preferred qualifications

■ A list of the job responsibilities based on information from the previously mentioned resources

3. Save the file as **Chap14-Assign1-YourLastName**. Submit it electronically or in print form to your professor.

ASSIGNMENT 2 Healthcare Informatics Education

■ **Directions**

1. Several professional healthcare organizations have identified the need for healthcare professionals to be computer, information, and informatics literate. Develop an outline identifying the basic concepts that should be included in your education so that you become computer, information, and informatics literate.

2. Review your educational program, and identify which content from your outline is or is not included in your program.

3. When content is not included, identify where it should be added to your program.

4. Based on your analysis, write a two-page position paper on healthcare informatics as part of healthcare education. Use Word to prepare your paper, formatting it as a table with the appropriate headings.

5. Save the document as **Chap14-Assign2-YourLastName**.

ASSIGNMENT 3 Healthcare Informatics

■ **Directions**

Many healthcare settings do not provide students with passwords and limit your access to the information systems used in health care.

1. Write a two- to five-page paper discussing how this limited access affects your learning and, in turn, your preparation for your role as a professional healthcare provider. Be sure to include, with appropriate documentation, references from published as well as gray literature. When possible, give examples from your own experience.

2. Make sure the paper is formatted according to APA style or a style approved by your school.

3. Save the file as **Chap14-Assign3-YourLastName**.

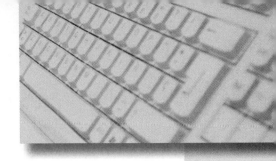

Glossary

Absolute Addresses: cell addresses in formulas that remain the same despite other changes in the worksheet; they are indicated by a dollar sign ($) preceding the part of the address that is to remain absolute in Excel.

Accessibility: refers to how easy it is to obtain information. Information is considered accessible if you can enter a search term looking for information, and the desired information is found in your search results.

Access Database: contains tables, forms, reports, queries, macros, and modules.

Access Providers: companies that provide access to an Internet host computer. They often supply the software needed to connect to the Internet as well as the appropriate connection equipment.

Account: an account is set up by the school or university so that the student can use the computer laboratory, the university's resources, the school's network, and have access to course materials made available through the Internet or that reside on course management software servers.

Active Cell: is the cell currently being used; it is outlined or highlighted so that it can be located quickly on the spreadsheet.

Add Function: permits placement of additional records into the database.

Administrative Information Systems: automate the management of data used in the daily operations of the institution as well as data used for strategic and long-range planning.

Adware: a specific type of spyware designed to collect data for targeted advertisements directed to your computer.

Aggregator: a software application or program that collects information from various online sources such as blogs, podcasts, and Web sites so that this information can be shown together in a single view.

AGP: the accelerated graphics port (AGP) bus is the default internal bus between the graphics controller and the main memory. It is dedicated to, and designed specifically for, video systems.

Alt, Ctrl, F4, and **Shift Keys:** special keys that modify normal operations. These keys, in combination with other keys, initiate commands or complete tasks.

Analytic Graphics: present data in graph form for analysis, understanding, and decision making. Presentation graphics, spreadsheet, or statistic programs can be used to create these graphs.

AND: this search strategy provides records that include both terms on either side of the AND.

Animated Files: include motion; they carry a .gif file extension. These files contain multiple images that are streamed together to produce the effect of animation.

Animations Tab: contains commands for previewing a slide show, adding animations, and adding the transitions between slides.

Answer Table: a temporary table in which the program stores search results.

Antivirus Software: scans the computer, email, and downloaded files to identify and disable virus software.

Application Key: displays the shortcut menu for the selected item.

Application Programs: meet specific task needs of the user; running these programs

to complete your work in an efficient and effective manner is the primary use of any computer system. Programmers use language software to write application programs such as Word, Excel, PowerPoint, and so forth.

Area Charts: present or emphasize the total quantity (volume) of several items over time.

ASCII: American Standard Code for Information Interchange.

Asynchronous: a communication exchange in which the people involved are communicating at different times. For example, email and discussion boards are asynchronous because the communicants do not need to be on the computer at the same time.

Attachments: files sent along with an email; they can be of any type from word to pdf to powerpoint.

AutoFill: a built-in, time-saving feature in which Excel automatically inserts data by following a pattern you have begun in a worksheet.

Automated Decision Support Systems: systems that process information, identifying and demonstrating pertinent interrelationships that can be used to support the decision making process of a care provider.

AutoReport Feature: creates a simple report showing all the fields in the table.

AutoSum: is the most commonly used function; it automatically adds a series of numbers in either rows, columns, or both in Excel.

Backspace Key: used to delete characters to the left of the cursor.

Bandwidth: describes the amount of data that can travel over a communications channel at one time.

Bar Graphs: compare data against some value at a specific point in time. The categories (similar to types of antibiotics) are arranged vertically in a column on the y-axis, whereas the values (rating effectiveness) are arranged horizontally on the x-axis. The emphasis with this type of chart is on the comparison, not time.

Bibliographic Database: a specific type of database designed to store information about articles, books, and other print materials.

Bit: the smallest unit of data, the lowest level; the term "bit" is an abbreviation for "binary digit."

Bitmapped Graphics: images are stored and represented as pixels (tiny dots). This form is commonly used for clip art images. Examples include the GIF, PCX, and TIF formats.

Blank Presentation: this is the default template used when PowerPoint opens. Slides that use this template have minimal design and no color applied to them.

Blank Slide: no placeholders in this slide.

Block: is a selected (highlighted) section of text that is treated as a unit.

Blog: a self-published Web site containing dated material, usually written in a journal format. Blogs may contain text, pictures, video, audio, and URLs of other relevant sites. They usually include a process for readers to post their comments and reactions. Mini-blogs called *tweets* are growing in popularity using a social networking service called *Twitter*. They are restricted to 140 characters.

Bluetooth: are special wireless port that competes with IrDA ports, although Bluetooth uses radio waves to communicate between the devices instead of infrared light waves. It uses the wireless protocol for exchanging data over short distances.

Bookmarks: (or favorites) saved URLs of frequently visited internet sites.

Boolean Searching: is one of the most commonly used features for searching any database; it provides the ability to narrow or expand a search as well as to eliminate some records.

Boot: to start the computer so that it can execute the necessary start-up routines. A cold boot means starting the computer when it has been powered off. A warm boot is the process of restarting a computer that is already on.

Bounce: failure of an email message to be delivered promptly. Emails can bounce for more than 30 reasons such as the email address is incorrect or has been closed; the recipient's mailbox is full, the mail server is down, the system detects spam or offensive content, and so on.

Brightness: refers to the visible light intensity of the screen and is measured in nits. The more nits, the brighter the picture.

Broadband Connections: such as DSL and cable, which are faster than dial-up access, provide an ongoing connection to the Internet.

Browser: see Web Browser.

Bulletin Board: a public area for messages; it is similar to its counterpart that hangs on a wall. Bulletin boards are typically organized around specific topics and may be part of an online service and accessed through Internet search engines.

Bullets (lists): small dots, squares, dashes, checks, or other graphics that begin a phrase or key points. Use them in documents, email, or presentations.

Byte: a string of bits used to represent a character, digit, or symbol. It usually contains 8 bits.

Cable: cable lines coming into most homes provide another option for a communications channel. This type of communication channel is faster than either dial-up or DSL, but degrades in speed as more people access the cable lines at the same time.

Cable Modem: a device that connects to the network using television cable services.

Cache Memory: stores frequently used instructions and data.

Calculated Fields: are generated by performing mathematical operations on selected fields.

Caps Lock Key: used to switch or toggle between all uppercase and lowercase letters.

Cascade Windows: works well if it is necessary to see all the open windows as all open windows will be cascaded from the top of the screen down, with the title bar of each open window being visible to the user.

Categories: labels given to the x-axis and y-axis.

Cell: is a placeholder for data in a spreadsheet. Each cell occurs at a specific intersection of a row and a column. Cells are labeled by the column letter followed by the row number.

Cell Address: (cell reference) is the label for each cell in a spreadsheet. It is used to reference the cell when creating formulas or using functions.

Change Function: permits the user to alter the contents of a record.

Chart Type: refers to the way the chart will display the data. Examples include pie and bar charts.

Chat: real-time communication between two or more users via a computer. Most Internet service providers have built-in chat features.

Chatiquette: similar to Netiquette in terms of the words and behavior acceptable while participating in a chat room.

Chat Room: a designated area or "room" where individuals gather simultaneously and "talk" to one another by typing messages. Everyone who is online usually sees the messages.

Chief Information Officer or Director of Information Services: is administratively responsible for the operation of the information services department.

Chip: a tiny piece of semiconducting material (usually silicon) that packs many millions of electronic elements onto an area the size of a fingernail. The circuit boards found in computers consist of many chips.

Click: (press) means to press and hold the mouse button down, as on a menu item to see the commands, or to scroll through a window until the desired command is selected.

Client–Server: Client–server computing architecture is the de facto model for network oriented computing. Generally clients are personal computers and servers hold the data accessed by client computers.

Clinical Information Systems: are used to process patient data and support patient care.

Clinical or Client Data: includes all data that are related to an individual client. A comprehensive collection of the client data is stored in the EHR.

Clip Art: a library of symbols (images) prepared by others for use with specific graphics programs.

Clipboard: is a holding area or buffer for copied or cut data for later use. Data placed onto a clipboard can then pasted into another document, another application, or another location within the original document.

Clock Speed: a function of the quartz crystal circuit that controls the timing of computer work.

Color: refers to whether the monitor is monochrome (one color, usually green or amber, on a black background) or colored. The number of displayed colors ranges from 256 to much higher numbers.

Column Graphs: show data changes over time or illustrate comparisons. The data or values are presented vertically (y-axis), whereas the categories appear horizontally (x-axis)— the reverse of bar charts.

Columns: go vertically down the spreadsheet. They are labeled from A to Z, going from left to right.

Communication: (also known as *connectivity*) refers to the electronic transfer of data from one place to another. It also refers to how people use the technology to enhance their communications with each other and with healthcare consumers.

Communication Device: any type of hardware capable of transmitting data and information from one computer to another.

Communications Channel: the transmission pathway that data take to arrive at the other end of a connection.

Comparison Layout Slide: includes a title placeholder, two text placeholders below it, and two content placeholders below them.

Compression Files: a compression utility is one that allows you to send or receive large or multiple files.

Computer: is a programmable machine capable of performing a series of logical and arithmetic operations and its function is to accept data and instructions from a user, process the data to produce information, store the data for later retrieval, and display the information.

Computer-assisted Communication: the computer enhances the communication process by either structuring the message or providing a channel through which to send and receive messages.

Computer-assisted Instruction Software: comprises a set of programs that help users learn concepts or specific content related to their discipline or area of study.

Computer Crimes: include a wide range of illegal activities, from computer intrusion into a computer system (i.e., hacking) to child pornography or exploitation.

Computer Information System: hardware (computers) and software plus people, data, communications (connectivity), and policies and procedures.

Computer Literacy: refers to the ability to use the computer to do practical tasks.

Computer Operator: refers to an individual who actually runs a mainframe or minicomputer; these individuals usually have minimal interaction with healthcare providers. Microcomputer operators, by comparison, work closely with users. They troubleshoot, upgrade, and repair computers as well as install software.

Confidentiality: deals with the healthcare provider's responsibility to limit access to information so that it is shared in a controlled manner for the benefit of the patient.

Consumer Information Systems: are applications that have been developed for the general public, patients, or clients, as opposed to the traditional care providers. These applications can be classified into three basic types: (1) Web pages and applications that provide health related information, (2) social services such as on line groups that provide emotional support and (3) applications that assist the general public in maintaining their personnel health data.

Content with Caption Slide: this layout features two text placeholders, one for a title and one for explanatory text. The third placeholder is intended to hold content.

Contextual Tab: occurs in a window that is available only in a certain context or situation.

Contrast Ratio: the ratio of the brightest color (white) to the darkest color (black) on the screen.

Cookie Files: designed to enhance the online experience by recognizing the visitor when he or she returns to a Web site and recording what was done at that site.

Copy Command: copies one, several, or all of the files from one place to another.

Course Management Software or System (CMS): a software application that is used by colleges and universities as well as corporations and government agencies to facilitate distance learning by centralizing the development, management, and distribution of instructional-related information and materials. A CMS provides faculty with a set of tools that allows the easy creation of course content—syllabi, course modules, lecture notes, assignments, tests and quizzes, and so forth—and is the framework faculty use to teach and manage their class. Two commonly used CMS programs are Blackboard and Moodle.

Cracker: a hacker who illegally breaks into computer systems and creates mischief.

Cradles or Docking Stations: input devices primarily used with PDAs, laptops, iPods, and cameras to input data from the mobile device to the desktop computer, and vice versa.

Current Cell Address: indicates the *active cell* and is displayed on the left side of the formula toolbar.

Cursor Movement Keys: (also known as arrow keys) generally take the form of a cluster of four keys that have directional arrows on them.

Custom Animations: apply a special visual effect or sound to text or other objects on the slide such as diagrams, clip art, and charts.

Cut (delete or move): removes the selection from the document and moves it to the clipboard; is the default option for the drag and drop method.

Cybercafe: internet access provided through local businesses such as hotels, coffee shops, or delis.

Cybercrime: the use of the Internet or other communication technology to commit a crime of any type.

Data: are raw facts. They exist without meaning or interpretation. Data are the attributes that healthcare professionals collect, organize, and name.

Database: is a collection of files that is analogous to a file cabinet; it holds related drawers of records.

Database Functions: allow users to create table structures, edit data or records, search tables, sort records, and generate reports.

Database Management System (DBMS): are the programs that enable users to work with electronic databases. They permit data to be stored, modified, and retrieved from the database.

Database Model: (or schema) refers to the structure of a database, which includes how that database is organized and used. These structures are generally stored in a data dictionary and many times are depicted in a graphical way.

Database Software: helps organize, store, retrieve, and manipulate data for the purpose of later retrieval and report generation.

Data Buses: comprise a collection of wires, and move data around in the computer.

Data diddling: a method of coding sensitive data to protect those data when they are sent over the Internet.

Data Mart: a subset or smaller-focus database designed to help managers make strategic decisions is termed a data mart. Sometimes it comprises a subset of a data warehouse.

Data Mining: this concept refers to database applications that look for patterns in already-created databases.

Data Projectors: display graphic presentations to an audience. Such a device takes the image on the computer screen and projects it onto a larger screen.

Data Relationships: how the data in the database are related.

Data Series: a group of related data points on a chart that originated from rows and columns in the worksheet. These values are used to plot the chart.

Data Tab: allows you to import external data, view linked spreadsheets (Connections group), sort and filter data, outline data, and use data tools.

Data Types: refer to the description of which data should be expected to appear in a field.

Data Warehouse: a collection of data designed to support decision making. Its purpose is to present a picture of the general conditions of the entity both at a particular time and historically.

Default: the setting the computer uses unless told otherwise.

Defragmentation Utility: a program that consolidates fragmented files and folders on the storage device so that each one is stored in a contiguous space.

Delete Command: removes files from the storage device; to remove some text, row, column, or slide from the document.

Delete Key: used to delete text to the right of the cursor.

Denial of service: any action or series of actions that prevents any part of an information system from functioning— for example, using several computers attached to the Internet to access a Web site so that the site is overwhelmed and not available.

Density per Inch (DPI): indicates the pixel density—that is, the number of dots (pixels) per inch. Resolution quality increases with larger DPI.

Design Tab: contains options for changing the page setup, themes, and background in the graphics presentation.

Desktop: the main window or screen that is seen after logging on to the computer.

Desktop Publishing Software: permits the user to create high-quality specialty publications such as newspapers, bulletins, and brochures.

Dialog Box: a special window that requires the suer to make selections to implement a command.

Dialog launcher: The Ribbon dialog launcher is a small icon that appears in the lower right corner of a group in Office 2007 programs. When the user clicks this icon, a custom dialog box opens.

Dial-up Modem: a device that prepares data for transmission over a telephone line. It converts digital data into its analog (wave) form and then reverses the process at the other end of the connection.

Dial-up Service: referred to as plain old telephone service (POTS). It uses telephone wires to access the network.

Digital Camera: used to take photographs and then upload them to the computer or to a special picture printer. They eliminate the need for both film and film development.

Directory: In the operating system, a simulated file folder on disk. Programs and data for each application are typically kept in a separate directory (spreadsheets, word processing, etc.). Directories create the illusion of compartments, but are actually indexes to the files which may be scattered all over the disk. The main directory on your hard drive is appropriately called the "root directory." Unix and DOS use the term directory, while the Mac and Windows use the term "folder."

Directory Site: On the Internet, it is a hierarchical grouping of WWW links by subject and related concepts; it is generally manually created and the links are prescreened.

Disk Cleanup: a program to remove any unwanted files. This utility is available only for cleaning the hard drive on a system; it is not applicable to removable storage devices.

Distance Education: the delivery of education when the student and the instructor are in physically different locations. In today's learning environment, this type of education is often delivered over the Internet using a variety of technical tools such as a course management software package.

Distributed Database: is stored in more than one physical place instead of in a single, central location.

Distribution List: (also called an *alias* or *mailing list*) an email application that is especially useful when sending a message to a group of people.

Documentation: handouts available in the computer laboratory or documents available online to read and/or print that provides helpful information for using computers and learning specific software programs.

Documentation Systems: collect assessment and patient status data from a variety of healthcare providers and are increasingly used as interdisciplinary communication tools.

Domain Name: an address, similar to that used by the postal service, that points to a computer with a specific IP address. It is a description of a computer's location on the Internet.

Dot Pitch: a measure (in millimeters) of the distance between the red, green, and blue phosphors that make up the colors of the monitor.

Double-click: means, with the cursor on an icon or option, to press and release the left mouse button twice in quick succession. Use a double-click to start an application program, to open a file or folder, or to select a word for editing.

Doughnuts: are variations of pie charts. They compare parts to the whole but can combine more than one data series.

Downloading: moving a file from one computer (generally a server) to another (generally a local PC).

Drag: to left-click an icon, menu option, or window border; then, without lifting the finger off the mouse button, roll the mouse to move the object to another place on the screen. This operation can change a window's size, copy a file or document, select text, or take something to the trash.

DSL Connection: makes a faster connection than dial-up service, usually through the phone system.

DSL Modem: a device that connects to the network over a DSL connection.

DVD: permitted storing videos—hence the name "digital video discs." As use of these discs increased as data storage media, DVD has come to mean "digital versatile disc." These discs can hold more data, such as a full-length movie, than can CDs.

Editing Features: inserting, deleting, and replacing items.

Electronic Discussion Group: an email service in which individual members post messages for all group members to read.

Electronic Health Records (EHRs): is a comprehensive collection of an individual's health-related data. Data from an individual's EHR can be stored in a clinical data repository, which can be conceptualized as a warehouse or large database where data elements from several different systems could be stored.

Electronic Mail (email) Software: permits the sending and receiving of messages from one person to one or many other people.

Email: a message that is composed and sent over a computer network to a person or group of people who have an electronic mail address. Email can be sent over a local area network or over the Internet.

Emoticon: a way to show an emotion via text on the computer. These symbols or combinations of symbols substitute for facial expressions, body language, and voice inflections.

Encryption: a method of coding sensitive data to protect those data when they are sent over the Internet.

End Users: are the healthcare providers who use computers as tools to assist them in delivering care and consumers who access healthcare information on the Internet and/or store their personal health records (PHR) on Internet-accessible servers.

Enter: refers to the Enter or return key and sends text to the next line.

Esc Key: generally backs out of a program or menu one screen or one menu at a time.

Ethernet Card: fits into a computer slot and provides connectivity to an internal network. Schools, offices, and businesses often use Ethernet cards to connect computers and peripheral devices to their network.

Exact Match: this search finds only entries that are an exact match for a specified word. Any minor difference results in exclusion of that entry from the results.

Existing Presentation: this option creates a copy of an existing presentation so that it can be changed without altering the original file.

Expansion Buses: internal collection of wires connected to the expansion slot which vary in speed and communication protocol.

Expansion Slots: places on the system board where one can add cards, adapters, or other computer boards.

Fiber-optic Cables: (such as those used in Verizon's FiOS service) are a broadband option for connecting to a network using the fiber-optic cable run to the home and businesses by some companies.

Field: (also called an attribute) is a space within a file that has a predefined location and length. Only one data item is placed in each field, a concept referred to as the use of atomic data.

Files: are collections of related records that contain data and are created by an application program; the place where the work or task is done.

File Formats: the way the program stores data such as in text, graphic, or image form which is an important consideration for importing or transferring files. Users must have an application program that can "read" the file format before the you can view it.

File Nomenclature: the file name, a delimiter, and a file extension.

File Transfer Protocol (ftp): a communications protocol and program that transfers files from one computer to another over the Internet.

Filter: a tool that automatically moves incoming emails into separate folders according to criteria that either you or your Internet provider have specified. Filters can also be included in a virus checker or a software program used to manage your email.

Filtering: allows you to select specific records for review. It does not rearrange data, but rather hides rows you do not want displayed.

Financial Data: includes all of the fiscal data related to the operation of the healthcare institution.

Find and Replace: to find, or find and replace, specific files or words within a folder or document.

Firewall: a piece of hardware or a software program used to protect computers from unauthorized access via the Internet as well as to secure the interactions between an organization's inside network of computers and the external computer environment.

FireWire: a special-purpose port that is similar to a USB port in that the user can attach multiple devices to it.

Flash Memory: a type of nonvolatile memory that the user can erase and rewrite, making it easier to update the memory contents.

Folder: is a storage place for files and other folders.

Font: defines a descriptive look or shape (font face or typeface), size, style, and weight of a group of characters or symbols.

Footer: is an information area that is placed consistently at the bottom of each page of a document.

Footprint: refers to how much space the monitor takes up on the desktop.

Formatting: is the process of editing the appearance of a document by using indentations, margins, tabs, justification, and pagination; format conditions affect the document appearance.

Format Painter: is used to copy formatting from one place and apply it to another.

Formulas: help you analyze the data on a worksheet. With formulas, it is possible to perform operations such as addition, multiplication, and comparison and to enter the calculated value on the worksheet. A *function* is a more complex preprogrammed formula.

Formula Toolbar: the data or formula entered appears in this location on the screen in Excel.

Function: are prewritten formulas in Excel that simplify the process of entering calculations; examples include SUM and AVERAGE.

Function Keys: special keys that application programs use to complete tasks.

Gadgets: special applications to customize your desktop. For example, the current weather or stock report.

Gaming Input Devices: light guns, joysticks, dance pads, and motion sensing controllers.

Get Started Tab: this group, which is found in the Home and Student versions of MS Office, helps the new user get started with Word 2007.

Grammar Checker: provides feedback to the user about errors in grammar.

Graphical User Interface (GUI): intended to take advantage of the computer's graphic and mouse capabilities and make it easier to use the commands and applications.

Graphics Software: facilitates the creation of a variety of graphics. Three types of graphics programs exist. *Presentation* graphics permit the user to create or alter symbols, display a variety of chart styles, make transparencies and slides, and produce slide shows. *Paint* programs permit users to create symbols or images from scratch. *Computer-aided drafting* programs meet the drawing needs of architects and engineers.

Gray Literature: includes works that are not formally reviewed and have not appeared in standard, recognized publications.

Groups: In Office 2007, commands organized in logical groups that are collected together under tabs in each ribbon.

Hacker: originally referred to a compulsive computer programmer; now this term has a more negative meaning and is often confused with "cracker."

Handheld Computers: fit in your hand. These models have full PC functionality but include much smaller screens and keyboards (sometimes specialized keyboards).

Handles: the squares that surround a selected image or block of text when it is viewed on screen.

Handouts: provided to the audience to outline the graphics presentation, define selected terms, or present complex information.

Hardware: for a computer system consists of input devices, the system unit (processing unit, memory, boards, and power supply), output devices, and secondary storage devices.

Hard Disks: (also known as *hard drives*) are fixed data storage devices in sealed cases that read stored data on platters in the drive. These magnetic storage devices store data in sizes ranging from gigabytes to the terabytes.

Hard Return: is a code inserted in the document by pressing the Enter key. It is usually placed at the end of a paragraph.

Header: is an information area that is placed consistently at the top of each page of a document. It can hold the name of the document, page number, date, or other identifying information.

Healthcare Informatics: the study of how health care data, information, knowledge, and wisdom are collected, stored, processed, communicated, and used to support the process of health care delivery to clients, providers, administrators, and organizations involved in health care delivery. It is concerned with the application of information and computer science concepts and theories to the delivery of health care and is an interdisciplinary science developed from the integration of information science, computer science, cognitive science, and the healthcare sciences.

Healthcare Information Systems (HISs): are often the backbone or primary system used to integrate or interface with the various applications throughout the organization. They communicate information between the point of care or clinical units and the various departments within the institution.

Health Literacy: the degree to which individuals have the capacity to obtain, process, and understand basic information and services needed to make appropriate decisions regarding their health.

Help: access the Help feature through the blue question mark on the ribbon or the Help option on a menu bar. Click the question mark, and a Word Help screen appears describing what is available in Help-either offline or online.

HIPAA: Health Insurance Portability and Accountability Act of 1996, which has as its goal the simplification of the administrative processes used to transmit electronic health information.

History List: keeps track of internet sites that have been visited over the past several days and offers a convenient means of redisplaying those pages.

Hits: a list of links that are returned as search results when a search engine is used.

Home Tab: (and its groups) Clipboard, Font, Paragraph, Styles, and Editing. These groups allow you to format the document.

Human Resources Data: includes all data related to employees as well as individuals who have a contractual relationship with the institution such as physicians, nurses, students, or volunteers.

Hyperlinks: are used to take the user someplace else or to provide additional information about a topic.

Hypertext Markup Language (HTML): provides a mechanism for displaying text- and graphics-based documents in Web browsers. HTML files are static Web pages in which the content is created at the time the page is created.

Hypertext transfer protocol: the communications protocol that is used for accessing and working with the World Wide Web. Do not confuse it with HTML, which is the tagging language.

Icons: represent applications, such as Internet Explorer and MSN, and special programs, such as the Recycle Bin.

Identity theft: a crime in which someone uses another person's private information to assume his or her identity.

Impact Printers: the printing mechanism touches the surface of the paper; that is, a mechanism strikes against a ribbon. Common examples include dot matrix and line printers or plotters.

Indent: means to establish tab settings that place subsequent lines of text the same number of spaces from the margin until the next hard return.

Informatics Specialists: are professionals who bridge the gap between the healthcare provider as end user and the technical expert. Their education and professional experience includes both health care and computer/information science.

Information: a collection of data that has been processed to produce meaning. Techniques that are used to process data include classifying, sorting, organizing, summarizing, graphing, and calculating.

Information Attributes: information from any source. These attributes used to develop criteria for evaluating the quality of information.

Information Literacy: the set of skills needed to find, retrieve, analyze, and use information.

Information Science: focuses on the study of information generation, transmission, and use.

Information System: produces information using an input/process/output cycle. A basic information system consists of four elements: people, policies and procedures, communication, and data.

Ink Jet Printers: are usually reasonably priced and less expensive to purchase than laser printers. They produce a better-quality output than do dot matrix printers, and serve as an excellent middle ground between laser and dot matrix printers.

Input Devices: hardware components that convert data from an external source into electronic signals understood by the computer.

Insert: means to add characters in the text at the point of the cursor, thereby moving all other text to the right.

Insert Key: serves as a toggle switch to move between typeover and insert modes; to add new text, slides, rows, columns, and so forth. In word processing programs, the insert mode is the default.

Insert Tab: consists of groups such as Pages, Tables, Illustrations, Links, Header and Footer, Text, and Symbols. You can add a cover page or insert a blank page, page break, table, chart, SmartArt or clip art using this tab.

Instant Messaging (IM): a communication service that permits you to send real-time messages via a private chat room to other individuals who are online.

Integrated Software: includes in one program multiple capabilities, such as word processing, database, spreadsheet, graphics, and communication programs.

Integrated Systems: share a common database.

Integrity: refers to the accuracy and comprehensiveness of data.

Intellectual Data: comprises the factual data that are stored in the various discipline- or subject-specific databases.

Interactive Whiteboards: display devices that connect to a computer and permit the user to interact with the computer through the whiteboard. This interaction can take place through remote controls, special pens, a writing tablet, or a finger.

Interfaced Systems: maintain their own database while sharing data across a network.

Internet: sometimes referred to as the information or global superhighway, is a loose association of millions of networks and billions of computers around the world, all of which work together to share information.

Internet/Application Buttons: control selected application functions such as email, documents, photos, gadgets, and Web access.

Internet Backbone: the main high speed lines that carry the bulk of the traffic are collectively known as the Internet backbone.

Internet Conferencing: a type of communication in which two or more persons interact over the Internet in real time, receiving more or less immediate replies. This communication can involve interaction via text, audio, or video.

Internet Front-end Software: the software with which the user interacts (the browser). It might be a comprehensive program, such as Firefox or Internet Explorer, or a program provided by the service provider.

Internet Protocol (IP): an address with a unique identification number that distinguishes each computer on the Internet.

Internet Service Providers (ISPs): sometimes called commerce service providers CSPs. Through their interconnection, these networks create high-speed communication lines for access to email and the Internet.

Invisible web: the part of the web that is not searched when using a search engine such as non-indexed pages or databases that require a password to enter them.

IrDA: an infrared light beam port connects wireless devices to the computer using light waves.

Justified: text that is aligned relative to both the left and right margins.

Kernel: the central module of the operating system; it is the part of the operating system that loads first and remains in memory as long as the computer is turned on.

Keyboard: an input device for typing data into the computer.

Keyboard loggers: either hardware or software installed on a computer to log the keystrokes of an individual. A keyboard logger can be used to monitor computer activities such as time spent on the Internet or to collect personal information such as passwords.

Keyword search: involves using terms or tags that were have been selected by the author, the publisher, or the developer of the database management system to search for a file or document.

Keyword Search Site: an Internet site that permits the user to type in "keywords" to retrieve links to sites that contain needed information; it comprises a server or a collection of servers dedicated to indexing Internet pages, storing the results, and returning lists of links that match particular queries.

Keywords: terms that may have been selected by the author, the publisher, or the developer of the literature database management system to identify the topic of the article.

Key Field: one or more fields with a unique identifier constitute key fields. Using key fields ensures that no duplicate records will appear in this.

Knowledge: a collection of interrelated pieces of information and data. In this aggregation, the interrelationships are as important as the individual items of information.

Labels: refer to the groups that represent the content of graph slides. They help the user to understand the graph (e.g., the names given to each pie wedge or bar).

Landscape Orientation: presents a document or slide in a wide or horizontal view.

Language: consists of a vocabulary and an accompanying set of rules that tell the computer how to work. Languages permit the user to develop programs to perform specific tasks. Popular languages include C, C++, C#, COBOL (Common Business Oriented Language), Java, and Visual Basic.

Laptops: (sometimes called notebooks) are generally more expensive than PCs, but have the same power and capabilities.

Laser Printers: produce high-quality print, are fast, and generate little noise.

Legend: the information that identifies the pattern or color of a specific data series or category.

Level 1 Data Sharing: involves integration of a specific institution service or function.

Level 2 Data Sharing: involves sharing data for an individual healthcare institution.

Level 3 Data Sharing: involves the sharing of data across all institutions within the larger organization, a type of system referred to as an enterprise-wide system.

Level 4 Data Sharing: involves sharing data outside of the institutions owned by the enterprise. These applications serve as regional or community health information networks.

Light Pen: a light-sensitive, pen-like device often used in hospital clinical information systems.

Line Graphs: present a large amount of data to show trends over time.

Link: a logical association between tables based on the values in corresponding fields; it is a connection between two tables in a relational database program.

ListServ: the trade name of a software program that manages automated discussion lists. This term is commonly used to refer to all mailing lists.

Literacy: the ability to locate and use printed and written information to make decisions and to function in society, both personally and professionally.

Local Area Network (LAN): a type of network with distance limitations. A building or small campus environment might use a LAN. LANs typically use a communications standard called *Ethernet.*

Lock Keys: lock part of a keyboard.

Logging In: accessing the system.

Logic bomb: a piece of program code buried within another program, designed to perform some malicious act in response to a trigger. For example, the trigger can involve entering a data or name.

Mailings Tabs: help you prepare envelopes, labels, mail merge letters, and recipient lists.

Mainframe: a large computer that accommodates hundreds of users simultaneously. It has a large data storage capacity, a large amount of memory, multiple input/output (I/O) devices, and speedy processor(s).

Material Resources Data: refers to all of the tangible resources used in the operation of the healthcare institution—everything from supplies that are purchased externally to supplies that are created internally.

Maximize Button: expands the window to fill the screen.

Media Control Buttons: make it easier to control the media player, access the DVD drive, and control the speakers.

Medical Identity Theft: occurs when someone uses another person's personal information without that individual's knowledge or consent to obtain or receive payment for medical care.

Memory: a form of semiconductor storage that resides inside the computer, generally on a motherboard, and that takes the form of one or more chips. It stores operating system commands, programs, and data.

Menus: are list of commands or tasks that are available to the user.

Message Area: in Excel shows which actions will occur when a function or button is activated. It may also show error messages. It is usually located in the -left corner of the status bar.

Meta-directory: (sometimes called a directory of directories or directories of directories) is a directory of links to other directories.

Metasearch sites: are not really search engines, but rather websites that work by taking the user's query and searching the Web with several different search engines at one time.

Metropolitan Area Network (MAN) and **Wide Area Network (WAN):** are high-speed networks that cover larger geographic distances. MANs may include a city or Internet service provider (ISP) that provides the connection for city agencies or individual users with access to the Internet. The best example of a WAN is the Internet, which uses the Transmission Control Protocol/Internet Protocol (TCP/IP) communications standard.

Microcomputer: a small, one-user computer system with its own central processing unit (CPU), memory, and storage devices. Also referred to as PCs and desktops, these models are growing in processing power, speed, and storage capacity.

Microcomputer Specialists: support personal computer users throughout the institution. They may install new software, troubleshoot or repair personal computers, answer user questions, and train users on new software.

Microphone: (voice input device) permits the user to speak into the computer so as to enter data or give instructions.

Microprocessor: a processor that fits on one integrated circuit chip.

Microsoft Office OneNote 2007: provides an electronic tool for organizing and storing information such as notes from class, reference materials, or Internet sources.

MIDI: a MIDI port permits the connection of musical instruments to the computer.

Midrange: (formerly called a minicomputer) describes a medium-sized computer that is faster and stores more data than a personal computer (PC). They are cheaper than mainframes, and in terms of size, they are between mainframes and PCs.

Minimize Button: places a button for the application on the taskbar and removes the window from the desktop; with this option, the program remains open, but runs in the background.

Mobile Devices: are laptops, PC tablets, handheld computers (also called ultra-mobile PCs), PDAs, and smart phones like the iPhone and BlackBerry.

Monitors: display graphic images from the video output of a computer. Other terms used for this device include display screen and flat panel.

Motherboard: (also referred to as the system board) is the main circuit board of the system unit. It contains slots for the processor chip, memory slots, and slots for adapter cards for video, sound, and connection to peripheral devices.

Mouse: input device. The traditional mechanical mouse has a ball on the underside of the unit. To use such a device, the user slides it over a mouse pad or desktop. Optical models that do not have a ball on the underside but rather sense changes in light reflection to detect mouse movement. An optical mouse has no moving mechanical parts.

Move Command: takes a file or folder from one place and puts it in another; it does not duplicate the file in the process; can also refer to placing data in another place in a document.

Movies: are video files that have extensions such as .avi, .mov, and .mpeg.

Multifunction Devices: all-in-one I/O devices. They typically incorporate a printer, scanner, copier, and fax machine into a single unit.

National Health Information Infrastructure (NHII): is a comprehensive network of interoperable network systems transmitting clinical, public health, and personal health information, with the goal of improving decision making by making health information available when and where it is needed.

NEAR: this search strategy is used when the terms should be located within the next few words.

Netiquette: the name given to electronic communication conventions.

Network: a collection of computers and other hardware devices such as a printer, scanner, and file server that are connected together using communication devices and transmission media.

Network Administrators: are responsible for planning and maintaining multiuser computer systems on a local area network.

Network Card: installed into a computer, enables a direct connection to a network.

Newsgroup: informational material and articles organized around a particular topic, such as Alzheimer's disease or child abuse. Newsreaders can post a message to the newsgroup for all to read and respond.

Nonimpact Printers: the printing mechanism does not touch the surface of the paper. Examples include laser, thermal, and ink jet printers.

Normal View: is used by default. It contains three parts: the slide, the notes pane at the bottom, and the left pane for seeing all of the slides or outline view.

NOT: this search strategy provides records that exclude the term following NOT.

Num Lock Key: used to toggle the numeric keypad on and off.

Objects: small pictures or graphic representations of icons, files, folders, and shortcuts found on the desktop.

Office Button: the Microsoft Office button replaces the File menu and provides access to the basic commands to open, save, and print a file.

Online Document Sharing: makes it possible for groups to work together on a common document even when the group members are separated in space. These applications let you upload files to a Web site where the group can work together.

Operating System (OS): the most important program that runs on a computer: It tells the computer how to use its own components or hardware. No general-purpose computer can work without an OS. The most common operating system for PCs is the Windows family (Windows Vista, XP, and Windows 7). Apple computers use the Macintosh operating system (OS 10).

Opt out: a number of measures designed to prevent users from receiving unwanted products or services. For example, if you signed up for a free journal on the Internet, you may want to opt out of receiving emails and product announcements from companies that advertise in this journal.

Optical Drives: an alternative to magnetic storage. They hold large amounts of data, which are usually written (pressed) once and accessed many times. The most common example is the CD-ROM (compact disc read-only memory).

OR: this search strategy provides records that have either term.

Outliner: is a feature of many word processing programs that enables the user to plan and rearrange large documents in an outline form.

Overtype: to replace the character under the cursor by the character typed.

Page Break: is the place where Word ends the text on one page before it continues text on the next page.

Page Layout Tab: (and its groups) Themes, Page Setup, Page Background, Paragraph, and Arrange. These groups help you select the font style and color, margins, paragraph indents and spacing, and allow you to add watermarks, add a page border, or change the page color or arrangement.

Page Tabs: (sometimes referred to as tabbed browsing) permit you to open a new Web site in a separate tab for quick access when you are working in multiple Web sites.

Page Up/Down, Home, and **End Keys:** used to move quickly from one place in the document or on the screen to other locations.

Pagination: consists of the numbers or marks that are used to indicate the sequence of the pages.

Parallel Ports: unidirectional ports that send data in parallel—that is, as groups of eight bits (one byte) of information in a row much like a parade. Parallel ports commonly connect the computer to a printer (one-way communication).

Password: a secret combination of symbols such as letters and numbers used to gain access to a restricted resource on a computer or network.

Patches: are generally fixes for problems discovered in the software after its original release. Many of these patches focus on fixing security problems inherent in the software that might make the user's computer vulnerable to hackers and viruses.

Pattern: this type of search permits the use of wild cards in place of a character.

PC Card: the PC card bus is used to move data from a digital camera through a PC card slot into the computer.

PCI/PCI-E: the Peripheral Component Interconnect (PCI) bus and the PCI-Express (PCI-E) bus are relatively new standards for connecting higher-speed devices such as the local hard drive, network cards, sound cards, and video cards. PCI-E is intended to replace the PCI and AGP buses.

PC Video Camera: an input device that the operator uses to capture video. It may be used to send video images as email attachments, to make video telephone calls (video conferencing), and to post live, real-time images to a Web server.

PDAs (personal digital assistants): or palmtop computers perform many of the same functions as PCs, but are meant to supplement PCs, not replace them. PDAs have a processor, an operating system (OS), memory, a power source (batteries), a display, an input device (newer ones use color touch screens), audio capability, I/O ports, and software, but no hard drive.

Personal Health Records (PHRs): are applications designed for patients to maintain copies of their own healthcare information.

Personal Software: programs that help people manage their personal lives. Examples include appointment calendars, checkbook balancing applications, money management applications, and calculators.

Personnel Systems: include a combination of systems that are used to track the characteristics of employees and/or the use of these employees within the institution.

PGP (Pretty Good Privacy): software that is used to encrypt and protect email as it moves from one computer to another. PGP can be used to verify a sender's identity.

Phishing: Pronounced "fishing"; the creation of a replica of a legitimate web page to hook users and trick them into submitting personal or financial information or passwords. It also refers to fraudulent email that solicits private information such as passwords or credit card numbers. It can result in identify theft.

Pictures: digital photographs that can be imported and used in a graphic presentation. They are generally in .jpg file format.

Picture with Caption Slide: this layout includes two text placeholders and one content placeholder that will accept only pictures.

Pie Graphs: compare parts to a whole or several values at one point in time. They also help to emphasize a particular part or to show relationships between sets of items.

Pitch: the number of characters printed in 1 inch (cpi).

Pixels: more formally, picture elements—are the tiny dots that make up the screen image. The more pixels used, the sharper the image (resolution).

Plagiarism: the act of stealing another person's ideas or work and presenting it as your own. The Internet has made it easier to plagiarize another's work and has created additional issues regarding attribution of sources.

Point: means to move the mouse so that the cursor is on or over a particular command or icon on the screen.

Pointer: a symbol used to represent the mouse location on the screen.

Pointer Shapes: the actual look of the printer.

Point Size: height of the font given in printing language, measured as 72 points per inch of height.

Policies and Procedures: outline the guiding principles related to information and technology use and give step-by-step directions for how the system works and how things are done to accomplish the end results.

Portrait Orientation: presents a document, spreadsheet, or slide in an upright or vertical view.

Ports: the highways that lead into, out of, and around the computer. They take the form of plugs, sockets, or hot spots that are found on the back, front, and sides of most system units.

Posters: used to present the results of a research study or to communicate ideas in a graphic presention. The poster handles the presentation while the presenter stands nearby, ready to field questions.

POST Test: (power-on self-test) which analyzes the buses, clock, memory, drives, and ports to make sure that all of the hardware is working properly.

Power Management Keys: provide the ability to place the computer in sleep mode and to power up the computer when it is currently in sleep mode.

PowerPoint: is the graphic presentation program provided as part of the Microsoft Office suite. It provides the user with the ability to design, create, and edit presentations.

Power Supply Box: converts the power available at the wall socket (120-volt, 60-MHz, AC current) to the power necessary to run the computer (+5 and +12 volt, DC current).

Presentation: the group of slides that makes up the actual material to be presented. It can vary from an unlimited number of slides to only a few.

Press Wheel Button: to click the wheel once and move the mouse on the desktop. This action causes the mouse pointer to scroll along the document automatically until the user presses the wheel button again.

Print Preview: shows the document as it will look when printed.

Print Screen Key: when used either in combination with the Alt key or alone, places the screen or active window onto the clipboard.

Privacy: refers to a person's desire to limit the disclosure of personal information.

Processor: the central unit in a computer that contains the circuitry for performing the instructions that computer programs provide. An older term for the processor is "central processing unit" (CPU).

Programmers: design, code, and test new software programs as well as maintain and enhance current applications.

Query: refers to the combination of terms that you enter into a search engine to conduct a search.

Quick access tool bar: The Quick Access Toolbar, located on the left of the title bar, is a customizable toolbar that contains a set of commands that are independent of the tab that is currently displayed. Commands can be added to the toolbar.

Quick Print: skips the dialog box and prints the document directly.

Random-access Memory (RAM): stores data that the computer needs to use temporarily. This type of memory is volatile—the data disappears from RAM when the power is off. The most common unit of measurement for RAM is the byte, which is the amount of storage space it takes to hold a character.

Range: (block - Excel) a group of cells in a rectangular pattern defined by the upper-left and lower-right corners is called a range or block of cells. For example, the range of cells from A1 to E6 would include all of the cells in columns A, B, C, D, and E in rows 1, 2, 3, 4, 5, and 6.

Range: (database) operators such as greater than, less than, equal to, or some combination of them are called logical operators.

Ranking: a process of indicating how relevant a hit may be. Many times a search engine will organize the search results by their ranking.

Readability statistics: the reading level of a word document is determined using the Flesh Reading Ease or the Flesh-Kincaid Grade Level tests. It is based on the number of syllables per word and the number of words per sentence.

Read-only Memory (ROM): memory that has been burned on the chip at the factory; the computer can read instructions from it but cannot alter them. This memory is permanent.

Record: a collection of fields related or associated with a focal point makes up a record.

References Tab: includes Table of Contents, Footnotes, Citations and Bibliography, Captions, Index, and Table of Authorities (cases, statutes).

Registers: temporary, high-speed storage spaces that the processor uses when it processes data. They are part of the processing unit, not the memory.

Relative Addresses: cell addresses in formulas that are designed to change when the formula is copied to other cells in Excel.

Rename Command: gives a file or folder a new name.

Replace: to substitute one thing for another; highlighting or selecting the text puts the application into the replace mode.

Resolution: describes the number of horizontal and vertical pixels (dots) found on the screen.

Response Time: refers to the time (in milliseconds) it takes to turn a dot on or off. Response times vary with monitors and can range from 3 to 16 milliseconds.

Restart Option: use when you are updating or installing new programs. The computer will turn off and then restart itself.

Review Tabs: used for proofing documents; for example, these groups help you check spelling and grammar, do a word count, track changes, insert comments, enable ScreenTips for showing a word in another language, or protect a document from changes by someone else.

RFID: (radio frequency identification) uses radio signals to communicate information found on a tag attached to an object or person first to an RFID reader and then to the computer.

Ribbon: MS Office 2007 uses a "fluent user interface" that is presented as a "ribbon." The tab names resemble menu names, and the ribbon resembles a toolbar, as in previous versions of Word.

Right-click: to press and release the right mouse button once. This operation is used to activate the shortcut menu.

Right-drag: to hold down the right mouse button, move the mouse to a different location, and then release the mouse button. This operation generally results in the appearance of a shortcut menu from which to select a command.

Robots: (also called *spiders* and *crawlers*) are used to create a database of links that are accessed when you conduct a search. These computer programs search the Web, locate links, and then index the links to create the results database.

Root Level: is the top level on which the folders reside. This level stores files the computer needs to access at start-up.

Rotate Wheel: to move the wheel forward and backward. Use this action to scroll up and down in a document or at a Web site.

Rows: run horizontally across the spreadsheet. Beginning with 1, they are numbered down the left side of the spreadsheet.

RSS (Really Simple Syndication): a scheme that makes it possible for users to subscribe to and receive information about a specific topic that has been published on blogs, podcasts, and other social networking applications.

Rules (Policies): All users of computer networked computer systems are subjected to acceptable use policies and procedures.

Sabotage: the purposeful destruction of hardware, software, and data

Salami method: a method of data stealing that involves taking little bits at a time.

Satellite Internet Connection: uses a satellite dish antenna and a transceiver (transmitter/receiver) that operates in the microwave portion of the radio spectrum.

Save As: to save a file to a file name, format, and location that you specify. It permits saving files in another format like a lower version of an application, as a PDF file, or as a Web page.

Scanner: an input device that converts character or graphic patterns into digital data (discrete coded units of data).

Scan Disk: use this error-checking tool to check the file system for errors and bad sectors.

Scatter Graphs: show trends or statistics, such as averages, frequency, regression, or distribution.

Scenarios: are a type of what-if analysis tool and a set of values that Excel saves and can substitute automatically in the worksheet. They are used to forecast the outcome of a worksheet model.

Screen Savers: moving or static pictures displayed on the desktop when no activity takes place for a specified period of time.

Screen Tip: when the mouse arrow is held over an option in the ribbon, a screen tip appears that describes its function. They are small windows that display descriptive text when you rest the pointer on a command or control.

Scrolling: is the process of moving around a document to view a specific portion of a page of text within a document.

SCSI: (Small Computer System Interface - pronounced "scuzzy") is a parallel port that supports faster data transfers than are possible with traditional parallel ports. SCSI ports permit attachment of as many as seven peripheral devices in a linked chain fashion.

Search Engines: software programs that are used to find and index information.

Search Sites: are places on the Internet where you go to find information.

Section Breaks: creates layout or formatting changes in the document.

Section Header: has two text placeholders. Use this layout when you have to break a presentation into separate parts.

Security: refers to the measures that organizations implement to protect information and systems.

Selecting Text: (or object) means to highlight the text or object, such as a word or a cell in a spreadsheet.

Select Fields: this type of search uses some mark to select the fields to be displayed in the search results. All of the fields or only selected ones may be chosen.

Serial Ports: (also known as "com" ports) arrange data in serial form, sending it to the destination one bit at a time.

Server: a computer that controls access to the software, hardware (like printers on the network), and data located on a network.

Setting-Specific Systems: include functions such as clinical, financial, and personnel information management; however, the functions are customized for the specific setting.

Shapes: predesigned forms used to enhance the look of the slide and include rectangles, circles, arrows, callouts, and so forth.

Shortcut: is a pointer to an object; it tells the computer where to find the object but is not the actual object.

Shut Down: the computer shuts down. Most computers today will turn off their system units automatically, but the monitor may need to be turned off separately.

Sidebar: the vertical bar on the right side of a Window's Vista computer.

Single-click: means to press and release the left mouse button once to activate a command or to select an icon or menu option.

Size: refers to the diagonal measurement from corner to corner of the display unit (monitor).

Slides: the individual screens that make up a presentation.

Slide Layout: refers to the way in which the placeholders for the text and images are arranged on the slide.

Slide Show Tab: has options for starting the presentation, setting it up, and determining how it will be displayed. These commands provide for inserting sounds, animation, special effects during transitions between slides, and automation.

Slide Show View: is the best way to view the slide show. Transitions from one slide to another or any special effects or sounds can easily be seen in this view.

Slide Sorter View: displays the entire presentation so that slides may be easily rearranged. This view gives you an opportunity to view the presentation in its entirety.

Slide Transitions: are animation-like effects that appear when moving from one slide to the next during an on-screen presentation.

SmartArt: is a new feature in Office 2007 that permits one to easily create a visual representation of your information. Use SmartArt to create graphic lists, show a process, or demonstrate hierarchies. SmartArt adds color and visual interest to slides.

Smart Cards: store data on a credit card-sized card that contains a microprocessor, input and output functions, and storage.

Smart Phones: devices such as the BlackBerry and the iPhone. They provide access to the Internet, email, phone, references, GPS, books, and games, to name a few resources.

Smart Tag: a pop-up that appears when you place the insertion point over certain text.

Social Networking Sites: Web-based services that allow users to construct a profile, identify a list of other users with whom they share a personal connection, and traverse that list of connections.

Software piracy: unauthorized copying of copyrighted software.

Software Programs: consist of step-by-step instructions that direct the computer hardware to perform specific tasks such as multiplying, dividing, fetching, or delivering data. All computers require software to function. Thee three major categories of software are operating systems (OS), languages, and applications.

Soft Return: the code inserted in the document automatically when the typed line reaches the right margin.

Solid-state Media: such as *flash memory cards* and *USB storage devices* consist of electronic components and have no moving parts.

Sorting: placing the data in a specific order like numeric or alphabetic.

Source: information on the Internet refers to both the author information and the location where the information is found on the Internet.

Space Bar: enters a space between words.

Spacing: proportional or fixed pitch. *Proportional* means a variable amount of space is allotted for each character depending on the character width. *Fixed space* or *monospace* means a set space is provided for each character regardless of the character width.

Spam: electronic junk mail. This type of email is unsolicited and/or not from an identifiable source.

Spamming: the act of sending unsolicited electronic messages in bulk. The most common form of spam is that delivered in email as a form of commercial advertising.

Speakers and Headsets: (headphones) come with most computers and reproduce high-quality sound.

Spell Checker: a program that checks words for correct spelling.

Spim: the spam of instant messaging. Part spam and part instant messaging, it is being used by an increasing number of advertisers.

Spreadsheet Software: permits the manipulation of numbers in a format of rows and columns. Spreadsheet programs contain special functions for adding and computing statistical and financial formulas.

Spyware: is a type of computer software designed to install itself on your computer and then send personal data back to a central service without your permission or knowledge.

Stacked and Side-by-Side: window arrangements to partition the screen into quadrants depending on the number of open windows.

Stand-alone Systems: do not share data or information with any other computer system.

Stand By Option: puts the computer into a low-power state, but will let the user quickly resume working. With this option, the computer looks like it is turned off, but the power lights remain on.

Standard Language: a set of terms that may have been accepted for indexing concepts or content. This is another term used to refer to a controlled vocabulary.

Statistics Software: permits statistical analysis of numeric data.

Status Bar: shows the page number, number of words in the document, some view buttons, and the Zoom slider.

Stop Word: a word that is ignored in a query because the word is so commonly used that it makes no contribution to relevancy. Examples include *and, get, the,* and *you.*

Storage: comprises a place or space for holding data and application programs.

Style: the vertical slant of the character— normal (upright), condensed, or italic (oblique).

Stylus or Digital Pen: used with a tablet to create an image on the tablet surface. The tablet then converts the marks or images to digital data that the computer can use.

Subfolders: are contained within other folders. They provide further division or structure to the organization of files.

Subject Terms: are standardized. Standard sets of subject terms are often referred to as a *controlled vocabulary.*

Suites: value packages that include a word processor, a spreadsheet, a database, a presentation graphics program, and sometimes a personal information manager.

Supercomputer: the fastest, most expensive, and most powerful type of computers available. They tend to focus on running a few programs requiring a lot of computations; by comparison, other types of computers typically run many programs concurrently. Uses of supercomputers include animation graphics, weather forecasting, and research applications.

Surfing: (or browsing) the Net refers to the process of clicking hyperlinks to go to another part of a document, to a different document, or to another site.

Surge Protector: a device that sits between the electrical outlet and the computer supply source. It protects the computer from low-voltage surges in electrical power by directing the extra power to the outlet's grounding wire.

Switch User Option: lets another user log on while keeping the previous user's programs and files open.

Symbols: the clip art or images that are available within, or can be imported into, a presentation program.

Symbol Set: the characters and symbols that make up the font.

Synchronous Communication: a situation in which people communicate with one another at the same time by using their computers. Chat rooms and Internet meetings are examples of synchronous communication, as all of the individuals involved are on their computers at the same time.

System: a set of interrelated parts.

System Unit: contains the control center or "brains" of the computer; it is not visible to the eye on most computers unless someone removes the cover of the computer.

Systems Analysts: work with users to define their information needs and design systems to meet those needs.

T1 and T3: communication connections used by large businesses. A telecommunications company generally provides these services.

Tab: a setting that places the subsequent text on that line a certain number of spaces or inches in from the left margin.

Tab Key: moves the cursor along the screen at defined intervals or to the next field in a dialog box.

Table: a structure consisting of columns and rows for holding and displaying data. Table structures are used in Word, Excel, Access, and PowerPoint.

Tagging: describes the process of indicating the appearance of contents of a Web page by specifying fonts and font-related attributes as well as location or layout of the text and graphics.

Tags: terms that function as keywords associated with online content such as blog postings, bookmarks, and Web sites. Tags make it possible for an aggregator to effectively search the Internet and group together related information.

Tape Drives: secondary storage devices that allow the backup or duplication of stored data on a hard disk.

Taskbar: contains the start button, quick launch toolbar, open applications, and notification area.

Taskbar: is the long horizontal bar at the bottom of the desktop unless moved to the top, right, or left of the screen.

Task Pane: a small window that displays additional options and commands for certain features.

Technical Professionals: are those who develop, maintain, and evaluate the technical aspects of information systems. They are generally responsible for the network, databases, software and hardware updates, security, communications, and so forth.

These are the people who respond to end user problems and questions.

Templates: predesigned (formatted) documents or files used as a starting point; used in Word, Excel, Access, and PowerPoint to save the user from having to redesign the document or file each time it is used.

Temporary Internet Files: sent to the computer for the purpose of speeding the loading of graphics files when a Web site is visited multiple times.

Theft of services: the unauthorized use of services such as those provided by a computer system.

Themes: (also called presentation styles in some programs) are professionally designed format and color schemes for a presentation.

Thermal Printers: press heated pins against special paper to produce the printed image; the quality of this output is low.

Thesaurus: a built-in feature that helps search for alternative words.

Threaded Discussion: an online information exchange that is similar to a bulletin board, except that topics within each interest area are identified and organized together so that users can access and read only the discussions pertaining to a particular interest area.

Time bomb: instructions in a program that perform certain functions on a specific date or time, such as printing a message or destroying data.

Title and Content Slides: layout includes one text placeholder, usually for the title, and one content placeholder.

Title Bar: horizontal bar at the top of a window.

Title Slides: introduce the presentation and to separate sections within the presentation.

Toggle: to switch from one mode of operation to another.

Touch Screen: allows commands or actions to be entered by pressing specific places on a special screen with a finger.

Transmission Control Protocol/Internet Protocol (TCP/IP): a base protocol (set of rules) that every computer on the Internet must use and understand for sending and receiving data.

Transmission Media: refers to the materials or substances capable of transmitting a signal. They are of two types: physical media and wireless media.

Transparencies: transparencies are thin sheets of transparent flexible material, typically cellulose acetate, onto which documents or slides can be printed. These are then placed on an overhead projector for display to an audience. This system is still found in schools, but is being largely replaced by LCD projectors.

Trapdoors: methods installed by programmers that allow unauthorized access into programs.

Triple-click: means to press and release the left mouse button three times. In word processing programs, this operation selects an entire paragraph.

Trojan horse: instructions in a program that add illegitimate functions; for example, the Trojan horse program may print out information every time information on a certain patient is entered.

Truncation: type the beginning of the term and then use a symbol to indicate that you are searching for any citation that includes a term beginning with these letters. The specific symbol will depend on the specific database management system in use.

Two Content Slide: layout includes one text placeholder for the title and two side-by-side content placeholders.

Typeface: the specific design of a character or symbol commonly referred to as the font face.

Uninterruptible Power Supply (UPS): is a device that provides electrical power generated by a battery in the event of a power outage. The battery keeps the computer going for several minutes after the outage occurs. During this time, the user can save data and properly shut down the computer.

Updates: are generally enhancements to the software that provide additional features or functions.

Upgrade: to enhance a piece of equipment or buy the newest release of a software program. Many computers are "upgradeable," meaning that the user may add more memory, additional storage devices, and so forth.

Uploading: transferring a file from a local computer to a remote server (the reverse direction from downloading); this process is used when moving local HTML files to a Web server for publishing on the Internet.

URLs: help a computer locate a Web page's exact location on the Web server. Although IP addresses and domain names locate the computer, they do not locate the Web documents on the server. The URL helps the computer find the actual Web pages.

USB Cellular Modem: a wireless adapter that connects a laptop to a cellular telephone system for data access and transfer.

USB (Universal Serial Bus): a port standard that supports fast data transfer rates (12 million bits per second).

Usenet: a form of an online bulletin board system. With this service, users read and post messages or articles in categories called newsgroups.

User Domain: is the location address for everyone who uses that mail system. This part of the address functions like the home address of a person in postal service mail delivery.

UserID: is the public name one uses to access a restricted resource such as an email system or network. No one else on that system will have the same userID.

Utilities: a group of software programs that help with the management or maintenance of the computer and protection of the computer from unwanted intrusion. Examples include hard disk managers, virus detectors, compression/decompression programs, spyware, firewalls, spam blockers, and viewers.

Vector Graphics: images created with lines, arcs, circles, and squares. This file format stores images as vector points. Examples include CGM and PGL.

Version: software programs are assigned unique numbers (sometimes names) as they are revised; the interface, commands, and functions can change with each version. Users may not be able to open newer files with older version software.

Video Conferencing: a conference involving a computer, video camera, microphone, and speakers. Along with hearing audio, whatever images appear in front of the video camera are delivered to the participant's monitor. A "virtual" conference can involve two participants or many.

View Tab: includes commands that allow you to view the document in print layout, full screen reading, Web layout, outline, or draft form.

Virtual Classroom: a learning environment that exists solely online in the form of digital content and online communication. The content is stored, accessed, and exchanged through networked computer and information systems. Everything in a virtual classroom occurs in a nonphysical environment, and students "go to class" by connecting to the network rather than by traveling to a real, physical classroom.

Virus: Computer viruses are small programs or scripts that can negatively affect the health of your computer. These malicious little programs can create files, move files, erase files, consume your computer's memory, and cause your computer not to function correctly. Most viruses duplicate themselves, attach themselves to programs, and travel across networks through external storage devices, email attachments, or downloaded files.

Virus definitions: a signature file used to ensure that your computer can detect the newest viruses. New viruses are being spread all the time and it is important to "update" the database of information on viruses through these signature files provided by the anti-virus software developer.

VoIP (Voice over Internet Protocol): the technology that makes it possible to transmit voice or sound via the Internet. With this protocol, your voice is converted into a digital signal that travels over the Internet.

Web 2.0: the second generation of Web utilization. This term does not refer to a change in technology, but rather a change in how Web technology and applications are now being creatively used to enhance and expand information sharing, communication, and collaboration. Examples of Web 2.0 include the evolution of Web-culture communities, social-networking sites, video-sharing sites, and blogs.

Webinar: an interactive presentation, lecture, workshop, or seminar delivered over the Internet. In many cases, the participants ask questions or offer comments via a chat or voice application.

Web Browser: the software program that is used to display Web pages on the World Wide Web.

Web Browser Security Settings. this protection can include a phishing filter, a pop-up blocker, notification that a Web site is trying to download files or software onto your computer, and notification if a program's digital signature is current and correct when you are trying to download a program or files.

Wiki: a Web page or a collection of Web pages that can be viewed and modified by anyone who has access to a browser and the Internet. Wikis are proving to be robust, open-ended collaborative group sites. One of the most commonly used wikis is Wikipedia, an online editable encyclopedia.

Windows: place on the desktop where the contents of application program, files, or folders, are displayed.

Windows Logo Key: displays or hides the Start menu.

Wireless Card: fits into a computer slot and permits the computer to access a wireless network via radio-based connection.

Wireless Connection: employs a microwave dish generally located outside the house.

Wireless Home Networks: part of the broadband services that many telecommunications companies offer. Each computer or device that connects to the wireless network must have a wireless network card or built-in wireless networking capabilities (found on many laptops).

Wireless Local Area Network (WLAN): does not use wires for communication between the "server" and the client computer or mobile device. Most WLANs physically connect to a LAN for the purpose of accessing resources on the LAN.

Wireless Modem: a device with an external or built-in antenna for use with mobile devices such as laptops and cell phones. Some mobile phones, smart phones, and PDAs can function as data modems.

Wireless Router: fiber-optic connections (such as the Verizon Fios service) rely on a wireless router to provide the connectivity between the computer, phone wire, and fiber-optic panel.

Wisdom: in health care, ethical decision making that ensures cost-effective quality care requires more than an empirical knowledge base. Knowing when and how to use this knowledge is referred to as wisdom. The development of wisdom requires not only empirical knowledge, but also ethical, personal, and aesthetic knowledge.

Wizards: step-by-step process of asking you questions to guide you through creating a document or file. It acts as a guide for creating a new document like a calendar or resume in Microsoft Word.

Word Processing Software: permits the creating, editing, formatting, storing, and printing of text. Most have spelling and grammar checkers.

Word Wrap: automatically carries words over to the next line if they extend beyond the margin.

Workbook: (notebook) is a collection of spreadsheet pages. Workbook pages are called worksheets in most programs.

Worksheet: (spreadsheet) is made up of labels (letters), values (numbers), lines or borders, and formulas. It can also contain charts, illustrations, tables, links, and special text like WordArt and text boxes.

World Wide Web (WWW): (also known more simply as the Web) is the part of the Internet where the graphical portion stores electronic files, called Web pages, on servers that are accessed from the user's computer.

Worm: A destructive program that can fill various memory locations of a computer system with information, clogging the system so that other operations are compromised.

X-axis: refers to the horizontal reference lines or coordinates of a graph.

Y-axis: refers to the vertical reference lines or coordinates of a graph.

Zoom: allows you to examine a part of the document more closely or to see a complete page of the document.

Index